PROTEIN PURIFICATION PROCESS ENGINEERING

BIOPROCESS TECHNOLOGY

Series Editor

W. Courtney McGregor

Xoma Corporation
Berkeley, California

1. Membrane Separations in Biotechnology, *edited by W. Courtney McGregor*
2. Commercial Production of Monoclonal Antibodies: A Guide for Scale-Up, *edited by Sally S. Seaver*
3. Handbook on Anaerobic Fermentations, *edited by Larry E. Erickson and Daniel Yee-Chak Fung*
4. Fermentation Process Development of Industrial Organisms, *edited by Justin O. Neway*
5. Yeast: Biotechnology and Biocatalysis, *edited by Hubert Verachtert and René De Mot*
6. Sensors in Bioprocess Control, *edited by John V. Twork and Alexander M. Yacynych*
7. Fundamentals of Protein Biotechnology, *edited by Stanley Stein*
8. Yeast Strain Selection, *edited by Chandra J. Panchal*
9. Separation Processes in Biotechnology, *edited by Juan A. Asenjo*
10. Large-Scale Mammalian Cell Culture Technology, *edited by Anthony S. Lubiniecki*
11. Extractive Bioconversions, *edited by Bo Mattiasson and Olle Holst*
12. Purification and Analysis of Recombinant Proteins, *edited by Ramnath Seetharam and Satish K. Sharma*
13. Drug Biotechnology Regulation: Scientific Basis and Practices, *edited by Yuan-yuan H. Chiu and John L. Gueriguian*
14. Protein Immobilization: Fundamentals and Applications, *edited by Richard F. Taylor*
15. Biosensor Principles and Applications, *edited by Loïc J. Blum and Pierre R. Coulet*
16. Industrial Application of Immobilized Biocatalysts, *edited by Atsuo Tanaka, Tetsuya Tosa, and Takeshi Kobayashi*
17. Insect Cell Culture Engineering, *edited by Mattheus F. A. Goosen, Andrew J. Daugulis, and Peter Faulkner*
18. Protein Purification Process Engineering, *edited by Roger G. Harrison*

ADDITIONAL VOLUMES IN PREPARATION

Recombinant Microbes for Industrial and Agricultural Applications, *edited by Yoshikatsu Murooka and Tadayuki Imanaka*

PROTEIN PURIFICATION PROCESS ENGINEERING

edited by
Roger G. Harrison

University of Oklahoma
Norman, Oklahoma

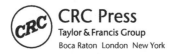

CRC Press
Taylor & Francis Group
Boca Raton London New York

CRC Press is an imprint of the
Taylor & Francis Group, an **informa** business

CRC Press
Taylor & Francis Group
6000 Broken Sound Parkway NW, Suite 300
Boca Raton, FL 33487-2742

First issued in paperback 2019

ISBN-13: 978-0-8247-9009-7 (hbk)
ISBN-13: 978-0-367-40225-9 (pbk)

Library of Congress Cataloging-in-Publication Data

Protein purification process engineering / edited by Roger G. Harrison.
    p. cm. -- (Bioprocess technology ; v. 18)
    Includes bibliographical references and index.
    ISBN 0-8247-9009-X
    1. Proteins--Biotechnology. 2. Proteins--Purification.
I. Harrison, Roger G.   II. Series.
TP248.65.P76P7654 1993   93-31555
660'.63--dc20   CIP

**Visit the Taylor & Francis Web site at
http://www.taylorandfrancis.com**

**and the CRC Press Web site at
http://www.crcpress.com**

Series Introduction

Bioprocess technology encompasses all the basic and applied sciences as well as the engineering required to fully exploit living systems and bring their products to the marketplace. The technology that develops is eventually expressed in various methodologies and types of equipment and instruments built up along a bioprocess stream. Typically in commercial production, the stream begins at the bioreactor, which can be a classical fermentor, a cell culture perfusion system, or an enzyme bioreactor. Then comes separation of the product from the living systems and/or their components followed by an appropriate number of purification steps. The stream ends with bioproduct finishing, formulation, and packaging. A given bioprocess stream may have some tributaries or outlets and may be overlaid with a variety of monitoring devices and control systems. As with any stream, it will both shape and be shaped with time. Documenting the evolutionary shaping of bioprocess technology is the purpose of this series.

Now that several products from recombinant DNA and cell fusion techniques are on the market, the new era of bioprocess technology is well established and validated. Books of this series represent developments in various segments of bioprocessing that have paralleled progress in the life sciences. For obvious proprietary reasons, some developments in industry, although validated, may be published only later, if at all. Therefore, our continuing series will follow the growth of this field as it is available from both academia and industry.

W. Courtney McGregor

iii

Series Introduction

Foreword

In the 20 years since the invention of genetic engineering, manufacture of recombinant proteins has become a mature industry impinging on almost every important aspect of our daily lives. Products range from extremely expensive diagnostic and therapeutic proteins to low-cost substances such as chymosin used in the manufacture of cheese. These latter substances compete successfully with traditional products in the commercial marketplace, on the basis of both quality and price. The number of commercial recombinant proteins continues to grow and both naturally occurring and genetically engineered molecules are now produced on a routine basis.

In order to maintain this remarkable momentum it is essential to solidify the technological base upon which this new industry is built. Almost obscured by the glamor surrounding these products is the simultaneous development of separation techniques needed for their production. Some of these techniques, such as large-scale cell disruption, exist only in biotechnology, and others have evolved into highly effective and specialized forms unique to protein purification. Rapid development of these processing techniques has given us little chance to consolidate and organize our understanding of them.

Although much information concerning protein purification is available, it has not been easy for the engineer or chemist to get the kind of detailed and explicit descriptions needed to develop effective expertise in either manufacturing or process development. It is particularly unfortunate that these newly important unit operations are being largely ignored in our educational institutions at all levels. A primary reason for this is the lack of reliable, readable, and well-organized texts.

Downstream processing, or recovery and purification, is particularly important because it typically accounts for nearly three-fourths of manufacturing costs in this new industry and because reliable and effective purification can be of the utmost importance to the user. Moreover, the developers of commercial purification processes must operate quickly and under heavy regulatory constraints. It is increasingly recognized that there must be effective communication among those engaged in research, process development, and manufacturing, from early stages of basic research through commercial production. At present, this is seldom the case.

Protein Purification Process Engineering is directed toward meeting these unfulfilled needs. The book begins with a basic overview of the facilities needed to work in this new area and the ways in which process development should be organized and implemented. The remainder of the text is devoted to individual separation and analytical techniques that are important to protein processing but are covered inadequately in other existing texts.

Analytical techniques are given strong emphasis. These techniques are essential in these systems, where the complexity of the product itself and the process streams can make it extremely difficult to close material balances and to characterize purity. Yields in the multistage purification chains characteristic of protein manufacture are usually low, and it is important to know where and why the losses occur, as well as to characterize the nature of the impurities. Moreover, analysis and quality control are expensive, often about one-third of total manufacturing costs in both upstream and downstream processing.

The most commonly used processing steps, described in the remainder of the text, all present unresolved engineering problems, and their effective use requires a great deal of judgment and experience. This is true for the humble but important mechanical rupture of cell walls as well as for more sophisticated techniques such as bioaffinity chromatography. Membrane filtration is an excellent example, as the potential economy and simplicity of these processes is clouded by poor understanding of boundary-layer behavior, fouling, and irreversible degradation. Liquid extraction is a potentially attractive process that suffers from both lack of suitable processing equipment and inadequate experience with solvent systems. Experience in the more conventional process industry cannot be simply translated into the complex chemistry and small flow rates of modern biotechnology.

The authoritative discussion of precipitation is also welcome. Selective precipitation is among the most powerful and potentially cheapest of all separation techniques, and it is widely used in selected protein purification processes. Extension to other applications is desirable, and the chief barrier is the complexity of this process for large unstable molecules such as proteins. The warning in the introductory chapter to pay close attention to biochemistry is highly appropriate, and success will require close cooperation between protein chemists and engineers.

The most difficult separation problems are almost always solved by some form of chromatography, and two chapters discuss these highly selective but complex and expensive processes. Chapter 7 is devoted primarily to the details of column design and operation, which tend to be neglected in similar monographs but are of great importance in day-to-day operations. This discussion provides both a useful qualitative introduction as well as an appreciation for orders of magnitude, and it should prove especially helpful for those new to protein processing technology. Chapter 8 deals with the highly selective and somewhat mysterious processes of biospecific adsorption. This chapter reinforces the introductory chapter's advice that system biochemistry must be understood as thoroughly as possible.

This ambitious and comprehensive text concludes with an eminently practical discussion of freeze drying, an important process but often neglected in discussions of downstream processing. Freeze drying is normally the last step in the manufacturing process, and the care with which it is carried out can have a great impact on product stability and quality.

The authors are all recognized leaders in their areas of expertise; all have had a great deal of experience. They have produced a coherent product with its own "personality," one which should fill an important niche. They have provided the book with detailed information and given it a practical emphasis. Moreover, the bibliographies are extensive, permitting readers to delve deeper into topics of their own interest. The text will supplement more theoretically oriented monographs and should prove to be highly useful.

E. N. Lightfoot
University of Wisconsin
Madison, Wisconsin

Preface

The biotechnology industry, which originated in the late 1970s, is now well into the commercialization stage. A significant segment of this new industry is dedicated to bringing to market purified proteins. The economics of the processes to produce these proteins tend to be dominated by purification—typically, 80–90% of the manufacturing cost is for downstream recovery and purification. Thus, it is essential that a very efficient protein purification process be developed in order for the overall process to be cost competitive.

Protein Purification Process Engineering focuses on providing guidance for the substantial effort required in developing protein purification processes for large scale, commercial operation. It is written primarily for those engaged in this or related efforts in the industry. Readers doing research on protein purification in both industry and academia will find this book very useful as they work to improve existing processes or develop new ones.

Chapters cover various aspects related to protein purification: process development, scale-up, mathematical descriptions of processes and phenomena, technology, and applications. These topics fall within the general field of process engineering. Most of the technologies currently used at the commercial scale are covered in this book. Some of the chapters, particularly those discussing precipitation and affinity chromatography, have greater emphasis on the basic science involved. This is primarily because these technologies require a deeper science base to understand and utilize them. The chapters are also of varying length because some fields of protein purification are newer and less developed than others. Included is a chapter on protein analytical methods by industrial practitioners, as these methods are essential to protein purification and should be in place before process development work begins.

The contributors were carefully selected, based on their substantial experience and expertise in their subject areas. The chapters are new, original treatments of the authors' respective subjects, thus constituting a new resource for those readers in the field.

I am grateful for the stimulating environment in purification process engineering at the Upjohn Company and Phillips Petroleum Company that helped lead to the idea for this book. Encouragement to pursue this project from colleagues in the School of Chemical Engineering and Materials Science at the University of Oklahoma is appreciated.

Roger G. Harrison

Contents

Series Introduction   *iii*
Foreword   E. N. Lightfoot   *v*
Preface   *ix*
Contributors   *xiii*

1 Organization and Strategy   1
   Roger G. Harrison

2 Analytical Considerations in the Development of Protein
   Purification Processes   11
   Vincent Anicetti and William S. Hancock

3 Cell Breakage   37
   Cady R. Engler

4 Crossflow Membrane Filtration   57
   Zhi-Guo Su and Clark K. Colton

5 Liquid-Liquid Extraction   87
   Dennis J. Kubek

6 Differential Precipitation of Proteins: Science and Technology   115
   Fred Rothstein

7 Conventional Chromatography   209
   John M. Simpson

xi

8   Biospecific Affinity Chromatography   259
      Nikos K. Harakas

9   Freeze Drying: A Practical Overview   317
      Larry A. Gatlin and Steven L. Nail

Index   369

Contributors

Vincent Anicetti Quality Control, Genentech, Inc., South San Francisco, California

Clark K. Colton Department of Chemical Engineering, Massachusetts Institute of Technology, Cambridge, Massachusetts

Cady R. Engler Department of Agricultural Engineering, Texas A&M University, College Station, Texas

Larry A. Gatlin Pharmaceuticals Department, Glaxo Research Institute, Research Triangle Park, North Carolina

William S. Hancock Department of Analytical Chemistry, Genentech, Inc., South San Francisco, California

Nikos K. Harakas Central Research Laboratory, Monsanto Company, St. Louis, Missouri

Roger G. Harrison School of Chemical Engineering and Materials Science, University of Oklahoma, Norman, Oklahoma

Dennis J. Kubek Biochemical Process R&D, Merck Sharp & Dohme Research Laboratories, West Point, Pennsylvania

Steven L. Nail Department of Industrial and Physical Pharmacy, Purdue University, West Lafayette, Indiana

Fred Rothstein Bio-Separations Consultants, Long Beach, California

John M. Simpson Medical Research Division, Department of Biochemical Engineering, Lederle Laboratories, American Cyanamid Company, Pearl River, New York

Zhi-Guo Su Department of Chemical Engineering, Dalian University of Technology, Dalian, People's Republic of China

1

Organization and Strategy

Roger G. Harrison
University of Oklahoma, Norman, Oklahoma

I. INTRODUCTION

During the development of a process to produce a protein, the initial emphasis of the work naturally is on the biological process. This focus on the biological process is often prolonged, because the time to develop this process can be lengthy. As a consequence, there can be a delay in shifting attention to the purification of the protein. However, it is important to realize that key organizational steps should be taken before experimental work on the purification process even begins, and that once the protein purification process development starts, the strategy to use in this development is crucial to the success of the project.

Several factors must be considered that relate to the organization of the work: The facilities and equipment must be appropriate for the job to be performed. The impact and applicability of the Current Good Manufacturing Practices (CGMP) regulations of the Food and Drug Administration (FDA) must be evaluated. The desirability of using a project team approach should be considered.

The complexity of most protein purification processes gives added importance to strategy considerations in the development of these processes. Purification processes for proteins nearly always involve more than one step and frequently involve a multitude of steps. Therefore decisions must be made about which individual unit operations to use and the order in which to use them. This effort is called process synthesis. The economics of the process should be evaluated at various times in the synthesis of the process in order to insure that the process is economically viable.

In addition to the strategy for the overall process synthesis, the strategy to apply in developing each individual process step is important. Four of these strategy considerations stand out, based on the author's practical experience.

In this chapter, elaboration of these organization and strategy considerations is given.

II. FACILITIES AND EQUIPMENT CONSIDERATIONS

Even before the actual process development work on purification begins, the issue of whether present facilities are adequate for the task needs to be addressed. Two situations need to be considered: laboratory scale work and pilot plant scale work.

For process development work at the laboratory scale, a good starting point is a typical protein chemistry laboratory. This would include a spectrophotometer with a UV lamp; a refrigerated centrifuge with centrifuging ability, expressed as relative g force times capacity in liters, on the order of 10,000–15,000; a wide variety of sizes of chromatography columns (glass or plastic) with adjustable plungers; a fraction collector with a UV monitor; a peristaltic chromatography pump; and a homogenizer for disrupting cells (1). Analytical equipment should include a system for analytical gel electrophoresis. In some cases, it may be highly desirable to have an analytical high-performance liquid chromatograph (HPLC) on hand for analyzing samples soon after they are taken.

Numerous operations for the purification of proteins need to be done at near 0°C to minimize proteolytic degradation and bacterial growth. The two options that arise for the lab scale are doing these operations in a refrigerated room and doing them in a chromatography refrigerator. The author has used only the latter option for lab process development work and found this to perfectly satisfactory. Chromatography refrigerators with glass doors, electrical outlets, and access portholes can be obtained with up to at least 75 cu. ft. of capacity.

The pilot plant is in essence a large-scale laboratory. Because of its larger scale, pilot plant equipment often must be constructed differently from laboratory equipment. Some equipment such as columns can be made of glass as in the lab. Other equipment such as vessels must be constructed of stainless steel or a plastic that has good chemical resistance, such as polypropylene. It is advantageous for each vessel to have its own pH probe for local and/or remote reading of pH. This is commonly done with an Ingold-type pH probe, which is made of glass and is capable of being sterilized. For applications involving food or pharmaceuticals, vessels should be of the "sanitary" design, which means that there are no threads on product contact surfaces and that surfaces must be smooth (150 grit or better finish). The sanitary equipment design standards usually employed are the "3A

Sanitary Standards" that are published by the *Journal of Food Protection*, Ames, Iowa.

Pumps are needed in the pilot plant for a variety of operations. All should have sanitary designs and, in some instances, should be able to be sterilized. For low-pressure and very low flow rate applications such as feeding a chromatography column, peristaltic tubing pumps are commonly used. Three of the most widely used sanitary pumps are centrifugal pumps, positive displacement rotary pumps, and flexible impeller pumps; factors in the selection of these pumps have been discussed in detail by Horwitz (2). A less frequently used pump is the diaphragm pump, which has the advantage of being able to be sterilized. This can be obtained with a double diaphragm so that the pump's hydraulic fluid will not contaminate the product when a diaphragm rupture occurs.

As to the means of keeping process liquids in the pilot plant refrigerated, one common practice is to use jacketed equipment with circulation of a suitable coolant (methanol-water, for example) through the jackets. However, pilot plants have been built with all or part of the equipment in cold rooms. Before using the cold room approach, the processes to be used should be analyzed to determine if the heat transfer will be adequate to maintain temperatures at near 0°C. Pilot plant processes that have appreciable heat generation will generally need to be done in jacketed equipment because the heat transfer coefficient for air in free convection is only a small fraction of the heat transfer coefficient for liquids in forced convection (3). Also, some operations such as precipitation with organic solvents must often be done below 0°C, which means that operation in a jacketed tank will be mandatory.

A number of utilities are needed in the laboratory and pilot plant. The ones required have been listed by Barrer (4). To provide flexibility in using equipment in the pilot plant, it is a good idea for utilities to be distributed to a number of locations, sometimes called utility stations, in the pilot plant. Each utility station contains appropriate outlets for many or all of the pilot plant utilities. If the equipment is modular and on casters, then a great amount of flexibility can be achieved in configuring pilot plant processes. The author both designed and used a pilot plant with utility stations and mobile equipment and found this concept to work out extremely well.

If solvents will be used in the pilot plant, then all the equipment should be designed to explosion-proof specifications. The National Electrical Code classification for electrical equipment and instrumentation is Class I, Group D for the solvents that would potentially be present in a pilot plant to purify proteins (5). If it is possible that solvents may be used at some point during the life of the pilot plant, serious consideration should be given to obtaining explosion-proof equipment initially because of the cost and inconvenience of converting non-explosion-proof equipment later.

III. GOOD MANUFACTURING PRACTICES

The Current Good Manufacturing Practices (CGMP) regulations issued by the FDA can have a large impact on how the purification process work is organized, depending on the end use of the product under development. In general, the CGMP regulations cover the design, validation, and operation of a pharmaceutical manufacturing facility. CGMP regulations have been issued in the United States *Code of Federal Regulations*, Title 21, which is published yearly. The most widely applicable CGMP regulations are those in Part 211 of Title 21 that govern the manufacture of drug products for administration to humans or animals (6). There are supplementary CGMPs for the manufacture of medicated animal feeds (part 225), medicated premixes (part 226), blood and blood components (part 606), and medical devices (part 820).

The FDA has issued helpful guidelines on how to apply and interpret the CGMP regulations. In 1991 a guide for inspection of bulk pharmaceutical chemical manufacturing was issued (7). Bulk pharmaceutical chemicals (BPCs) are defined as being made by chemical synthesis, recombinant DNA technology, fermentation, enzymatic reactions, recovery from natural materials, or combinations of these processes. On the other hand, finished drug products are usually the result of formulating bulk materials whose quality can be measured against fixed specifications. Thus BPCs are components of drug products. This guideline states that "there are many cases where CGMP's for dosage form drugs and BPC's are parallel." The guidelines goes on to say that "in most other cases it is neither feasible nor required to apply rigid controls during the early processing steps....At some logical point in the process, usually well before the final step, appropriate CGMP's should be imposed and maintained throughout the rest of the process." A useful interpretation of these guidelines has been done recently by Moore (8).

In 1991 the FDA issued a very helpful guideline on practices and procedures for the preparation of investigational new drug products that constitute acceptable means of complying with the CGMPs (9). The FDA recognizes that manufacturing procedures and specifications will change as the trials of a new drug advance. However, when drugs are produced for clinical trials in humans or animals, compliance with the CGMPs is *required*. According to this guideline, this means that "the drug product must be produced in a qualified facility, using laboratory and other equipment that have been qualified, and the processes must be validated." In contrast, the CGMP regulations do not apply for the preparation of drugs used for preclinical experimentation (such as toxicity studies on laboratory animals). Furthermore, like drugs approved for marketing, investigational drugs have always been subject to the FDA's inspectional activities.

Each company that is developing processes for protein drug products must carefully design its process development laboratories and pilot plants to be capable of adhering to the CGMPs when required. It is highly desirable that some labs be designated as CGMP labs and others as non-CGMP labs. This type of designation can be done for pilot plants also. However, some smaller firms have only one pilot plant, and for this situation it is not a good idea to be switching back and forth between CGMP and non-CGMP use. It is better to stick with CGMP operation entirely to avoid confusion and to make sure that CGMP procedures are followed when they are supposed to be. Likewise a lab should not be switched back and forth between CGMP and non-CGMP use.

IV. PROJECT TEAMS

Bringing a new protein to market is often extremely complex, involving a number of professionals from different disciplines who are involved in tasks that frequently must occur simultaneously. There is almost always pressure to bring the product to market as soon as possible. Competition with other companies is often intense. Furthermore, more time will be left on the product's patent life if the time required to reach the market is relatively short.

A good way to coordinate the various activities in product development is by a project team. For example, the author was on a project team in Phillips' Biotechnology Division for a new peptide with a molecular biologist, a microbiologist, an analytical chemist, and a marketing professional. This group met often to articulate goals, plan strategy, and discuss results obtained by group members. The project at Biogen on human gamma interferon for use as a pharmaceutical had a team of a group of individuals representing the laboratory research, regulatory affairs, quality control and quality assurance, clinical research, process development, and marketing functions of the company (10). This group met both as a complete team and also in smaller groups.

Since purification usually cannot begin until the protein has been synthesized, the question may arise as to when the purification professional should become involved in the process development effort. Strong arguments have been made that the scientists and engineers involved in purification scale-up should take an active part in the decision making from the *start of the process development* (11–13). One example involving recombinant products is the choice of the expression system. This choice probably will have more impact upon the purification system than any other single factor. Purification scientists and engineers can contribute to this decision by evaluating the following factors: equipment available, characterization of the protein or peptide, and consideration of the experience with the group on the various types of protein purification.

V. PROCESS SYNTHESIS

The creation of a processing scheme to purify a protein is called process synthesis. A common approach to process synthesis is the use of rules of thumb, or heuristics, in making the decisions on which separation steps to use and the order in which to use them. The most important heuristics for protein purification have been identified by Prokopakis and Asenjo (14) and Asenjo and Patrick (15) as follows:

1. Choose separation processes based on different physical, chemical, or biochemical properties.
2. Separate the most plentiful impurities first.
3. Choose those processes that will exploit differences in the physicochemical properties of the products and impurities in the most economical manner.
4. Use a high-resolution step as soon as possible.
5. Do the most expensive step last.

Prokopakis and Asenjo rate rules 1 and 3 as the most important and point out that these rules rely heavily on property information that is incomplete and only qualitative most of the time.

Because each protein is different, it is often worthwhile to focus on a property or properties that make the protein unique. An example is the Phillips process for the purification of alcohol oxidase, which the author helped scale up (16). This process was based on the discovery by a biochemist at Phillips, T. R. Hopkins, that alcohol oxidase could be crystallized when the ionic strength was lowered to a certain point (17). The scaled-up process was very simple and consisted of cell lysis, removal of cell debris by crossflow microfiltration, concentration by ultrafiltration, and crystallization by lowering the pH.

One tool that can be very useful in the synthesis of protein purification processes is computer simulation of the process. Software to do this simulation specifically for bioprocesses is now commercially available (for example, by Intelligen, Inc., Westfield, New Jersey). It may be helpful to do this simulation with available laboratory data before the development of the process has proceeded very far. Later on in the development of the process, the economics of the process can be evaluated conveniently using the simulation program to determine the feasibility of the process and to pinpoint those steps in the process that are most in need of improvement. The computer simulation and economic evaluation of the purification process for porcine growth hormone have been well documented (18).

The use of artificial intelligence in the synthesis of protein purification has been a subject of research in the last few years. It is likely that artificial intelligence will become well enough developed in the near future to be used routinely as an aid in the synthesis of protein purification processes. Progress in this field has been reviewed by Prokopakis and Asenjo (14).

VI. PRACTICAL CONSIDERATIONS IN THE SCALE-UP OF INDIVIDUAL STEPS

In scaling up individual purification process steps, four points especially stand out as worth remembering and adhering to, based on the author's experience:

1. Do careful material balances.
2. Pay attention to the biochemistry involved.
3. Initially look at wide ranges of variables and examine narrower ranges as time permits.
4. Be prepared to do engineering analysis.

An elaboration of these points follows.

A common tendency of those working in protein purification is to follow only the main product stream in terms of specific activity (desired protein activity/total protein weight) and total protein concentration. A better approach is to analyze *each stream* in a given step for the desired protein (and for the impurities, if possible). Closure of the material balance should always be checked. Failure of the material balance to close can mean that product inactivation is occurring, which could lead to a study of ways to prevent this from happening or to minimize the inactivation. Because of assay errors, it is often desirable to obtain an average material balance for a number of runs using the same procedure.

Good material balances are possible only if a good quantitative assay is being used. Ideally, the development of a reliable quantitative assay should *precede* the start of the scale-up work.

Careful attention should always be paid to the biochemistry of the process. Often, the process times become longer and different materials are used as the process is scaled up. Both of these factors can lead to unwanted biochemical reactions that can reduce yield and purity. Longer processing times can give more proteolytic degradation, especially if the process has to be partially carried out at a higher temperature than at the previous scale of operation, which is often the case. Different processing materials (such as column packings, materials of construction, or chemicals used in the process) can give reactions that bind or denature the product or convert it to undesired by-products. When these undesired events occur, it is often a good idea to go back to the laboratory and simulate what is happening at the larger scale.

Looking at a wide range of variables is a good idea at the start of the process development and can sometimes lead to unexpected results that possibly can be patented. One should always keep in mind that each protein is different and has the potential to behave in a manner very different from the norm.

Engineering analysis should never be overlooked as a tool to understand what is going on. This can take a myriad of forms, from the simple calculation of a Reynolds number, which can differentiate laminar from turbulent flow, to more complex analysis. An example of more complex analysis is in the scale-up from laboratory scale to pilot plant scale of a whole broth adsorption process that was done by the author (19). In this process the whole broth passes through a series of columns where the adsorbent resin is mixed. Mass transfer correlations for the lab and pilot plant columns were found to be widely different. This led to the experimental determination of the residence time distribution for the pilot plant column. The result was that the mixing in the column was far from ideal. The mixing was well modeled by a plug flow region in series with a back-mixed region connected to a stagnant zone. The process was successfully modeled on a computer when the mass transfer correlation was corrected for nonideal mixing.

REFERENCES

1. Scopes, R. K. (1987). *Protein Purification*, 2d ed., Springer-Verlag, New York, p. 2.
2. Horwitz, R. P. (1985). Factors in the selection of sanitary pumps, *Pharm. Manufact.*, Oct.:19.
3. Bird, R. B., Stewart, W. E., and Lightfoot, E. N. (1960). *Transport Phenomena*, John Wiley, New York, p. 393.
4. Barrer, P. J. (1983). Critical factors in the design of a pilot plant, *Bio/Tech.*, *1*:661.
5. Crowl, D. A., and Louvar, J. F. (1990). *Chemical Process Safety: Fundamentals and Applications*, Prentice-Hall, Englewood Cliffs, New Jersey, p. 227.
6. Harrison, F. G. (1985). Current good manufacturing practices for biotechnology-oriented companies, *Bio/Tech.*, *3*:43.
7. Food and Drug Administration (1991). Guide to inspection of bulk pharmaceutical chemicals, Washington, D.C.
8. Moore, R. E. (1992). FDA's guideline for bulk pharmaceutical chemicals—A consultant's interpretation, *Pharm. Tech.*, *16*:88.
9. Food and Drug Administration (1991). Guideline on the preparation of investigational new drug products (human and animal), Washington, D.C.
10. Kelley, W. S. (1986). Issues in the development of biotechnology products, *Pharm. Tech.*, *10*:48.
11. Bonitz, S. (1988). Product success depends on early decisions in bioprocessing scale-up, *Gen. Eng. News*, July/Aug.:20.
12. Van Brunt, J. (1985). Scale-up: The next hurdle, *Bio/Tech.*, *3*:419.
13. Fish, N. M., and Lilly, M. D. (1984). The interactions between fermentation and protein recovery, *Bio/Tech.*, *2*:623.
14. Prokopakis, G. J., and Asenjo, J. A. (1990). Synthesis of downstream processes, in *Separation Processes in Biotechnology* (J. A. Asenjo, ed.), Marcel Dekker, New York, p. 571.
15. Asenjo, J. A., and Patrick, I. (1990). Large-scale protein purification, in *Protein Purification Applications. A Practical Approach* (E. L. V. Harris and S. Angal, eds.), IRL Press, Oxford, p. 1.

16. Harrison, R. G., and Nelles, L. P. (1990). Large scale process for the purification of alcohol oxidase, U.S. Patent No. 4,956,290.
17. Hopkins, T. R. (1985). Alcohol oxidase from *Pichia*-type yeasts, U.S. Patent No. 4,540, 668.
18. Petrides, D., Cooney, C. L., Evans, L. B., Field, R. P., and Snoswell, M. (1989). Bioprocess simulation: An integrated approach to process development, *Computers Chem. Engng.*, *13*:553.
19. Harrison, R. G. (1981). Antibiotic adsorption process using a non-ionic macroporous resin, American Institute of Chemical Engineers National Meeting, Houston, April 5–9.

2

Analytical Considerations in the Development of Protein Purification Processes

Vincent Anicetti and William S. Hancock

Genentech, Inc., South San Francisco, California

I. INTRODUCTION

A key challenge in biotechnology is the production of proteins by large-scale cell culture in a cost-effective manner. The challenge is that of any mature industry: to produce large amounts of material at a competitive cost while ensuring that product quality is maintained. Although the practice of large-scale cell culture includes the manufacture of long-established products such as alcohol and antibiotics, the production of protein pharmaceuticals, commodities (for example, industrial enzymes), and monoclonal antibodies are better examples of the leading edge of the industry today. Recent protein therapeutics produced through biotechnology and approved for marketing include vaccines, interferons, growth factors, and a variety of monoclonal antibodies. In addition to these pharmaceuticals, commodity products are now routinely produced through genetic engineering. Beta-Amylase, used in the manufacture of starch, and chymosin, used in the manufacture of cheese and aspartame, are recent examples of proteins or peptides produced through genetic engineering. These recombinant DNA derived proteins compete successfully on a cost and quality basis with the products derived from traditional sources. As the biotechnology industry matures, recombinant pharmaceuticals will drive the development of larger-scale production systems, both to meet increasing market demands and to compete on a cost basis.

In addition to the traditional scale-up challenge, process development scientists will be presented with the need for rapid and simplified purification techniques and strategies. The large R and D investment in biotechnology over the past decade has resulted in many new candidate molecules being produced for clinical studies. Although some of the initial public excitement and publicity surrounding the production of recombinant proteins has diminished, a second generation of both naturally occurring proteins and truly "engineered" molecules has quietly moved from the research labs into large-scale development. Techniques in molecular biology have advanced to the point where chimeric molecules, hybrid proteins crossing species and/or function, are produced on a routine basis. The rate of delivery of these products to the clinic will depend in part on the ability to quickly develop and implement scalable production and purification processes.

The development of efficient and reproducible separation processes for proteins and peptides relies, in large part, on the availability of suitable analytical methods. The complexity of proteins, relative to small molecule drugs, requires that a spectrum of methods be used to ascertain quality, quantity, and activity. Most analytical methods can only explore a particular aspect of the protein. Therefore methods should be used in a corresponding fashion to complement one another (1–3). For example, biological assays are generally the best reflection of potency, but as a group these methods are imprecise compared to most other techniques. Therefore bioassays are best used as qualitative assessments of the product and should be combined with more precise physical/chemical methods of quantitation.

Most analytical strategies seek to describe the following attributes of proteins: identity, quantity, activity, and purity. Identity methods have limited application in process scale-up as they are not quantitative. However, such tests can be valuable for ensuring that product cross contamination does not occur, especially in a multiuse facility. *N*-terminal sequence determination, isoelectric focusing, and spectral analysis are good examples of such methods. Quantitative methods are obviously much more useful in process development. An immunoassay, for example, can provide both product identity and quantitation. Advances in the HPLC analysis of complex biological samples have resulted in the growing use of this technique for process monitoring and development (4,5). More recently, the potential of high-performance capillary electrophoresis (HPCE) has been demonstrated (6,7), for example in a report where the different steps of the production of a hepatitis vaccine were successfully followed by HPCE (8).

Protein potency and purity can only be expressed according to narrow definitions dependent on the type of activity assayed or the presence of a particular impurity. Thus a number of methods that measure particular impurities or activities are needed to make strong statements about the overall activity or purity of the molecule. While such methods serve a quality control function, they are also key process development tools to guide steps that increase yield, activity, and purity. Analytical studies are particularly important in process scale-up, as subtle changes can occur either to the product or to its associated impurities from an apparently minor process change.

Potency is a term used to indicate the amount of biological activity for a given mass of product (specific activity). The ideal potency assay should be one that reflects the desired activity of the product for the intended application. This is because many proteins and peptides are modulators of biological activities, with the potential to cause different and perhaps opposite biological effects based on concentration and/or the target tissue. The use of biological assays, if they can be made cost-efficient and precise, is a significant asset in process development, first to identify biologically active forms of the desired product and second to determine if losses in specific activity occur during the process. In a recovery scheme, denaturation of the target protein is often observed, where there is typically a loss of biological activity without significant change in the amount of material.

The analysis of product purity is by necessity multifaceted, because the protein purity can be described in as many ways as there are distinct and analyzable impurities. Impurities may be intrinsic to the desired protein, for example deamidation products or proteolytically cleaved material, or substances extrinsic to the product, such as growth medium constituents. In fact, intrinsic product purity is a meaningful term only if it is assessed by a number of analytical methods that are orthogonal, through methods based on different physicochemical properties, while extrinsic impurities are measured through a variety of broad spectrum biological or chemical methods.

Finally, a discussion regarding application of analytical methods to process scale-up must include method validation. Analytical results can only be interpreted in relation to the quality and validity of the method used, and the credibility of the data obtained is as much a function of the method itself as it is of the product. This is particularly true of methods designed to analyze process-specific impurities. In this chapter we will define some of the analytical strategies useful in assessing protein purification processes and demonstrate the importance of the analytical method development in all aspects of process development.

II. METHOD VALIDATION

The interpretation of data from any method must be made within the context of its accuracy and precision, including variation associated with the sample preparation procedures. This knowledge is critical for the establishment of specifications governing what is an acceptable degree of process variation and product quality. The degree to which process variation can be accurately characterized will depend on the variability inherent in the analytical method. Analytical methods validation generally concentrates on certain key performance characteristics and reagent considerations. The most common performance characteristics evaluated are precision, accuracy, sensitivity, and specificity. The following is a brief discussion of the key assay validation criteria. For a comprehensive discussion of most of these parameters, *Statistics for Analytical Chemists* is an excellent text (9).

A. Key Terms

Precision refers to the variability associated with repeated determinations of an identical sample. There are two contributing assay components to the precision error: intraassay and interassay variation. Interassay variation is also commonly referred to as reproducibility.

For convenience, an assay should be considered to be the sample group size that can be processed with a single set of critical reagents, equipment, and physical operations. An example would be a single microtiter plate ELISA, with a unique standard curve and buffer set. Precision errors are generally quantified as the relative standard deviation (RSD) or percent coefficient of variation (%CV). Poor intraassay precision suggests that several replicates should be run, just as poor interassay precision suggests determinations across several assay runs. Among the primary factors contributing to precision errors are reagents, equipment, analyst technique, sample selection, and preparation.

Accuracy commonly refers to the degree that the test value approximates the true value and will, in practice, be affected by the intraassay precision error. With the availability of highly purified recombinant proteins, the accuracy of most methods can be tested directly using either the spiked placebo recovery or the standard addition technique in which pure proteins are added back into the appropriate sample matrix. The availability of pure proteins has also allowed the routine use of quantitative amino acid analysis as the preferred reference method to establish protein concentration. Amino acid analysis provides a quantitation based on an expected protein composition and thus may not require the use of a reference material. The selection of a "pure" reference material representative of the purification process can prove difficult early in the development cycle due to limited knowledge of the process. Methods of quantitation using such reference materials often result in circular errors because of the poorly characterized or first-generation reference materials.

Accuracy can be affected by substances that interfere in the assay, cross-reactive materials, or variant forms of the product. Common examples of interfering substances are salts or detergents. The presence of interfering substances can be detected by testing samples of the reference material added back into process buffers or growth medium. To determine the potency of interfering substances, the analyst should determine the minimum dilution of the buffer or medium containing constant levels of product required to circumvent the interference. However, the mandatory dilutions of the sample may be so large as to reduce assay sensitivity to an unacceptable level, as well as introducing more sample handling error, and therefore methods of sample pretreatment are often required.

Sensitivity is commonly defined as the "detection limit of the assay." This term is often used to define the theoretical limit of detection in the method. However, a pragmatic goal might be stated as, "The lowest concentration of product in the sample matrix that can be routinely determined to be significantly different from a sample lacking product." This definition of assay sensitivity reflects the reality that the minimum detectable concentration is quite likely to change from day to day and to be dependent on variation in assay parameters and sample preparation. This practical definition is often referred to as the "limit of quantitation" and reflects the lowest level at which acceptable accuracy can be obtained from an assay. While sensitivity is not generally a concern for product quantitation, it is often a critical issue in the detection of product variants or process impurities.

Specificity refers to the ability of the method to detect only the product of interest. The assay specificity is often inferred by measuring the extent to which other materials cross-react in the assay. Bioassays, in particular, may demonstrate an identical assay response for different proteins. While exceptions exist, generally bioassays and protein dye binding assays are less specific than immunoassays or chromatographic procedures. However, no method is foolproof; for example, antibody based methods may not be sensitive to chemical differences such as deamidation or oxidation. It is particularly important to assess the specificity of methods intended to measure very small (i.e., parts-per-thousand to parts-per-million) levels of product variants or impurities. Other key parameters to be defined in the validation effort are the linearity and range of method and the ruggedness of the technique. Ruggedness is a catch-all term used to describe studies assessing variables such as instrumentation, operators, reagents, and individual laboratories, that may affect the method.

Sample pretreatment procedures are often required to remove interfering substances or concentrate samples prior to analysis. Pretreatment steps are an important variable in the analytical method and a frequent source of error. The variation associated with a sample pretreatment, for example the extraction of proteins from bacterial inclusion bodies, should be determined by parallel extractions of the reference material in the same sample matrix. If available, radiolabeled product can provide a valuable aid to quantitation of any pretreatment steps.

For most immunoassays, the usual pretreatment procedure is sample dilution. Very often the protein product is present at mg/mL concentrations and the immunoassay is performed in the range of ng/mL. While simple in theory, in practice a dilution series can result in a significant cumulative error over five or more tenfold dilution steps. A number of technical details, if included in the assay, can greatly reduce such errors. For example, dilutions should be performed in the same assay buffer as used to prepare the standard curve. The laboratory may prepare or store its own assay buffer, yet lot-to-lot differences in assay buffer can have significant effects on the assay background. The preparation and inclusion in each sample batch of a control sample (which has been aliquoted and stored at a concentration similar to typical process samples) can be used to maintain a historical database of sample preparation and assay variation. Alternatively, extensive dilution series can be avoided through the development of methods with greater detection ranges. However, the effect of interfering substances, such as salts or detergents, may increase and require the development of sample pretreatment steps for their removal.

A variety of approaches exist for the removal of interfering substances, in particular for chromatographic analysis (10). If the target protein is large enough, techniques that separate based on size are widely available and extremely useful. Dialysis is effective but slow and difficult with small volumes. The use of centrifugal concentrators with membranes of particular molecular weight exclusions are available as low as 3000 daltons. However, protein recovery from these devices can vary between the main protein species and its variants (proteolytic or others). Other alternatives include differential precipitation using acids, bases, or organics, or equalization of the salt content and pH between samples and standards. The product of interest can be separated by exploiting its nonpolar properties that allow binding of the product to C4, C8, or C18 bonded stationary phases, while salts and inhibiting components flow through. The product is then eluted from the column with an appropriate nonpolar solution. This general approach can also be used with ion exchange pretreatments. Again, recoveries are often variable, and proper experiments to quantify and control this are essential.

III. ANALYSIS OF BIOLOGICAL ACTIVITY

The preservation of biological activity while increasing product purity is the essential objective in the process development mode and during subsequent scale-up. Biological activity can be affected by components of the harvest material, changes in processing time, or heat or shear forces (11), all of which are parameters that may change in the scale-up operation.

Unlike small molecules, for which activity can be assured through physical or chemical structural analyses, proteins and peptides require methods that directly access bioactivity. Proteins or peptides may lose activity through a variety of chemical changes. Proteolysis, in particular, can produce significant changes in activity. Both prokaryotic and eukaryotic cells contain a variety of digestive enzymes such as nucleases, polysaccharide hydrolases, phophatases, and proteases. These enzymes are also present in medium components such as fetal calf serum or hydrolyzed yeast extracts. Although process steps can be optimized to minimize proteolytic activity (12), activity measurements are an important tool in the control of these processes.

In addition, other physical changes such as oxidation, deamidation, or aggregation may have a significant effect on the biological activity. For example, aggregation is associated with a loss of activity in the case of human growth hormone (hGH). Isolation and analysis of the dimeric form of recombinant growth hormone has shown it to be inactive in a bioassay based on the growth of hypophysectomized rats (13).

The analysis of biological activity can be further complicated because the product may display more than one biological activity, and thus a number of potential assays may be used. It is common for many classes of proteins, for example, the cytokines, to possess different modulatory effects at different concentrations or in different biological systems. Stimulatory activities may be observed at certain concentrations or in particular cell lines, while inhibitory effects are observed at other concentrations or in other cell lines. Transforming growth factor beta (TGF-β) is an excellent example of a growth modulator. In general, TGF-β will inhibit cell culture proliferation, for example epithelial derived cells, lymphocytes, and hepatocytes, but it will stimulate the growth of mesenchymal cells (14).

A. Approaches to the Development of Bioactivity Methods

The extension of biological activity measurements from the in vitro system to the in vivo system is complex. In vivo, molecules rarely act individually but are affected by other, often poorly understood, factors. A conservative approach would suggest that whole animal assays are the best reflection of potency. However, animal models are very expensive, quite variable, and often require special facilities (2). A current area of active research in analytical biotechnology is the replacement of whole animal assays with cell culture or analytical chemistry methods.

Human growth hormone is a good example of a protein pharmaceutical in which the potency is measured by a whole animal assay. While this assay does provide information that the hormone is biologically active, it is very imprecise and wasteful. In this example a growth-hormone-specific cell based bioassay has not been developed, but replacement approaches through methods based on receptor binding or size exclusion have been proposed.

Insulin is an example of a protein pharmaceutical where the traditional bioassay, based on the lowering of blood glucose levels in rabbits, has been partially replaced with an HPLC assay, which is complemented by a bioidentity test using fewer animals than the traditional method.

1. Receptor-Binding Assays

A difficult question that arises in analytical method development is assessment of the three-dimensional structure of the protein and its relationship to bioactivity. One solution to this concern is the development of "biological" assays that infer bioactivity by demonstrating that the product can bind to its receptor in a quantifiable and reproducible fashion; for a recent review see Strosberg and Leysen (15). Once a protein has been purified, it is possible that its receptor can be isolated using the purified protein as a ligand in an affinity based separation. This, of course, is often technically very difficult and assumes that the receptor is intact and soluble when removed from the cell surface. In addition, this approach assumes that the product will select for a single, authentic receptor. Commonly, receptors will exist as a number of subtypes, and a single natural agonist will often interact with a number of different receptors. The receptor can then be directly used for assays or, after transvection, be expressed on the surface of a continuous cell line. The latter approach is advantageous in that transmembrane portions of the receptor can be left intact, as the removal of highly hydrophobic transmembrane portions is often required for purification of the receptor and subsequent analytical work. Truncated receptors (lacking the transmembrane domains) generally are more successful in the development of solution based direct binding assays.

Assay systems that measure direct binding of the receptor and ligand (the product) in solution are the least expensive, most automatable systems. These approaches must meet the general requirements of traditional antibody binding assays, in that the free and receptor complexed product can be separated prior to quantitation, or that the assay signal is only obtained from the receptor-product complex.

Separation methods generally require an immobilization of the receptor on resins, beads, or microtiter plates. Binding of the product to the immobilized receptor is detected though the use of labeled product or labeled antibody against the product. The microtiter plate format provides very high throughput and can be used in any lab performing ELISA or RIA methods. If a competitive binding reaction is performed by the inclusion of soluble receptor during sample incubation, a binding constant can be calculated. These methods require that the receptor be immobilized without loss or change in its ability to bind the product, and they also require one or more steps to separate free from receptor complexed product.

An alternative methodology that does not require separation of free and receptor complexed product is the scintillation proximity assay (SPA) technology (16). This technique can use receptor-coated fluormicrospheres, to which radiolabeled ligand will bind. The fluor is activated by the bound ligand(s) to produce light and is not activated by the free ligand. Competitive assay systems that can measure large numbers of samples without a separation step can be conveniently performed with this technology.

Finally, an alternative approach that also does not require immobilization of receptor or radiolabels is based on a modification of the gel chromatography method of Hummel and Dreyer (17). In this procedure, a known amount of receptor, in stoichiometric excess, is mixed with the product. The receptor-product complex is then separated from free receptor by size exclusion chromatography. This approach can potentially serve as a bioactivity assay for human growth hormone (hGH), as it will distinguish monomeric and dimeric hGH (18), the latter reported to be inactive in a rat weight gain bioassay (13). The method is advantageous in that it allows relatively rapid and precise determinations of the receptor binding in solution phase at high concentrations of product. There is also the advantage of confirmation of the complex formation by measurement of molecular size shifts. However, the method is limited to reactants that are sufficiently different in molecular weight to be differentiated by size exclusion chromatography and is only useful at process steps where the product is highly pure.

2. Cell-Bound Receptor Systems

Expression of the receptor on the cell surface may be necessary for proper folding of the receptor and thus product binding. Organs rich in cells expressing the desired receptor are occasionally used as a convenient reagent source. Human placental cells, for example, provide a rich source of human-insulinlike growth factor I (IGF-I) receptor (19). These cells can be adhered to a solid support and a competitive assay established using a radiolabeled product. Recent advances in automated harvesting devices and beta-particle counting that use the 96 well microtiter plate format have greatly automated and reduced the expense of cell based assays (15). Often, the cellular membranes containing the receptor can be isolated and used in place of immobilized cells. This can be advantageous if it is difficult to immobilize the receptor directly. However, this approach may also lead to more nonspecific reactions with the disrupted, denatured, and generally hydrophobic cell membranes.

The reproducibility of the cell preparations or membranes containing receptor can be a significant variable in these assays. Receptor density may vary from individual to individual, and the isolation, storage, and processing of the preparation can be extremely variable. Thus it is not uncommon to observe a large variability in these methods over time or with a change in critical reagents. An alternative approach is the use of continuous cell lines that express the specific receptor naturally or after transfection with the receptor gene. The use of continuous cell lines provides greater reproducibility of reagents and performance and provides greater safety from infectious agents. The use of a continuous BALB/c 3T3 mouse embryo fibroblast cell line for IGF-I radio-receptor assay development is a recent example of the advantages of this approach (20).

3. Cell Culture-Based Assays

The most widely utilized bioassay systems are in vitro methods based on continuous cell lines. This approach avoids the expense, waste, and poor reproducibility of whole animal systems or primary cell culture. The cell line can be banked (i.e., aliquots of cells frozen in liquid nitrogen at a particular passage number) to ensure a consistent supply of this crucial reagent. Bioassays can be developed based on most cellular responses to the product, if the response correlates with concentration. Ideally, the assay response should be linear and directly related to the desired biological activity. For example, nerve growth factor (NGF) added to pheochromocytoma cell line (PC 12 cells) will cause differentiation to sympatheticlike neurons, where the cells stop dividing, sprout neurites, and become electrically excitable (20). This is an excellent bioassay to reflect the neurotrophic activities of NGF and is widely used.

The NGF PC 12 system is also a good example of the numerous effects that can be observed in a particular cell culture as the result of interaction with a single protein. NGF will change cell surface topography, nutrient uptake, oncogene induction, and the production of neuro-specific proteins (21). Any of these effects might form the basis for a bioassay. However, not all effects that correlate with an observed morphological change are part of a common biochemical pathway. In the PC 12 system, an increase in sodium channel expression parallels the morphological changes that lead to neurite outgrowth. An attractive opportunity for automation is provided because changes in sodium current can be quickly measured by highly automated fluorescent activated cell sorters. However, a synthetic glucocorticoid, dexamethasome, will inhibit increases in sodium current and density but not neurite outgrowth, suggesting the neurite outgrowth does not depend on sodium channel effects (21). Conversely, neurite outgrowth in PC 12 cells can be induced by other factors such as basic fibroblast growth factor (FGF), and FGF is commonly found in serum, which is a typical medium component.

Many bioassay systems rely on general effects such as inhibition or enhancement of cell growth. These assays are attractive for process development work because they can be developed relatively quickly and lend themselves to objective methods of signal quantitation. A very common endpoint in growth enhancement assays is the measurement of tritiated thymidine uptake as an indicator of DNA synthesis and thus cell proliferation. The use of radiolabeled thymidine allows the cells to be harvested and separated from the culture medium, which would contain thymidine that was not taken up by the cells. The amount of radiolabel within the cells can be measured in a scintillation counter. High-throughput filter based cell harvesting devices are widely available, as are rapid, high-throughput beta counting instruments for 96-well plates.

4. Biochemical Methods

Products that have enzymatic activity provide the opportunity to establish in vitro assays for potency. These methods are well established and typically much more precise and less expensive than animal, cell culture, or receptor based systems. Furthermore, these systems can be readily adapted to the microtiter plate or centrifugal analyzer formats to provide large numbers of determinations. The general approaches for enzyme activity determinations and preservative of activity are well known (12). When available, biochemical methods to assess product activity are generally preferred for process development work.

B. Interference in Bioassays

Typically assays for bioactivity and yield are the most important early in process development and especially upstream in the process, while purity is a more important concern later in the development cycle. However, samples obtained from upstream process steps will contain more cross-reactive or interfering substances. A cell proliferation assay, for example, will respond positively to most mitogens. IGF-I, IGF-II, and insulin all act through a common receptor, the alpha 2, beta 2 type I receptor, and these growth factors are common components of serum widely used in cell culture processes.

These same mitogenic effects of growth factors will cause an apparent decrease in the activity of antiproliferative agents when measured in cell growth assays. An example of this effect is shown in Fig. 1. Increasing con-

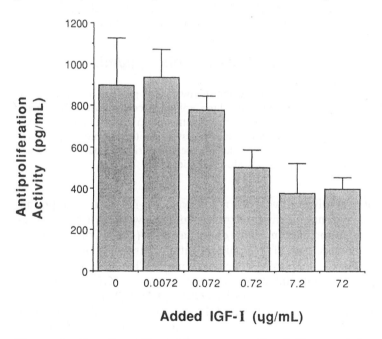

Figure 1 The effect of increasing amounts of insulinlike growth factor I (IGF-I) on the apparent activity of transforming growth factor β (TGF-β) in a cell culture assay using mink lung epithelial cells. TGF-β is an inhibitor of cell growth in this line. Increasing amounts of IGF-I, a growth factor commonly found in serum, will artificially decrease the apparent activity of TGF-β.

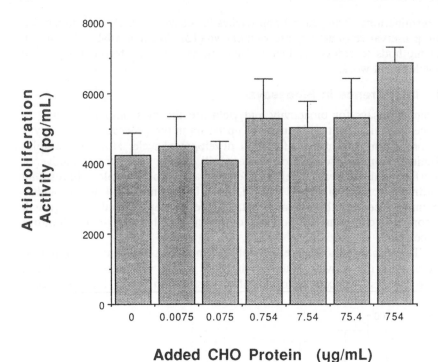

Figure 2   The effect of CHO (Chinese hamster ovary) cell proteins on the apparent TGF-β antiproliferative activity on mink lung epithelial cell culture.   Increasing amounts of CHO cell proteins inhibit cell profileration in this system and are a good model for the potential effects of upstream process impurities on bioassays.   Such assays should be tested for the effect of likely process impurities as part of the assay qualification prior to use for process scale-up studies.

centrations of insulinlike growth factor I, a common mitogenic compound, decreases the apparent bioactivity of transforming growth factor beta (TGF-β), a growth inhibitor of mink lung epithelial cells (14).   Conversely, an example of an enhancement of the apparent antiproliferative activity of TGF-β is shown in Fig. 2.   Increasing concentrations of Chinese hamster ovary (CHO) cell proteins were added to a constant amount of TGF-β, causing an apparent increase in the antiproliferative activity of TGF-β. It is clear from this data that the specific activity of TGF-β or similar growth modulators could be miscalculated upstream in the process due to the effects of host cell proteins or medium constituents in poorly validated assays.

It is not unusual for the source of culture medium components to change during process scale-up as a consequence of efforts to reduce costs or move to more reliable vendors. The new medium may have components that alter the bioassay performance. The amount of such components can vary, and each lot of serum should be characterized prior to use. In addition, cell lines will often produce autocrine growth factors in response to extracellular stimuli, or serum and cells may contain binding proteins that neutralize the bioactivity of many growth factors. Preservatives, pH variations from neutrality, and high ionic strength are all common inhibitors of cell growth.

Similarly, the presence of mitogens is also a problem in growth inhibition assays as they mask the activity of the product, while growth inhibitors can result in greater apparent activity. Other interfering substances in these assays are less obvious. Conditioned media may contain enzymes that act on the cells directly or on the amino acid nutrients in the medium, an example of which is arginase (22). These enzymes may result from mycoplasma contamination of the cells. Mycoplasma will produce arginine deaminase, which has been shown to inhibit cell culture systems (23). Assays that utilize the uptake of tritiated thymidine can be affected by tissue derived kinases and mycoplasma derived phosphorylases, which can degrade thymidine (24). While growth proliferation and inhibition assays are among the least specific bioassays, similar problems will exist to some extent in most bioassay systems. It is therefore essential that a bioassay system be validated for use at each step and scale of the process.

IV. ANALYSIS OF PURITY

The purity requirements for protein or peptide products will vary dependent upon the intended use of the material. Proteins intended as bulk commercial grade reagents, for example detergent enzymes, will have much lower purity requirements than pharmaceuticals, for which the purity requirements are rigorous and highly regulated (25,26).

In general, proteins or peptides intended as bulk reagents are held to functional purity requirements, in that they must be pure enough to work as intended and remain stable over the stated shelf life. However, recombinant DNA technology allows the production of consistent and highly pure proteins. As a result, recombinant DNA derived proteins are often held to purity requirements of approximately 95% or greater for many commercial applications. This level of purity analysis can be quickly and cheaply performed by SDS-PAGE, using Coomassie brilliant blue stain for most proteins. This approach, however, will not detect impurities of similar molecular weight to the target protein. Peptides are normally more difficult or impossible to analyze by SDS-PAGE, and therefore techniques such as reversed phase HPLC or TLC are more applicable.

When commercial grade reagents are used for applications where safety or stability is a concern, the purity requirements will rise. Materials that contact humans, for example detergents or cosmetics, may contain deleterious impurities that could cause allergic reactions in some individuals. Therefore these products are generally held to higher purity standards. The current state of the art in protein purity requirements exists in the pharmaceutical industry, where products are often intended for long term and frequent in vivo use. These products are necessarily held to the highest purity standards.

A. Types of Impurities in Protein Pharmaceuticals

Recent strategies for protein characterization and purity analysis have focused on pharmaceutical products (2,3,26). Often, the most discriminating analysis of a purification scheme comes from the final product impurity profile. This is because there are many sources of potential impurities. Impurities are materials that result from the product or process itself, while contaminants are adventitious agents accidentally introduced into the product. Commonly employed categories of impurities are *innocuous*, which do not pose a health concern, or *deleterious*, which might represent a health or safety risk. Impurities are also grouped by quantity. Major impurities are present at 0.5% or greater, while minor impurities are below the 0.5% level. The absolute amounts of impurities may not relate directly to their deleterious effects.

Specific methods should be developed for impurities that are endogenous to a given process and have a predictable presence in the product. Contaminants and impurities of poorly defined composition, however, must rely on methods that employ a broad spectrum and less specific approach to

Table 1 Typical Impurities in Protein Pharmaceuticals

Impurity	Detection methods
Endotoxin	Rabbit pyrogen test, Limulus Amebocyte Lysate test
Host cell and media proteins	SDS-PAGE, immunoassay
Monoclonal antibodies and defined proteins used in production system	SDS-PAGE, immunoassay
DNA	Hybridization assays, antibody or binding protein sandwich assays
Infectious agents	Reverse transcriptase assay, cell culture cytopathic effects (CPE), electron microscopy
Product variants	
Deamidation products	Isoelectric focusing
Oxidation products	HPLC-tryptic mapping, and/or
Amino acid substitutions	HPLC-mass spectrometry
Aggregated forms	SDS-PAGE, size exlusion HPLC
Proteolytic products	SDS-PAGE, HPLC
Highly conserved or homologous host cell species proteins	Monoclonal antibody based immunoassays

their detection. A general breakdown of typical impurities in a rDNA pharmaceutical are shown in Table 1.

Common examples of *major impurities* are product variants, which contain some chemical or conformational difference from the protein product. These forms may include protein degradation products such as deamidation, oxidation, or unintentional substitutions in the primary structure, such as the substitution of norleucine for methionine.

Minor impurities such as host cell proteins, DNA, or endotoxin may pose potential health hazards and therefore should be reduced to part-per-million levels or less. Residual protein impurities can result from the source material for the drug, for example the host cell organism, components of the fermentation medium, or the components of natural sources from which the product is extracted. In addition, proteins used as process raw materials, such as a monoclonal antibodies, are also potential product impurities.

The production of peptides by chemical synthesis will often use hazardous chemicals and organics, for example fluoride and acetonitrile, during their production. These components must be essentially eliminated from the final product.

The purity requirements for protein pharmaceuticals are an area of continual review because protein purity can only defined by the resolution and sensitivity of the currently available analytical methods. In addition, the intended use of the product will greatly influence its individual purity requirements (26). However, the following strategies for purity analysis will be applicable in most cases.

B. General Strategies for Analytical Methods

In general, impurities can be grouped as either related to the target protein, typically product variants, or as impurities unrelated to the product. The pattern of impurities must be defined for any given product or process. In general, product variants are relatively defined impurities, which are known, restricted families of molecules to which the analyst can apply specific assays based on electrophoretic, chromatographic, or monoclonal based immunochemical methods. By contrast, unrelated impurities are generally unknown or exceedingly heterogeneous populations of complex materials, for which specific assays cannot be developed.

1. Impurities Related to the Product

Clearly, as proteins become more complex in their composition and structure the number of potential impurities related to the product will increase. A well-known example of a structurally heterogeneous glycoprotein is recombinant DNA-derived tissue plasminogen activator (rt-PA). A highly purified preparation will contain many variants that may be very similar to one another. These variants will result from either the inherent heterogeneity of the molecule due to the carbohydrate side chains or the degradative reactions such as deamidation or proteolysis. Despite this complexity it is

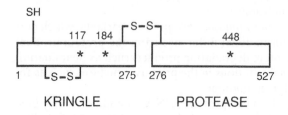

Figure 3 A stylized structure of recombinant tissue plasminogen activator (rt-PA). Glycosylation sites are indicated by asterisks.

often necessary to be able to monitor the level of different variants to demonstrate consistency in the manufacturing process.

Recombinant t-PA has four major forms due to glycosylation and proteolysis (27). As is shown in Fig. 3, the molecule has glycosylation sites at positions 117, 184, and 448. The 184 site is not always glycosylated, however, so that approximately 50% of the molecules contain three carbohydrate groups (Type I) and 50% two groups (Type II). In addition, rt-PA can exist in a 2-chain form as the result of a proteolytic cleavage between residues 275 and 276, which is believed to be related to the bioactivity of the molecule (see Fig. 3). Therefore a preparation of rt-PA will contain four populations (Type I, 1 chain; Type I, 2 chain; Type II, 1 chain; Type II, 2 chain) characteristic of the culture conditions and the recovery process. Secondary processes such as deamidation and proteolysis will introduce additional heterogeneity into each of these populations, although these variants are typically present in low levels in the purified product. Since all of these variants contain the essential features of the rt-PA molecule, polyclonal antibody based assays and biological assays cannot discriminate these forms, and electrophoretic or chromatographic methods are required.

Electrophoretic methods such as isoelectric focusing (IEF) gel electrophoresis or SDS-PAGE are extremely powerful general purpose methods for purity analysis, which generally require little development time. While these methods will rarely define a new impurity, they are very often the first methods where impurities are observed, even in established processes.

Furthermore, these methods can be used at early stages of the recovery process, as they can be used with crude preparations and are simple enough for routine in-process use. IEF is very useful for the detection of relatively subtle variants such as deamidated forms of the product. The use of the SDS-PAGE with silver stain provides extremely sensitive detection of proteolytically cleaved or aggregated variants of the product and protein impurities from the production organism or medium. This analytical method is used extensively throughout the purification process, as well as for final product analysis. An example of the ability of SDS-PAGE, silver stain, to

EVALUATION OF PRODUCT CONSISTENCY

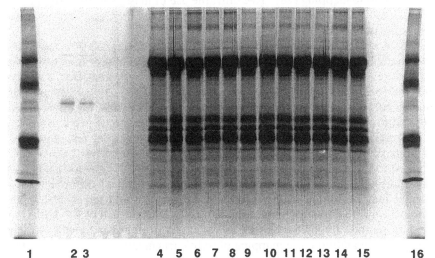

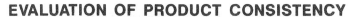

LANE

Figure 4   SDS-PAGE, silver stain, analysis of lot-to-lot consistency of final product rt-PA. This gel is a good example of a relatively simple, broad spectrum, yet very sensitive, analysis of a fairly complex protein. Lanes 1,16: MW markers; Lanes 2,3: 2 and 5 ng BSA staining intensity markers; Lanes 4 and 15: various lots of rt-PA.

provide broad spectrum, highly sensitive analysis of rt-PA consistency is shown in Fig. 4. Most proteins are routinely observable at approximately 2 to 5 ng levels in 20 μg loads providing a detection limit for the variants on the order of parts-per-thousand (w/w). Silver stain does not produce reliable quantitation and therefore must be interpreted in relation to a reference material. The in-process information obtained from these methods can be used to minimize side reactions by modifying the fermentation conditions or to devise a purification step that removes the variant. The success of these steps must then be confirmed by suitable final product analyses.

Once observed, these variants can be identified and characterized through more sophisticated techniques such as mass spectrometry. The use of high-powered analytical methods is necessary, as qualitative techniques such as SDS-PAGE silver stain or IEF analysis do not provide detailed structural information. At present the majority of these high-powered methods are chromatographic, although recently high-performance capillary electrophoresis (HPCE) and so called "hyphenated techniques" that combine methods such HPLC, HPCE, and mass spectrometry are increasingly used. For example, the detection of deamidation can be greatly complicated in IEF analysis by the presence of carbohydrate side chains that contain terminal sialic acid residues. The sites of deamidation can be determined by HPLC based peptide mapping (28). Recently, the use of mass spectrometry on-line with HPLC has become an important technique for the rapid characterization of protein variants (29).

Size exclusion chromatography is a relatively low-resolution analytical technique but provides the advantages of accurate quantitation, insensitivity to charge, and can be used with detergents. In a protein that contains disulfide bridges, the analysis can be performed after reduction of the protein and separation of the protein fragments. In this case the size based separation provides a quantitative method for estimation of proteolysis.

Reversed phase HPLC (RP-HPLC) is a chromatographic technique that is primarily sensitive to differences in hydrophobicity and has been widely applied to the analysis of proteins and peptides (4,30). As a consequence of the three-dimensional structure of proteins, the chemical difference of a variant may be buried in the interior of the protein and not available for interaction with the chromatographic support. Thus the use of RP-HPLC to analyze peptide fragments as well as the intact protein has become widely accepted. In addition, the mapping of tryptic fragments is recognized as the best general analytical technique to monitor the primary sequence of a protein. As trypsin cleaves at frequent intervals in the polypeptide chain (at relatively abundant arginine and lysine residues), the resulting peptides are usually of 2 to 20 residues in length. Therefore an amino acid substitution or cleavage of the polypeptide backbone would be expected to generate a shift in retention time, as would deamidation or oxidation. Peptide maps can be complex but highly resolving; for example, the tryptic map for rt-PA includes over 50 peptides that are separated in a single chromatographic analysis. Recently, electrospray mass spectrometry has been used on-line with HPLC separation and allows the detection of coeluting peptides by mass analysis (31,32). In Fig. 5 the monitoring of a tryptic map by both UV and total ion current (TIC) is shown to give a similar result in monitoring the complex elution profile (29). A mass scan of 300 to 2400 Da is performed each 7 seconds, with the result that a mass can be readily calculated for each of the chromatographic peaks. In addition, the complex elution profile of glycopeptides can be examined by the use of selected ion monitoring, which can be used to define the retention time of each glycopeptide (29).

At present, quality control procedures are focusing on the amino acid sequence of a protein rather than the carbohydrate portion. This has partly been determined by the excellent analytical methods available for monitoring protein sequence, while methods available for quantitative carbohydrate analysis have been much more time-consuming and less effective. The high degree of site dependent microheterogeneity known in many glycoproteins and the lack of methods are barriers to routine carbohydrate analysis. Although such an analysis must of necessity be incomplete in terms of defining actual product heterogeneity, new methods such as high-pH anion exchange chromatography have allowed impressive separations of oligosaccharides after cleavage from the peptide backbone (33). At present, such methods are more suitable for research applications than for routine product monitoring.

2. Impurities Unrelated to the Product

Impurities unrelated to the product include components added to the culture medium or those used as raw materials in the purification process. Media supplements such as insulin, transferrin, antibiotics, and neoplastic agents are common potential impurities arising from the cell culture process. Such impurities may possess significant biological activity or immunogenic poten-

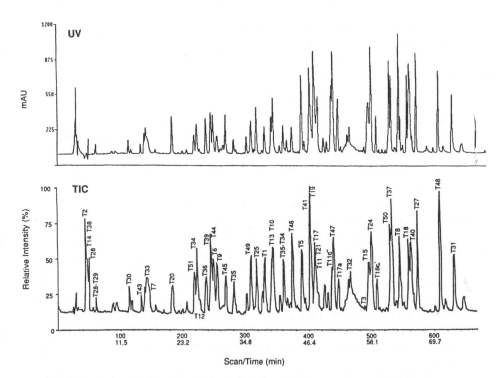

Figure 5 RP-HPLC tryptic map of recombinant tissue plasminogen activator (rt-PA) with UV monitoring at 214 nm (upper trace) or total ion current (TIC) as measured by the electrospray mass spectrometer (bottom trace). The tryptic peptides, as determined by mass spectrometry, are numbered from the *N*-terminus with T-1 containing the *N*-terminus and T-51 containing the *C*-terminus. Three peptides contain a site not readily cleaved by trypsin, and so the uncleaved peptides are observed (T28-T29, T29-T30, T34-T35). In addition, fragments of T18 (lacking the residues ILIGK) and carbohydrate peptide T11 (lacking the residues SGR) are observed and are denoted as T18C and T11C (C for chymotrypticlike cleavage). T17a refers to the nonglycosylated form. The elution positions of the peptides are recorded as both retention time (min) and scan numbers.

tial and must be removed to part-per-million levels. To demonstrate the achievement of such purity requires a combination of highly sensitive assays and process validation. Clearance of each impurity can be determined by assay at each step in the process up to the stage where the impurity is no longer detectable. Further clearance factors for the impurity are calculable by adding known amounts of the impurity to the product pool before each process step. The prestep pool and the poststep pools are then assayed and the removal factor for each process step determined. This approach to process validation has been particularly useful for low-level impurities, for example to validate the removal of media components and viral material (34,35).

Purification processes that employ immuno-affinity chromatography may result in antibody-derived impurities. Antibodies and their fragments possess significant immunogenic potential at most therapeutic doses and particularly if they are nonhuman in origin. Furthermore, immune complexes may be carried through the process, making the analysis difficult, and the antibody preparation itself may contain significant impurities. Fetal calf serum, bovine immunoglobulins, and Protein A or Protein G are examples of impurities that are often associated with monoclonal antibodies. The leakage rate of the immunoaffinity column and the subsequent clearance from the product by the purification process must be demonstrated as part of the process validation effort (36).

3. Approaches for Assay of Unrelated Impurities

Knowledge about the precision, specificity, and accuracy of the analytical method are of particular concern in the detection and quantitation of undefined impurities. Unlike a process derived impurity in a well-developed purification scheme, undefined impurities may vary in both quantity and composition from one production run to another. Broad spectrum assays that detect a general biological effect or an assay signal from any of a family of components are generally used. However, reference methods are rare given the lack of specific analytes. Therefore these methods can only be validated by rigorous control of assay reagents and careful design of the assay.

Increasingly, mammalian cell culture is the preferred production system for proteins. In these systems, cells must be taken from a well-characterized cell bank to allow for a careful examination of the presence of virus or viruslike bodies in the cells. Typical testing on the cell bank will include electron microscopy to detect and quantitate potential viral particles, reverse transcriptase activity, and characterization of the cells' ability to support the replication of a wide range of animal viruses. In addition, it is likely that each lot of harvested cell culture fluid would require assay for adventitious virus via cytopathic effects on at least three different cell lines and for mycoplasma by one or more standard methods (35). Bacterial sterility testing is also mandatory (37).

Host cell DNA is another undefined impurity that must be measured in every lot of drug produced. The widely accepted dot blot assay relies on the hybridization of cellular DNA from the sample with specific ^{32}P-labeled DNA probes obtained from the DNA of the host cell, although new assay methodologies for DNA detection have recently been introduced (2,26).

Endotoxin and other pyrogenic materials are a group of poorly defined impurities of major concern in pharmaceutical manufacture. A combination of the USP rabbit pyrogen assay and the Limulus Amoebocyte Lysate (LAL) assay are considered the most conservative and appropriate approaches for the testing of recombinant biologics (2). The rabbit pyrogen assay is highly variable and may result in false positives due to infection, antigenicity of the product, or handling practices. In addition, some of the recombinant cytokines, such as tumor necrosis factor, are themselves natural pyrogens and will be cross-reactive in the whole animal model. The LAL method is subject to interference by a number of substances and assay conditions, such as low pH.

Assays for the detection of host cell proteins require part-per-million sensitivity and the detection of large numbers of proteins, requirements that have mandated the development of immunoassays to measure process-specific protein impurities. These assays can be made more sensitive and selective if the population of antibodies raised against process-specific host cell proteins are further selected by affinity chromatography. An ELISA method is then developed in which the host cell contaminants are quantitated as a group (38,39).

A number of technical problems occur in the development of these assays, of which the most difficult usually involves selection of a reference material that contains a representative mixture of the host cell proteins. Other key parameters are the method for production of antibodies to this protein mixture and the validation of the assay. The isolation of the reference protein mixture may be attempted from in-process material by immunoabsorption of the product away from the protein impurities. These immunoabsorption procedures, however, are very difficult to perform and validate because all of the product and product fragments must be removed without the loss of any of the impurities. Any residual product will produce antibodies during the immunization and render the assay nonspecific.

An alternative to the product depletion approach is the performance of a "blank run," which consists of a fermentation of the host cell lacking the product gene. The harvest is then purified through one or more steps of the process depending on the purity and yield achieved at each step. Two key assumptions are made. The first is that the lack of product expression does not significantly affect the population of in-process impurities; the second is that the lack of product does not significantly affect the chromatography of the impurities. Performing the blank run at manufacturing scale and isolating the impurities upstream in the process will also help both to mimic the growth conditions of the host cell and to alleviate somewhat the subtle variations in chromatography due to the presence of the product.

Finally, the design and development of these assays present a number of problems. The development lead times are very long, and validation of these assays can only be approached by demonstrating internal consistency of the method and the quality of the reagents. Furthermore, because each assay is process specific, any subsequent process step and scale changes are major considerations. If the process undergoes a scale-up, this event usually requires a requalification of the method to ensure that the reagents are still capable of detecting and quantifying the major impurities. If it is found that the process impurity profile has changed significantly, then a new assay will need to be developed, which will require substantial resources.

V. SUMMARY

Successful and rapid process development requires the availability of suitable analytical methods at all stages of the development cycle (see Tables 2 and 3). The methods should be selected first to ensure the identity, potency, and purity of the product and second to facilitate the process development. Some assays are particularly valuable early in the recovery process (and early in the development cycle) because they are typically robust and can be used with crude samples that contain many components. Popular examples include SDS-PAGE, IEF, and immunoassay, which allow the process scientist simply to monitor the yield and removal of impurities on a broad scale. Each step should be monitored with a biological assay, so that the specific activity of the target protein can be followed and steps that cause a loss of activity can be quickly detected. At the end of the recovery process (and

Table 2 Analytical Methods Evolution in Process Development and Scale-Up

Stage	Primary methods	Analytical goals
Early development or upstream analysis	Immunoassay	Yield analysis
	SDS-PAGE	High-throughput methods
	IEF	Gross product and impurity profile
	Bioassay/immunoassay	Ratio bioactivity/specific protein
Fixed process or final product	Chromatographic methods	Product variant detection/elimination
	Mass spectrometry	
	Protein impurity immunoassay	Process-specific impurity to ppm level
	Bioassay	Exact specific activity, large number of determinations per sample

Table 3 Evolution of Purity Analysis Methods Capable of High
Sample Throughput

Method	Approximate level of purity analysis (%)
Immunoassay/total protein assay	10
SDS-PAGE, Coomassie blue stain	10–95
Fast RP-HPLC(5)	99.9
SDS-PAGE, silver stain	>99.9
Immunoassay	>99.99

Note: Each of the methods listed has limitations, and these techniques are best used in a complementary fashion. For example, gel electrophoresis techniques will not detect impurities with molecular weights similar to those of the product. Silver stain has a very limited linear range of protein concentration, and the slope and range of the assay vary greatly from protein to protein, although well-characterized systems with internal markers of protein stain intensity can provide relatively accurate estimations. Impurity immunoassays are highly process-specific and lack the ability to detect new impurities.

development cycle) more sophisticated analytical methods, for example RP-HPLC and mass spectrometry, are used to detect and characterize variants of the desired product. Highly process-specific assays, such as host cell impurity ELISAs, are developed at this point, and the key methods for process monitoring and final product characterization are selected. While each process development project is distinct, in all cases the use of well-validated complementary analytical methods will provide greater assurance of a timely and successful project.

ACKNOWLEDGMENTS

The authors would like to thank Dr. Stu Builder, Dr. Dan Gold, and Dr. David Giltinan for their helpful advice and comments.

REFERENCES

1. Canova-Davis, E., Teshima, G. M., Kessler, T. J., Lee, P. J., Guzzetta, A. W., and Hancock, W. S. (1990). Strategies for analytical examination of biological pharmaceuticals, *Analytical Biotechnology Capillary Electrophoresis and Chromatography* (C. Horvath and J. G. Nikelly, eds.), American Chemical Society, Washington, D.C., p. 90.
2. Garnick, R. L., Solli, N. J., and Papa, P. A. (1988). The role of quality control in biotechnology: An analytical perspective, *Anal. Chem.*, *60*: 2546.
3. Geisow, M. J. (1991). Characterizing recombinant proteins, *Bio/Technology*, *9*: 921.
4. Frenz, J., Hancock, W. S., Henzel, W. J., and Horvath, C. (1990). Reversed phase chromatography in analytical biotechnology of proteins, *HPLC of*

Biological Macromolecules (K. M. Gooding and F. E. Regnier, eds.), Marcel Dekker, New York, p. 145.

5. Nugent, K., and Olsen, K. (1990). Applications of ultafast protein analysis for real time process monitoring, *BioChromator, 5*: 101.

6. Kuhr, W. G. (1990). Capillary electrophoresis, *Anal. Chem., 62*: 403R.

7. Frenz, J., and Hancock, W. S. (1991). High performance capillary electrophoresis, *TribTech, 9*:243.

8. Hurni, W. M. and Miller, W. J. (1991). Analysis of a vaccine purification process by capillary electrophoresis, *J. Chromatogr., 559*: 337.

9. Caulcatt, R., and Boddy, R. (1989). *Statistics for Analytical Chemists*, Chapman and Hall, London.

10. Wehr, C. T. (1987). Sample preparation and column regeneration in biopolymer separations, *J. Chromatogr., 418*: 27.

11. Knight, P. (1989). Downstream processing, *Bio/Technology, 7*: 777.

12. Scopes, R. K. (1987). *Protein Purification: Principles and Practice*, Springer-Verlag, New York, pp. 221–278.

13. Riggins, R. M., and Farid, N. A. (1990). Analytical chemistry of therapeutic proteins, *Analytical Biotechnology Capillary Electrophoresis and Chromatography* (C. Horvath and J. G. Nikelly, eds.), American Chemical Society, Washington, D.C., p. 113.

14. Miyazaki, K., and Hario, T. (1989). Growth inhibitors—molecular diversity and roles in cell proliferation, *In Vitro, 25*: 866.

15. Strosberg, D., and Leysen, J. E. (1991). Receptor-based assays, *Current Opinion in Biotechnology, 2*: 30.

16. Bosworth, N., and Towers, P. (1989). Scintillation proximitry assay, *Nature, 341*: 167.

17. Hummel, J. P., and Dreyer, W. J. (1962). Measurement of protein-binding phenomena by gel filtration, *Biochem. Biophysis. Acta, 63*: 530.

18. Cunningham, B. C., Ultsch, M., DeVos, A. M., Mulkerrin, M. G., Clauser, K. R., and Wells, J. A. (1991). Dimerization of the extracellular domain of the human growth hormone receptor by a single hormone molecule. *Science, 254*: 821.

19. Marshall, R. N., Underwood, L. E., Voina, S. J., Foushee, D. B., and Van Wyk, J. J. (1974). Characterization of the insulin and somatomedin-C receptors in human placental cell membranes, *J. Clin. Endocrinol. Metabl., 39*: 283.

20. Karey, K. P., Riss, T. L., Burleigh, B. D., Parker, D., and Sirbasku, D. A. (1988). Human recombinant insulin-like growth factor I. II. Binding characterization and radioreceptor assay development using BALB/c 3T3 mouse embryo fibroblasts, *In Vitro Cell. Develop. Biol., 24*: 1107.

21. Pollock, Krempin, and Rudy, J. (1990). Differential effects of NGF, FGF, EGF, cAMP, and dexamethasone on neurite outgrowth and sodium channel expression in PC 12 cells, *J. Neurosci, 10*: 2626.

22. Teryama, H., Koji, T., Kontani, M., and Okumoto, T. (1982). Arginase as an inhibitory principle in liver plasma membranes arresting the growth of various mammalian cells in vitro, *Biochem. Biophysis. Acta, 720*: 188.

23. Sasaki, T., Shintani, M., and Kihara, K. (1984). Inhibition of growth of mammalian cell cultures by extracts of arginine-utilizing mycoplasmas, *In vitro, 20*: 369.

24. Dent, P. B., Liao, S. K., Ettin, G., and Cleland, G. B. (1978). Characterization of an inhibitor of thymidine uptake produced by cultured human melanoma cells, *Oncology, 35*: 235.
25. Hancock, W. S. (1986). Significance of purity in manufacture of recombinant DNA-derived proteins, *Chromatogr. Forum, 1*: 57.
26. Anicetti, V. R., Keyt, B. A., and Hancock, W. S. (1989). Purity analysis of protein pharmaceuticals produced by recombinant DNA technology, *Trends in Biotechnology, 7*: 342.
27. Vehar, G. A., Spellman, M. W., Keyt, B. A., Ferguson, C. K., Keck, R. G., Chloupek, R. C., Harris, R., Bennett, W. F., Builder, S. E., and Hancock, W. S. (1986). Characterization studies of human tissue-type plasminogen activator produced by recombinant DNA technology. *Cold Spring Harbor Symposia on Quantitative Biology, Vol. LI*, Cold spring Harbor Laboratory, Cold Spring Harbor, New York, p. 551.
28. Johnson, B. A., Shivokawa, J. M., Hancock, W. S., Spellman, M. W., Basa, L. J., and Aswad, D. M. (1989). Formation of isoaspartate at two distinct sites during in vitro aging of human growth hormone, *J. Biol. Chem., 264*: 14262.
29. Ling, V., Guzzetta, A. W., Canova-Davis, E., Stults, J. T., Hancock, W. S., Covey, T. R., and Shushan, B. I., (1991). Characterization of the tryptic map of recombinant DNA derived tissue plasminogen activator by high-performance liquid chromatography-electrospary ionization mass spectrometry, *Anal. Chem., 63*: 2909.
30. Mant, C. T., Zhou, N. E., and Hodges, R. S. (1989). Correlation of protein retention times in reversed phase chromatography with polypeptide chain length and hydrophobicity, *J. Chromatogr., 476*: 363.
31. Caprioli, R. M., Fan, T., and Cottrell, J. D. (1986). Continuous-flow sample probe for fast atom bombardment mass spectrometry, *Anal. Chem., 58*: 2949.
32. Covey, T. R., Bonner, R. F., Shushan, B. I., and Henion, J. (1988). The determination of protein, oligonucleotide, and peptide molecular weights by ion-spary mass spectrometry, *Rapid Commun. Mass Spectrom, 2*: 249.
33. Spellman, M. W. (1990). Carbohydrate characterization of recombinant glycoproteins of pharmaceutical interest, *Anal. Chem., 62*: 1714.
34. Jones, A. J. S., and O'Connor, J. V. (1985). Control of recombinant DNA produced pharmaceuticals by a combination of process validation and final product specifications, *Developments in Biological Standardization: Vol. 59* (F. T. Perkins and W. Hennessen, eds.), S. Karger, Basel, p. 175.
35. Wiebe, M. E., Becker, F., Lazar, R., May, L., Casto, B., Semense, M., Fantz, C., Garnick, R., Miller, C., Masover, G., Bergmann, D., and Lubiniecki, A. S. (1989). A multifaceted approach to assure that recombinant tPA is free of adventitious virus, *Advances in Animal Cell Biology and Technology for Bioprocesses* (R. E. Spier, J. B. Griffiths, J. Stephenne, and P. J. Crooy, eds.), Butterworth, London, p. 68.
36. Lucas, C., Nelson, C., Peterson, M. L., Frie, S., Vetterlein, D., Gregory, T., and Chen, A. B. (1988). Enzyme-linked immunosorbent assays (ELISAs) for the determination of contaminants resulting from the immuno-affinity purification of recombinant proteins, *J. Immunol Methods, 113*: 113.
37. Committee for Proprietary Medicinal Products Ad Hoc Working Party on Biotechnology/Pharmacy (1987). Guidelines on the production and quality

control of medicinal products derived by recombinant DNA technology, *Trends Biotechnol., 5*:61.

38. Anicetti, V. R., Fehskins, E. F., Reed, B. R., Chen, A. B., Moore, P., Geier, M. D., and Jones, A. J. S. (1986). Immunoassay for the detection of *E. coli* proteins in recombinant DNA derived human growth hormone, *J. Immunol Methods, 91*: 213.

39. Anicetti, V. R. (1989). Improvement and experimental validation of protein impurity immunoassays for recombinant DNA products, *Analytical Biotechnology Capillary Electrophoresis and Chromatography* (C. Horvath and J. G. Nikelly eds.), American Chemical Society, Washington, D.C., p. 127.

3

Cell Breakage

Cady R. Engler
Texas A&M University, College Station, Texas

I. INTRODUCTION

Commercial production of proteins and peptides until recently was limited to a relatively small number of enzymes produced by microorganisms or extracted from plant or animal tissues. However, recent advances in recombinant DNA (rDNA) and tissue culture technology have made it possible to consider large-scale production of a wide variety of proteins and peptides that previously were difficult to obtain in large quantity. Many of these are important health care products such as interferons, antibiotics, and vaccines. Others are microbial enzymes, mostly intracellular, which have only recently been studied for commercial application.

In most cases, isolation and purification of a protein is simplified if the protein is excreted by the producing organism into the surrounding medium. However, this frequently is not possible if the protein is to retain its biological activity. For example, most rDNA products are complex structures that must be assembled intracellularly to obtain the desired biological activity. When the host cells are made to excrete these products, biological activity often is lost. Therefore most rDNA products to date have been intracellular products.

For isolation and purification of any intracellular product, an efficient cell breakage process will be required. Normally, such a process will follow cell harvesting and washing to remove any residual culture medium. For cells that are surrounded only by a cell membrane, such as mammalian cells and hybridomas, breakage is easily accomplished by placing the cells in a medium of low osmotic pressure or by relatively low levels of shear. In fact, maintaining the integrity of these types of cells during culture is a significant problem. On the other hand, cells that are surrounded by a polymeric cell wall structure, such as microbial cells, are difficult to disrupt. The purpose of this chapter is to address the problem of large-scale cell breakage or disruption of these latter types of cells.

II. METHODS OF CELL DISRUPTION

A variety of disruption techniques have been developed for laboratory-scale solubilization of intracellular proteins. The more commonly used methods, based on either physically or chemically breaking the cell wall structure, are summarized in Table 1 and have been reviewed in several previous articles (1–3). Several of these methods have been adapted for large-scale use, with the most applicable being high-pressure homogenization and high-speed agitator bead milling. Unless the product is extremely sensitive to mechanical stress or heat, these currently would be the methods of choice. Several previous discussions of large-scale cell disruption processes have been presented (1,4,5).

Although chemical methods should be relatively easy to scale up, most subject the cell contents to harsh conditions that damage many proteins. However, enzymatic lysis, which utilizes mild conditions and has high specificity for degradation of cell wall structures, is one of the best for retaining biological activity of proteins. Unfortunately, different lytic enzymes are required for different organisms, and the sensitivity of an organism to enzymatic lysis varies considerably with its physiological state. Since most lytic enzymes currently are not available commercially, costs for large-scale applications are prohibitive. Large-scale production of enzymes and immobilization to facilitate recycling could reduce the cost (6–8), but it seems likely that this method will be limited primarily to high-value products that are severely damaged by mechanical processes.

Among the physical methods of disruption, ultrasonication is one of the most widely used in the laboratory. Large-scale ultrasonic equipment currently is in use in the chemical industry for continuous homogenization of liquid-liquid dispersions and size reduction of agglomerates (9). However, ultrasonication does not appear to be particularly good for large-scale cell

Table 1   Cell Disruption Methods

Physical	Chemical
Ultrasonication	Enzymatic lysis
French press	Detergents
High-pressure homogenizer	Solvents
High-speed agitator bead mill	Acid hydrolysis
Freezing and thawing	Alkali hydrolysis

disruption. Problems include transmission of sufficient power to large volumes of cell suspension (10), formation of free radicals that can destroy biological activity of proteins (11), dissipation of the large amount of heat generated (12), and generation of very fine cell debris (13).

III. GENERAL PROCESS CONSIDERATIONS

Cell disruption is an intermediate step in the production of intracellular products from microorganisms. Therefore interactions with both upstream and downstream processes must be carefully analyzed during the design phase. Upstream processes will influence disruption primarily through the physiological state of the organism being produced, whereas downstream processes must take into account removal of cell debris created by the disruption process, contamination of the product with other cellular proteins, and possible denaturation of the product.

Studies with both high-pressure homogenizers and high-speed agitator bead mills have shown that susceptibility to disruption varies from one organism to another and, for a given organism, with conditions under which the organism is grown. Disruption studies comparing different organisms have shown *Candida utilis* to be more difficult to disrupt than *Saccharomyces cerevisiae* in both a high-pressure device (14) and a bead mill (15); *Bacillus subtilis* was as easily disrupted as *S. cerevisiae* in a high-pressure device (14); but *Brevibacterium ammoniagenes* was more difficult to disrupt than *S. cerevisiae* in a bead mill (5).

Disruption studies of the same organism grown under different conditions have shown a strong dependence of disruption on the physiological state of the organism. For example, studies have shown that cells grown on a complex medium are more robust than those of the same strain grown on a simple medium (16); recombinant organisms appear to be easier to disrupt than nonrecombinant organisms of the same type (17), and limited growth (i.e., lower specific growth rate) due to nutrient limitations or stress causes cells to reinforce the cell wall structure making disruption more difficult (5,14). However, there is no way to predict a priori what the dependency of disruption on cell physiological factors will be. Therefore experimental studies should be carried out when there are no previous data available for a particular organism.

Biologically active proteins normally are denatured by temperatures in the range of 50 to 100°C or extremes of pH and also may be sensitive to shear or other mechanical stresses. When cells are disrupted, all proteins are mixed together. The desired product(s) may then become the target for proteolytic enzymes released from the same cell. Disruption processes must be designed to minimize product exposure to undesirable conditions. Since mechanical disruption processes generate large amounts of heat, substantial cooling normally will be required. Additionally, it may be necessary to limit processing time in the disruption step.

   The size of cell debris generated by the disruption process is another factor that must be considered. Disruption usually is followed by a solid-liquid separation process to remove cell debris. Otherwise, the debris will clog chromatography columns or foul adsorbents used in protein purification steps. Typical processes used are filtration and centrifugation. Both of these depend on particle diameter to the second or higher power. Therefore creation of very small cell wall fragments will substantially decrease the performance of these solid-liquid separation processes.

IV. HIGH-PRESSURE HOMOGENIZERS

Two different types of high-pressure homogenizers are available for cell disruption. The most widely studied is the Manton-Gaulin APV type, which uses a spring-loaded valve originally developed for milk homogenization. The second type utilizes interaction between two high-velocity submerged jets of cell suspension to disrupt the cells. Characteristics of the two types of systems are somewhat different; therefore they will be described separately.

A. Valve-Type Systems

Valve-type systems consist of a positive displacement pump with one or more plungers coupled to an adjustable, restricted orifice discharge valve unit (Fig. 1). Several valve designs (Fig. 2) have been evaluated, with knife-edge or similar designs giving the best results (Fig. 3) (18,19). Also, materials of construction are important, particularly when multiple passes are required, since inclusion bodies and cell debris apparently are highly abrasive (20). A valve made of a wear-resistant ceramic is offered by one manufacturer to combat this problem (19). Two homogenizer manufacturers, APV Gaulin and Rannie, offer systems designed specifically for cell disruption.

   The extent of cell disruption is a strong function of operating pressure and number of passes through the valve, as well as valve design. Temperature has a weak effect on extent of disruption. Disruption is independent of the concentration of cells in the feed up to concentrations of 60–80% wet wt/v (18–24% dry wt/v), but at higher concentrations the amount of disruption decreases (18,21).

   The amount of disruption (R) has been shown to be first order with respect to the number of passes through the valve (N) and a power function of operating pressure (P) (18):

$$\ln(1 - R) = -kNP^a \qquad (1)$$

The value of the parameter a varies according to type of organism and growth conditions as shown in Table 2. Although the data in Table 2 were not all obtained using the same type of disruption device, they do indicate that considerable variation can be expected. It also has been shown that the value of a is not constant over extremely wide ranges of operating pressure (23,24).

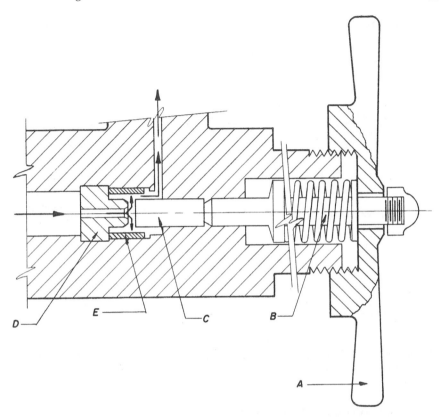

Figure 1 High-pressure homogenizer valve. (A) Handwheel for pressure control, (B) spring-loaded valve rod, (C) valve, (D) valve seat, (E) impact ring. (Redrawn from Ref. 18 by permission of the Institution of Chemical Engineers.)

The extent of disruption (R) usually is determined from the amount of soluble protein released, and in most studies, the maximum amount of soluble protein released has been found to be independent of operating pressure. However, two studies have indicated that the maximum soluble protein after disruption increases with increasing operating pressure (25,26). In those studies, the cell rupture valve design in Fig. 2 was used, which may account for the observed difference in behavior.

Valve-type homogenizers have been used successfully for disruption of both yeasts and bacteria. However, very small bacteria with thick cell walls apparently are not ruptured (5). Generally, these systems are not suitable for disruption of mycelial organisms, such as *Aspergillus niger*, due to blockage of the homogenizing valve by mycelial pellets (10,27).

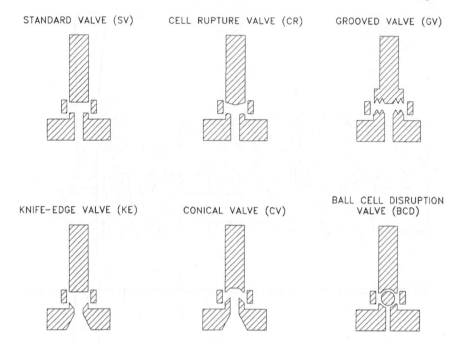

Figure 2   Homogenizer valve configurations evaluated for disruption of microbial cells. (Redrawn from Ref. 19 by permission of APV Gaulin, Inc.)

B. Fluid Interaction Systems

The second type of high-pressure homogenizer, manufactured by Microfluidics Corporation, uses a ceramic interaction chamber rather than a spring-loaded valve to disrupt cells. In the interaction chamber, the cell suspension is forced through two parallel channels having dimensions of 2 × 100 μm (17). The suspension is accelerated to extremely high velocity in these channels, and the streams are then directed toward one another as they exit the channels to form submerged jets. A schematic of the flow path through the interaction chamber is shown in Fig. 4.

For the fluid interaction homogenizer, disruption was not found to have a simple first-order dependency on the number of passes but could be correlated by the equation (17)

$$\ln(1-R) = -kN^b P^a \qquad (2)$$

The value of the parameter b was found to vary with specific growth rate and type of cells being disrupted and the concentration of feed to the homogenizer. No systematic effect of organism type or growth rate on the value of parameter a was observed.

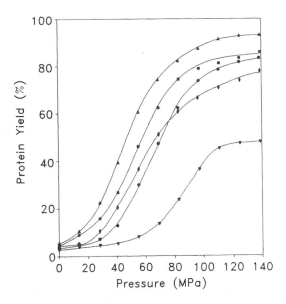

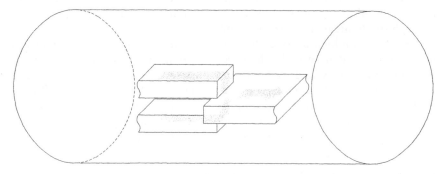

Figure 3 Protein release from baker's yeast as a function of pressure for various homogenizer valve configurations: (▲) knife-edge valve, (■) cell rupture valve, (●) standard valve, (♦) conical valve, and (▼) grooved valve. (Redrawn from Ref. 19 by permission of APV Gaulin, Inc.)

Figure 4 Schematic showing the pathway for fluid flow through the disruption chamber of a fluid interaction system. (Adapted from Ref. 17 by permission of John Wiley, ©1989 John Wiley.)

Table 2   Values of Parameter *a* for Eq. (1)

Organism	*a*	Ref.
Baker's yeast[a]	2.9	18
Bacillus brevis[a]	1.8	22
Escherichia coli[a]		
Synthetic medium	2.2	16
Candida utilis[b]		
Continuous culture, $\mu = 0.1$ h^{-1}	1.77	14
Batch culture, $\mu = 0.5$ h^{-1}	1.17	14
Spent brewery yeast[b]	1.87	14
Saccharomyces cerevisiae[b]		
Continuous culture, $\mu = 0.1$ h^{-1}	0.86	14
Bacillus subtilis[b]		
Continuous culture, $\mu = 0.2$ h^{-1}	1.07	14

[a]Manton Gaulin-APV homogenizer.
[b]Impingement disruption device.

Although there have been fewer studies of this type of cell disrupter reported, the available literature indicates that it is suitable for all types of cells, including mycelial organisms. The interaction chamber, however, contains very small channels for fluid flow, so there is potential for blockage by mycelial pellets.

C. Product Denaturation

For either type of high-pressure homogenizer, essentially all the pressure energy imparted to the fluid is dissipated as thermal energy. Assuming the specific heat of the process stream to be the same as for water, a temperature increase of 10°C will occur per 42 MPa pressure dissipated (20). To minimize thermal denaturation of products, cooling of the homogenizer effluent should be provided. This is particularly critical if multiple passes through the homogenizer are required.

Studies with high-pressure homogenizers have shown that enzymes are not appreciably denatured by the process at temperatures below 30°C, even after prolonged recycling through the homogenizer (28). As pump designs are improved to allow increased maximum operating pressures, effluent cooling will become more important to minimize product exposure to high temperatures. For heat-sensitive products, the maximum pressure at which the homogenizer can be operated may be dictated by the temperature increase that occurs.

D. Scale-Up of High-Pressure Processes

The important factors that affect the degree of disruption in high-pressure homogenizers are summarized in Table 3. As discussed previously, organism-related factors are important, and some generalizations regarding their ef-

Table 3 Factors Affecting Disruption in High-Pressure Homogenizers

Valve design
Operating pressure
Number of passes
Cell concentration
Temperature

fects can be made: e.g., limited growth usually produces cells with stronger walls, and recombinant organisms usually have weaker walls. However, we cannot predict a priori the operating conditions required to achieve a given level of disruption for a particular organism, even if we know the conditions under which it was grown. Therefore experimental data relating disruption to operating conditions must be obtained to provide a basis for scale-up.

Once the dependency of disruption on pressure and number of passes is known for an organism, scale-up of the process becomes straightforward. For vale type homogenizers, capacity can be increased over a wide range by increasing the capacity of the high-pressure pump that feeds the disruption valve. Increased throughput causes the valve to open wider and remain open for a greater fraction of time, but it does not appear to have any detrimental effect on performance (18). Thus disruption obtained with larger units should be the same as that obtained with a laboratory unit. Once the maximum throughput for the valve is reached, additional capacity is obtained by adding more units rather than changing the valve design. Although fewer data are available for fluid interaction units, disruption does not appear to be a function of capacity in these units, either.

As seen from Eqs. (1) and (2), increasing the operating pressure can reduce the number of passes needed to achieve a given amount of disruption. This has the benefits of increasing the throughput of the system or reducing the number of homogenizers required and also of reducing the further disintegration of cell debris on repeated passages through the homogenizer. Increased disruption per pass, however, must be balanced against higher discharge temperatures, which may be detrimental to the process stream.

Homogenizer manufacturers have recognized the benefits of higher operating pressures for cell disruption and now offer production and pilot-scale units with higher pressure ratings than those used for milk homogenization. Valve-type systems are available in production-scale units capable of processing up to 4,500 L/h at a pressure of 70 MPa and in pilot-scale systems with a capacity of 133 L/h at a pressure of 105 MPa (20). Fluid interaction systems are available in production units with capacities up to 11,000 L/h operating at 110 MPa and in pilot systems that can process 340 L/h at 124 MPa with an option to increase pressure to 206 MPa. Design of high-pressure disruption processes also must include provisions for cooling of the homogenizer effluent and high-pressure pump. Although higher feed temperatures have been shown to increase disruption rates (18), protein stability is decreased. In most cases, rapid removal of heat generated in the homogenizer will be beneficial to retention of biological activity of the product. When multiple passes are needed, cooling becomes critical to prevent exposure of the product to excessive temperatures. Additional cooling is needed for pump plungers and packings to allow operation at the high pressures required for disruption.

For most applications, discharge of aerosols containing microorganisms into the workplace cannot be tolerated; therefore a final consideration in high-pressure disruption process design is containment of aerosols. Fluid circulating behind the main seals of the pump to cool the plungers may assist in purging leakage from that part of the system. In many cases, however, total enclosure of the system will be required to assure that there is no leakage.

V. HIGH-SPEED AGITATOR BEAD MILLS

High-speed agitator bead mills originally were developed for comminution of pigments used in the paint and lacquer industry, and various designs have been investigated for microbial cell disruption. These mills consist of either a horizontal or a vertical grinding chamber enclosing a central agitator shaft on which impellers are mounted. The grinding chamber is filled to the desired level with glass beads, which provide the grinding action. These are retained in the chamber during continuous flow operations by some type of dynamic opening, e.g., a narrow slot formed between a rotating disk and a stationary plate, which reduces fouling and allows the system to operate in a continuous flow mode. A typical bead mill arrangement is shown in Fig. 5.

A. Process Kinetics

Batch disruption in bead mills can be described as a first-order process (29,30):

$$\ln(1-R) = -kt \tag{3}$$

where t is the batch time. The value of the rate constant k depends on several of the operating parameters including impeller speed and design, bead loading, bead size, and cell concentration.

For continuous disruption processes, mixing in the grinding chamber must be taken into consideration. A CSTR-in-series model has been used to describe kinetics in this case (29):

$$\frac{1}{(1-R)} = 1 + \left(\frac{kt}{j}\right)^j \tag{4}$$

where t is the mean residence time in the mill (total volume divided by total throughput, V/Q) and j is the number of CSTRs in series, which may include

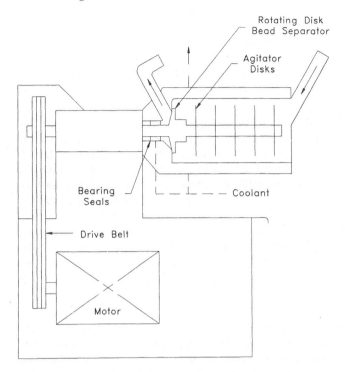

Figure 5 Typical bead mill arrangement. Fluid inlets and outlets are above tank level, and the rotating disk is used to retain beads in the grinding chamber. (From W. A. Bachofen, Basle, commercial literature.)

a fractional CSTR. Values of j must be obtained experimentally from residence time distribution studies. Again, the value of the rate constant depends on various operating parameters.

Table 4 Factors Affecting Disruption in High-Speed Agitator Bead Mills

Chamber design
Agitator speed
Agitator design
Bead size
Bead loading
Cell concentration
Feed rate
Temperature

B. Design Considerations

The extent of cell disruption in high-speed agitator bead mills is influenced by numerous design parameters and operating conditions. The most important factors are summarized in Table 4. In addition, organism-related factors are important as discussed previously.

1. Chamber Design

Although both vertical and horizontal arrangements of bead mills are available, previous studies indicate that the horizontal arrangement is more effective for disruption (5,31,32). In the vertical arrangement, fluid flow is in the upward direction, which tends to fluidize the beads and reduce the grinding efficiency. Horizontal mills are advantageous if high bead loadings and small bead sizes are used, which generally is the case for cell disruption (32).

Commercially available bead mills have varying length-to-diameter ratios, with the optimum considered to be between 2.5 and 3.5 (5). Since laboratory mills frequently have different L/D ratios than pilot- or production-scale units, extrapolation of laboratory data to predict large-scale performance is difficult.

2. Agitator Speed

The rate of disruption tends to increase with increasing tip speed of the agitator impellers up to a point and then it appears to level off as shown in Fig. 6. The exact behavior depends on the organism being disrupted and on the agitator design. Smaller organisms such as bacteria have higher optimum tip speeds than do larger organisms (5). The actual rate of disruption many continue to increase with increasing tip speed, but a simultaneous increase in dispersion in the grinding chamber may negate this effect (29).

3. Agitator Design

The impellers attached to the agitator shaft should be designed to give optimal transfer of kinetic energy to the grinding elements. Although a variety of designs have been studied, there has not been a systematic attempt to relate disc design to agitation or disruption efficiency. The impellers can be mounted either centrically or eccentrically, perpendicularly or obliquely. They may be grooved or have openings cut in them to aid agitation. Various configurations are shown in Fig. 7 and orientations with respect to the shaft, in Fig. 8. At lower speeds an open agitator design was found to cause greater back-mixing, which reduced efficiency, but at high speeds the open design gave greater agitation and had increased power consumption (23). Oblique mounting of impellers on the shaft improved the agitation efficiency at lower speeds but required greater power input and more cooling to maintain the desired operating temperature (15).

4. Bead Size

Special lead-free glass beads, which range in diameter from 0.2 to 1.5 mm or larger, are normally used as the grinding elements. The optimum bead size

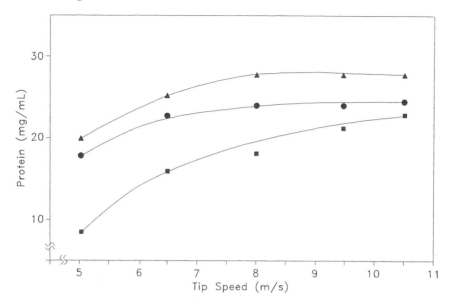

Figure 6 Effects of agitator tip speed and bead loading on protein release from baker's yeast. Bead loadings (% chamber volume): (■) 70%, (▲) 80%, (●) 85%. (Redrawn from Ref. 33 by permission of Butterworth-Heinemann.)

for disruption depends on both the size of the organism and the location of the product being released. The smallest-diameter beads have been found most effective for disruption of bacteria (5,33), whereas larger-diameter beads are optimum for yeast cells. For large-scale processing, the need for continuous separation of cell suspension from beads places a lower limit on bead diameter of about 0.4 mm (5).

Location within the cell of the product being released also affects optimum bead size, as seen in Fig. 9. The optimum bead diameter for release of enzymes located primarily in the periplasmic space (e.g., α-glucosidase) is larger than that for release of enzymes located in the cytoplasm (e.g., glucose-6-phosphate dehydrogenase). For release of enzymes located in the periplasmic space, complete disintegration of cells may not be necessary.

5. Bead Loading
The optimum bead loading, which is expressed as the percentage of free chamber volume nominally occupied by the beads, generally is in the range of 80% to 90%. If the bead loading is too low, shear forces and frequency of collision will not be sufficient to provide good disintegration. If the loading is too great, interference among the grinding elements prevents the establishment of effective velocity profiles. Larger-diameter beads generally require a somewhat lower loading than do smaller beads (33). Temperature

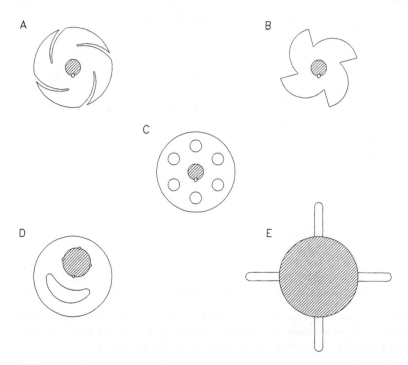

Figure 7   Disk configurations used in agitator bead mills: (A) Slitted disk, closed design; (B) slitted disk, open design; (C) perforated disk; (D) eccentric disk; and (E) pin agitator. (Adapted from Ref. 32 by permission of Marcel Dekker, Inc.)

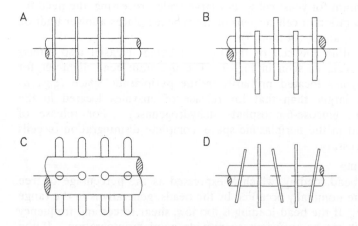

Figure 8   Disk arrangements used on bead mill drive shafts: (A) Concentric disks, (B) eccentric disks, (C) pin agitator, and (D) oblique mounting. (Adapted from Ref. 32 by permission of Marcel Dekker, Inc.)

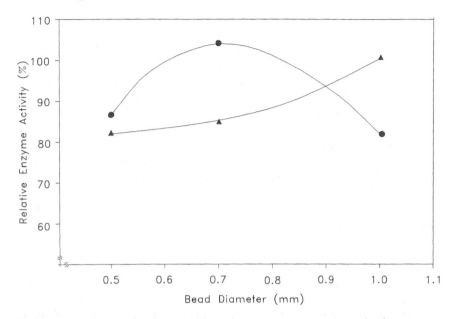

Figure 9 Effect of bead diameter on enzyme release from *Saccharomyces cerevisiae.* The optimum bead size is smaller for glucose-6-phosphate dehydrogenase (●), which is located in the cytoplasm, than for α-glucosidase (▲), which is located in the periplasmic space. (Reproduced from Ref. 5 by permission of the American Institute of Chemical Engineers, ©1987 AIChE.)

and power consumption both increase markedly with increasing bead loading (5,29,33).

6. Cell Concentration

Cell concentration generally has been found to have only a small effect on disruption (29,30,33), although a decrease in disruption with increasing cell concentration between 30 and 60% (wet weight) has been reported (23). Heat generation decreases with decreasing concentration, but energy consumption per unit weight of cells increases. The optimum cell concentration appears to be between 30 and 50% (wet weight) (5).

7. Feed Rate

The amount of disruption decreases with increasing flow rate, and a first-order relation between disruption and the inverse of flow rate has been suggested (30):

$$\ln (1 - R) = - \frac{k}{Q} \tag{5}$$

However, flow rate also affects the residence time distribution within the bead mill, with higher flow rates producing less back-mixing and giving narrower residence time distributions (5). Thus the net influence of feed rate on disruption frequently is not given by the simple first-order relation in Eq. (5) (5,15,30,33). For most situations, the optimum feed rate will depend on agitator speed, bead loading, and other operating conditions as well as mill design and organism properties.

8. Temperature

Operating temperatures for disruption generally are limited to a narrow range to prevent thermal denaturation of solubilized proteins. Within a range of 5 to 40°C, temperature has been shown to have only a limited effect on disruption, with somewhat greater disruption occurring at lower temperatures (29,34). Typically, the range of operating temperatures for disruption is limited to 5 to 15°C.

C. Product Denaturation

Temperature is difficult to control precisely in bead mills because of the large amount of heat generated by the process. As with high-pressure homogenizers, virtually all the energy supplied to bead mills is converted to heat. For example, in a Netzsch LME 20 mill with a power consumption of 7.5 kW, heat generation was reported to be 7 kW (5). For small mills, a cooling jacket on the grinding chamber usually is sufficient to remove the generated heat. For larger mills, however, additional cooling is necessary. This is provided on the Netzsch LM20 by a patented system for cooling the agitator shaft and disks (4).

In bead mill processing, not only may thermal denaturation be a problem but also denaturation caused by shear and other mechanical forces. For example, enzymes have been shown to be detectably inactivated by bead milling, even at temperatures below 5°C (35). For less stable enzymes, plots of activity as a function of time during batch disruption may show a maximum indicating damage to the enzyme caused by shear or other stresses (32).

D. Scale-Up of Bead Mills

High-speed agitator bead mills are commercially available with grinding chamber volumes up to 250 L, with larger units having been built for special cases (32). Feed rates of up to 2000 L/h may be used with a 250-L mill. Results obtained using laboratory units having volumes of 50 mL to 2.5 L can be used to estimate operating conditions for larger-scale units. However, many of the laboratory systems are not geometrically similar to their large-scale counterparts, so that some experimental verification is usually required for scale-up (5,32).

VI. CONCLUSIONS

Large-scale disruption of microorganisms can be accomplished efficiently with either high-pressure homogenizers or high-speed agitator bead mills. Both types of equipment are available commercially in models designed specifically for cell disruption. Bead mills are most suitable for disruption of yeasts, mycelial organisms and microalgae (4,32), whereas high-pressure homogenizers are more suitable for bacteria and some yeasts (4). High-pressure homogenizers have fewer design and operating parameters to consider, and they can be scaled up directly from laboratory data. Bead mills have more design and operating parameters, which gives them more flexibility for special applications but makes scale-up more difficult.

Evidence has shown that denaturation of proteins during disruption generally is not a serious problem, with the exception of membrane-associated enzymes and multienzyme complexes, which may be damaged by mechanical forces. For these types of products, enzymatic lysis or other gentle means of breaking open the cell are required. The fact that the physiological state of the cell influences its susceptibility to disruption may be used to advantage in selecting fermentation conditions for products that require cell disruption.

REFERENCES

1. Engler, C. R. (1985). Disruption of microbial cells, *Comprehensive Biotechnology* (M. Moo-Young, ed.), Pergamon Press, Oxford, vol. 2, p. 305.
2. Coakley, W. T., Bater, A. J., and Lloyd, D. (1977). Disruption of microorganisms, *Adv. Microb. Physiol., 16:* 279.
3. Hughes, D. E., Wimpenny, J. W. T., and Lloyd, D. (1971). The disintegration of micro-organisms, *Methods in Microbiology* (J. R. Norris and D. W. Ribbons, eds.), Academic Press, New York, vol. 5B, p. 1.
4. Chisti, Y., and Moo-Young, M. (1986). Disruption of microbial cells for intracellular products, *Enzyme Microb. Technol., 8:* 194.
5. Kula, M.-R., and Schütte, H. (1987). Purification of proteins and the disruption of microbial cells, *Biotechnol. Prog., 3:* 31.
6. Asenjo, J. A., and Dunnill, P. (1981). The isolation of lytic enzymes from *Cytophaga* and their application to the rupture of yeast cells, *Biotechnol. Bioeng., 23:* 1045.
7. Galas, E., Bielecki, S., Antczak, T., Wieczorek, A., and Blaszczyk, R. (1981). Optimization of cultivation medium composition for lytic enzyme biosynthesis, *Advances in Biotechnology* (M. Moo-Young, ed.), Pergamon Press, Toronto, vol. 3, p. 301.
8. Dunnill, P. (1972). The recovery of intracellular products, *Fermentation Technology Today* (G. Terui, ed.), Society for Fermentation Technology, Japan, p. 187.
9. Grange, A. (1982). Ultrasonic homogenizers—their development and application, *4th European Conference on Mixing*, BHRA Fluid Engineering, Cranfield, England, p. 423.

10. Lambert, P. W. (1983). Industrial enzyme production and recovery from filamentous fungi, *The Filamentous Fungi* (J. E. Smith, D. R. Berry, and B. Kristiansen, eds.), Edward Arnold, London, vol. 4, p. 210.
11. Doulah, M. S. (1977). Mechanism of disintegration of biological cells in ultrasonic cavitation, *Biotechnol. Bioeng., 19*: 649.
12. Lilly, M. D., and Dunnill, P. (1969). Isolation of intracellular enzymes from microorganisms—The development of a continuous process, *Fermentation Advances* (D. Perlman, ed.), Academic Press, New York, p. 225.
13. Wang, D. I. C., Cooney, C. L., Demain, A. L., Dunnill, P., Humphrey, A. E., and Lilly, M. D. (1979). *Fermentation and Enzyme Technology*, John Wiley, New York.
14. Engler, C. R., and Robinson, C. W. (1981). Effects of organism type and growth conditions on cell disruption by impingement, *Biotechnol. Let., 3*: 83.
15. Rehacek, J., and Schaefer, J. (1977). Disintegration of microorganisms in an industrial horizontal mill of novel design, *Biotechnol. Bioeng, 19*: 1523.
16. Gray, P. P., Dunnill, P., and Lilly, M. D. (1972). The continuous-flow isolation of enzymes, *Fermentation Technology Today* (G. Terui, ed.), Society for Fermentation Technology, Japan, p. 347.
17. Sauer, T., Robinson, C. W., and Glick, B. R. (1989). Disruption of native and recombinant *Escherichia coli* in a high-pressure homogenizer, *Biotechnol. Bioeng., 33*: 1330.
18. Hetherington, P. J., Follows, M., Dunnill, P., and Lilly, M. D. (1971). Release of protein from bakers' yeast (*Saccharomyces cerevisiae*) by disruption in an industrial homogenizer, *Trans. Inst. Chem. Eng., 49*: 142.
19. A. P. V. Gaulin. (1985). *Cell Disruption with APV Gaulin High Pressure Homogenizers*, Technical Bulletin No. 74, APV Gaulin, Everett, Mass.
20. Engler, C. R. (1990). Cell disruption by homogenizer, *Separation Processes in Biotechnology* (J. A. Asenjo, ed.), Marcel Dekker, New York, p. 95.
21. Brookman, J. S. G. (1974). Mechanism of cell disintegration in a high pressure homogenizer, *Biotechnol. Bioeng., 16*: 371.
22. Augenstein, D. C., Thrasher, K., Sinskey, A. J., and Wang, D. I. C. (1974). Optimization in the recovery of a labile intracellular enzyme, *Biotechnol. Bioeng., 16*: 1433.
23. Dunnill, P., and Lilly, M. D. (1975). Protein extraction and recovery from microbial cells, *Single Cell Protein II* (S. R. Tannenbaum and D. I. C. Wang, eds.), MIT Press, Cambridge, Mass., p. 179.
24. Engler, C. R., and Robinson, C. W. (1981). Disruption of *Candida utilis* cells in high pressure flow devices, *Biotechnol. Bioeng., 23*: 765.
25. Whitworth, D. A. (1974). Assessment of an industrial homogenizer for protein and enzyme solubilization from spent brewery yeast, *Compt. Rend. Trav. Lab. Carlsberg, 40*: 19.
26. Whitworth, D. A. (1974). Hydrocarbon fermentation: Protein and enzyme solubilization from *Candida lipolytica* using an industrial homogenizer, *Biotechnol. Bioeng., 16*: 1399.
27. Zetelaki, K. (1969). Disruption of mycelia for enzymes, *Process Biochem., 4*(12): 19.
28. Follows, M., Hetherington, P. J., Dunnill, P., and Lilly, M. D. (1974). Release of enzymes from bakers' yeast by disruption in an industrial homogenizer, *Biotechnol. Bioeng., 13*: 549.

29. Limon-Lason, J., Hoare, M., Orsborn, C. B., Doyle, D. J., and Dunnill, P. (1979). Reactor properties of a high-speed bead mill for microbial cell rupture, *Biotechnol. Bioeng., 21*: 745.

30. Mogren, H., Lindblom, M., and Hedenskog, G. (1974). Mechanical disintegration of microorganisms in an industrial homogenizer, *Biotechnol. Bioeng., 16*: 261.

31. Rehacek, J., Beran, K., and Bicik, V. (1969). Disintegration of microorganisms and preparation of yeast cell walls in a new type of disintegrator, *Appl. Microbiol., 17*: 462.

32. Schütte, H., and Kula, M.-R. (1990). Bead mill disruption, *Separation Processes in Biotechnology* (J. A. Asenjo, ed.), Marcell Dekker, New York, p. 107.

33. Schütte, H., Kroner, K. H., Hustedt, H., and Kula, M.-R. (1983). Experiences with a 20 litre industrial bead mill for the disruption of microorganisms, *Enzyme Microb. Technol., 5*: 143.

34. Currie, J. A., Dunnill, P., and Lilly, M. D. (1972). Release of protein from bakers' yeast (*Saccharomyces cerevisiae*) by disruption in an industrial agitator mill, *Biotechnol. Bioeng., 14*: 725.

35. Marffy, F., and Kula, M.-R. (1974). Enzyme yields from cells of brewers' yeast disrupted by treatment in a horizontal disintegrator, *Biotechnol. Bioeng., 16*: 623.

4

Crossflow Membrane Filtration

Zhi-Guo Su

Dalian University of Technology, Dalian, People's Republic of China

Clark K. Colton

Massachusetts Institute of Technology, Cambridge, Massachusetts

I. INTRODUCTION

Filtration is a process for separating components of a fluid mixture according to their size by pressure-driven flow through a porous medium. Conventional filter media such as woven cloth or steel mesh are not suitable for the separation of dissolved molecular solutes or even living cells. The introduction of synthetic polymeric membranes (1,2) has opened a vast field of applications for filtration to be used in downstream processing of biological products (3–5). There are three main classes of membrane filtration that are arbitrarily distinguished according to their nominal pore diameter (NPD). Microfiltration (MF) membranes have NPD between about 0.1 and 10 μm and are used, for example, in the removal of particulates such as cells or cell debris from culture suspensions or cell homogenates (6). Ultrafiltration (UF) membranes, with NPD between about 0.001 and 0.1 μm, are used for concentrating macromolecules such as proteins or polysaccharides (7). Reverse osmosis (RO) applies to membranes with NPD < 0.001 μm that are used for the separation of microsolutes, such as inorganic salts, from water (8). Table 1 lists a general classification of membrane filtration processes. The boundary between MF and UF is blurred. Henry (9) suggested that MF deals with suspensions containing particles while UF deals with solutions containing dissolved macrosolutes. However, very small particles such as inclusion bodies and viruses are often

Table 1   Membrane Filtration Processes in Biotechnology

Type of filtration	Typical retained species	Nominal pore diameter
Microfiltration (MF)	Cells, cell debris	$0.1–10\ \mu m$
Ultrafiltration (UF)	Proteins, polysaccharides	$0.001–0.1\ \mu m$
Reverse osmosis (RO)	Ions, microsolutes	< 1 nm

separated with UF membranes; UF membranes are sometimes used to concentrate cells, especially with process streams that lead to fouling of MF membranes. Another view is that MF membranes have pores or interstices that can be visualized by light microscopy, whereas UF membranes do not.

In all crossflow membrane filtration processes, fluid shear is used to minimize accumulation of retained species at the membrane surface, resulting in significantly higher filtration rates than can be attained in a dead-ended system. This technique has been termed "crossflow" because the feed suspension or solution flows tangentially across the membrane surface and perpendicularly to the direction of filtrate flow through the membrane.

Conventional filtration, in which relatively coarse particles are separated from a fluid using an inexpensive filter medium, can be operated in crossflow mode. Conversely, membrane filtration can be conducted in conventional dead-end mode. The choice depends upon process economics (10,11). Crossflow filtration requires additional energy in order to generate a high fluid shear rate near the membrane surface. In general, the use of crossflow in membrane filtration has resulted in significant filtrate flux increases and economic benefits (9,12). The term crossflow appears to have been coined more than 20 years ago (13). Other names that have appeared in the literature for the same concept include dynamic filtration (14,15), tangential flow filtration (16), and delayed cake filtration (17).

Reverse osmosis may be increasingly used in the future to concentrate antibiotics and small organic molecules because of the energy savings realized over the use of evaporative techniques and because of a lower processing temperature for temperature sensitive products (18,19). However, microfiltration and ultrafiltration have found more applications than reverse osmosis in downstream processing of biological products and will be the subject of the remainder of this chapter.

II. MEMBRANES AND EQUIPMENT

A variety of MF and UF membranes and crossflow filtration modules are marketed by filter manufacturers around the world (20,21). It is important for a particular application to choose an appropriate membrane and filter module.

A. Membrane Structures and Materials

Membranes are thin, porous sheets, usually less than 0.1 mm in thickness. Most membrane materials are fabricated from synthetic organic polymers, although membranes have also been fabricated from inorganic substrates such as ceramics and metals. There are some important differences in structure between MF membranes and UF membranes. Nearly all UF membranes are anisotropic with a thin barrier layer or skin on one surface which contains the smallest pores that determine the rejection characteristics and hydraulic permeability. Below the skin is a matrix consisting of much larger pores that acts as a support for the thin skin and usually determines the diffusive permeability. Once a molecule passes through the barrier layer, it will encounter relatively little resistance in flowing through the rest of the matrix. This structure minimizes blockage of internal membrane pores, a potentially serious problem with isotropic membranes. Most MF membranes, however, are isotropic with relatively homogeneous pore structure. In some cases, a thin skin is present, but its pores are comparable in size to that of the interior. Virtually all MF membranes, except nuclear-track-etch membranes, have irregular, tortuous, and interconnected pores that have a distribution of size. Because there is a distribution of pore sizes throughout the membrane, MF membranes can be more susceptible to a decay of hydraulic permeability (fouling) than UF membranes. Some asymmetrical MF membranes have also been developed (22,23). Nuclear-track-etch membranes provide straight-through pores with a narrow size distribution, but their pore density is very low, resulting in low filtration rates.

Manufacturers usually provide some characterization of the pore size or retention properties of their membranes. MF membranes are characterized by a nominal pore diameter determined by one of the several possible physical measurement techniques. UF membranes are classified by a nominal molecular weight cutoff (NMWC), which typically represents the molecular weight of a macromolecule that has a rejection coefficient of about 90 or 95%.

Rejection of solutes or particles by UF or MF membranes is a complex phenomenon that depends upon the size distribution of pores and their shape, the size and conformation of the solute, and the presence of any interaction (e.g., charge) between solute and membrane. A layer of concentrated rejected solute at the membrane surface may serve as a dynamically formed membrane that increased the rejection of smaller solutes (24,25).

Polymeric membranes are made from two classes of materials, cellulosics and noncellulosics (20,26). Cellulosic membranes include regenerated cellulose and cellulosic derivatives such as cellulose nitrate and cellulose acetate. Cellulose and the mono- and diacetate derivatives are hydrophilic, which helps to minimize protein adsorption that is a cause of membrane fouling. Cellulosic membranes lack resistance to chemical, mechanical, and thermal stresses, thus preventing them from being used for most large-scale industrial applications.

Noncellulosic membranes include those made from polysulfone, polyamide, polyacrylonitrile, polycarbonate, and polypropylene. They are stronger and more resistant than cellulosics to extreme pH, most chemicals, and heat. They have found applications in industrial processes where steam sterilization and periodic cleaning with detergents and other chemicals are necessary. These membranes are usually hydrophobic, which can result in fouling due to protein adsorption and denaturation on the surface. Proper surface treatment is desired to render these membranes less protein adsorptive.

B. Filtration Modules and Systems

A variety of membrane module designs have been developed for various practical applications (27,28). Membranes are fabricated in two broad classifications, tubular and flat sheets. The tubular configuration is further divided into two classes based on internal diameter. Hollow fibers are small membrane tubes with internal diameters in the range of about 0.2–2 mm. They are made by spinning technology similar to that used in the production of synthetic fibers for textiles (20). Tubular membranes of larger internal diameter are usually cast inside of a porous, cylindrical support.

Hollow fibers are usually bundled together, encased in a cylindrical shell, and potted at each end to form a cartridge similar to that of a multitube heat exchanger. A barrier layer or skin, if present, is usually on the internal lumenal surface so that filtration is carried out from the lumen to the shell side. An advantage of the hollow fiber cartridge is the large membrane area per unit volume of module. A disadvantage is the possible occurrence of fiber clogging by particles in crossflow microfiltration (29). Consequently, hollow fibers may require prefiltration with some particulate suspensions. Large-bore tubular membranes are usually installed as an integral component of a long plastic or steel cartridge. These modules have a low surface-to-volume ratio, but they can be operated in turbulent flow, do not clog with particulates, and can be cleaned easily.

Flat sheet membranes are installed in either a plate-and-frame or a spiral wound module for largescale applications. In a plate-and-frame module, flat membranes are stacked in parallel with a spacer between every two membranes. One type of spacer has flow channels for feed, the other has supporting grids or screens for filtrate flow. Some designs are similar to the conventional plate-and-frame filter press, except that the membrane filters are designed for crossflow with an outlet for concentrated solutions or suspensions.

In a spiral wound module, a sandwichlike arrangement of membranes and spacers similar to that of the plate-and-frame design is rolled around a central perforated hollow tube to form a cylindrical module. Feed flows in the axial direction between alternating membrane layers. Filtrate is directed to the central hollow tube from which it exits the module. The spiral wound module has a high surface to volume ratio, but it is susceptible to blockage of the feed channel with feed streams containing particulates.

In order to carry out crossflow membrane filtration, one or more membrane modules is connected with a pump, tubing, and valves to form a complete system. The feed is pumped into the membrane module where it is separated into two streams (1) the filtrate (or permeate) and (2) the retentate in which the retained species has been concentrated. In applications where the flow of filtrate is small compared to that of the feed, a single pass through the module may not be sufficient to achieve a substantial degree of concentration of the retained species or a high recovery of the products in the filtrate. Therefore the retentate can either be completely recirculated back to the feed tank as a batch operation without retentate output or partially recirculated back as a continuous operation with some retentate output. Continuous operation, without recirculation of retentate, is also possible with a multiplicity of membrane modules and pumps in a cascade arrangement.

The aforementioned pumped systems, i.e., systems in which crossflow is generated by pumping the feed through a static conduit containing the membrane, have been widely used in many applications. There are, however, some problems inherent in such systems. First, the pressure of the flowing feed stream decreases along the flow path due to frictional losses. Second, the velocity decreases and the concentration of the retained species increases along the flow path as a consequence of filtration. These effects result in a nonuniform shear rate in the module. Furthermore, the shear rates attainable in such systems are limited by constraints on pressure drop, pumping capacity, and mechanical strength of the membrane module.

Efforts have been made in recent years to circumvent the limitations of pumped systems by moving the membrane or elements of the filter hardware in order to generate high shear rate. This concept has led to several designs of rotary high shear filter configurations. (1) A rotating body (e.g., a disk in a housing) installed close to the membrane surface rotates at a high speed to generate a high shear rate at the membrane surface. This arrangement is similar to that of a laboratory stirred cell in which a flat membrane is placed on a supporting screen at the bottom of the cell, and a magnetic bar stirring the liquid is placed just above the membrane (30). (2) A rotating cylindrical support covered by a membrane is installed inside a cylindrical housing. The inner cylinder rotates around the central axis at a high speed to generate a high shear rate at the membrane surface. The filtrate is drawn out through the inner-rotating cylinder (31). (3) In a system geometrically similar to that described in (2), a membrane is placed on both the inner rotating cylinder and the outer stationary cylinder. This design has been called a dynamic filter (14,15). Feed is pumped tangentially into one end of the narrow, annular gap between the two cylinders and flow out from the other end. When the inner cylinder rotates at a sufficiently high speed, as in case (2), Taylor vortices form which greatly enhance the shearing action of the fluid at the membrane surfaces. Results with this type of filter for UF and MF processes have achieved significant improvement in filtrate flux (15,31). These configurations bear some similarity to designs (32,33) that rotated the filter medium for increased filtration rates in conventional filtration. The disadvantages of these rotating membrane filters are low membrane surface area per unit volume, difficulties in replacing the membrane, and a high capital equipment cost.

III. PERFORMANCE CHARACTERISTICS

The performance of crossflow membrane filtration processes is usually characterized in terms of two parameters, filtrate flux and solute rejection coefficient. Filtrate flux J is defined by

$$J = \frac{Q_f}{A} \tag{1}$$

where Q_f is filtrate flowrate and A is the area of the membrane. The observed (measured) solute rejection coefficient R is

$$R = 1 - \frac{C_f}{C_b} \tag{2}$$

where C_f and C_b are the concentrations of the species of interest in the filtrate and bulk feed solution, respectively. If $R = 1$, the species concentration is 0 in the filtrate. If $R = 0$, the species passes through the membrane without any retention.

The actual flux and rejection characteristics observed are influenced by concentration polarization and by membrane fouling. Concentration polarization is the increase in concentration of completely or partially rejected species near the membrane surface. Membrane fouling is observed as a decrease in filtrate flux with time, all operating parameters remaining the same, and usually a simultaneous increase in rejection coefficient(s). These phenomena are in turn influenced by the membrane and module type employed, the properties of the solution or suspension being filtered, and the operating conditions.

A. Concentration Polarization

Concentration polarization refers to the formation of a concentration gradient of rejected species close to the membrane surface in all crossflow filtration processes including UF and MF. The concentration is maximal at the membrane surface and decreases with distance from the membrane over the concentration boundary layer thickness. The existence of concentration polarization has been visualized in ultrafiltration of a protein solution (34) and microfiltration of a cell suspension (35).

If a pure solvent or a solution containing no rejected solutes is filtered, the filtrate flux is a linear function of the transmembrane pressure difference (TMP) with a proportionality constant equal to the phenomenological hydraulic permeability of the membrane. In the presence of rejected species, the flux departs from linearity versus TMP, and the departure increases with increasing TMP. At high TMP, the flux becomes asymptotic to a maximum, pressure-independent value. At low TMP, the flux is said to be membrane limited, whereas at high TMP it is limited by phenomena in the concentration polarization boundary layer.

Models have been developed to account for the phenomenon of concentration polarization. The simplest is the equivalent stagnant film model with constant physical properties, which can be described as follows. Following a step change in TMP, the concentration of the retained species at the membrane surface C_w increases with time as a result of the convective transport of that species toward the membrane. The rejected species also diffuses back to the bulk stream as a result of the concentration gradient developed within the mass transfer boundary layer. C_w continues to increase until steady state is attained, at which point the convective transport toward the membrane is balanced by back diffusion away from the membrane. Under these conditions, the flux through the membrane J can be expressed as

$$J = k \ln\left[\frac{C_w - C_f}{C_b - C_f}\right] \qquad (3)$$

where k is the mass transfer coefficient, equalling D/δ, in which D is the rejected species diffusion coefficient and δ is the thickness of the concentration polarization boundary layer; C_w is the solute concentration at the wall or membrane surface; C_f is the solute concentration in the filtrate; and C_b is the solute concentration of the bulk feed stream. If the solute is completely rejected, then $C_f = 0$ and Eq. (3) is simplified to

$$J = k \ln\left(\frac{C_w}{C_b}\right) \qquad (4)$$

As TMP increases, C_w increases asymptotically until it reaches some maximum value associated with, for example, a solubility limit, a gel formation, a maximum packing concentration, or a very steep increase of osmotic pressure with concentration. When C_w attains a value that is insensitive to further increases of TMP, Eqs. (3) and (4) represent the maximum pressure-independent filtrate flux.

This simple model can be tested by measuring the maximum pressure-independent filtrate flux at different bulk feed concentrations and plotting the flux at steady versus ln C_b. If the data yield a straight line, C_w is determined by extrapolation of the line to obtain the intercept on the ln C_b axis where $J = 0$, and k is determined by the slope of the line.

The approximate validity of Eqs. (1) and (2) has been demonstrated for ultrafiltration of a large number of macrosolutes and colloidal species (24,25,36,37), usually together with use of the Leveque solution (38) for estimating k under conditions of laminar flow where the concentration boundary layer is not yet fully developed at the feed stream outlet. In at least one study (39), the value of C_w obtained by linear extrapolation of the plot of flux versus ln C_b gave estimates that increased when C_b was increased, thereby indicating that the maximum value of C_w obtained in this way was not necessarily a constant for a particular solute.

The notion is now well established that the steady state, maximum, pressure-independent filtrate flux is determined by the rate of back transport of rejected species from the membrane surface through the concentration boundary layer to the bulk feed stream. Nonetheless, there must exist other mechanisms that can accommodate this imposed flux limitation by reducing the effective pressure driving force across the membrane. That reduction can be accomplished by having a sufficiently large osmotic pressure difference across the membrane or by adding an additional hydraulic resistance (40). The flux-pressure relationship may be described by

$$J = \frac{\Delta P - \Delta \pi_w}{R_m + R_p} \tag{5}$$

where ΔP is the TMP, $\Delta \pi_w$ is the osmotic pressure difference of the solutions in contact with either face of the membrane, R_m is the effective membrane hydraulic resistance (including any additional resistance caused by adsorption of proteins on the membrane surface), and R_p is the hydraulic resistance of the concentration polarization boundary layer, including any layer (e.g., gel or cake) that deposits on the membrane surface. The reduction of filtrate flux can be associated with osmotic pressure and/or hydraulic resistance effects. If the dependence of osmotic pressure on solute concentration is sufficiently strong, as is the case for highly charged low-molecular-weight proteins, like albumin, then the high osmotic pressure associated with C_w can account for the requisite reduction in driving force (34,41,42). For example, when ΔP is increased, any increase in flux causes the concentration at the membrane surface C_w to increase. This will result in an increase in osmotic pressure $\Delta \pi$ so that the overall driving force $\Delta P - \Delta \pi_w$ does not increase proportionally. When π increases very sharply with C, a further increase in ΔP may incur virtually an equal increase in $\Delta \pi_w$ with a very small increase in C_w, in which case the flux cannot be increased any further by an increase in ΔP. This concept effectively explains the observation that the flux increases with ΔP in the low-pressure range but cannot increase perceptibly when ΔP is high (43). Conversely, with a macromolecular solution exhibiting a small increase in osmotic pressure with concentration, a compressible layer (e.g., a gel or cake) having a large hydraulic resistance that increases with TMP must be invoked in order to be consistent with experimental observation.

The equivalent stagnant film concentration polarization model has been widely used as an approximate model for the ultrafiltration of macrosolutes. In all cases, the Brownian motion molecular diffusivity has been used in the theoretical expression for the mass transfer coefficient. However, use of the same approach for microfiltration of particulate suspensions underpredicts the filtrate flux (24) and gives the wrong dependence on shear rate. The discrepancy between the model prediction and experimental results arises from the inappropriate use of the Brownian-motion diffusivity for particles in crossflow microfiltration (44) at all but extremely low bulk concentration. At the high particle concentrations typical of a concentration polarization boundary layer, the particle diffusivity is significantly augmented by fluid shear as a result of collisions between particles, and flux can be predicted with reasonable accuracy by incorporation of an appropriate expression for the shear-augmented diffusivity into the concentration polarization model (45,46).

Because they exert negligible osmotic pressure, solutions of particulates must exhibit a region of hydraulic resistance while undergoing filtration. Deformable cells, such as red cells, can pack to very high volume fraction (e.g., close to 100%) under compressive pressure. The resulting low porosity offers high hydraulic resistance (47). Consequently, there results a pressure boundary layer, the region where hydrostatic pressure decreases from its bulk value, which is embedded within the concentration boundary layer (48). Relatively nondeformable cells, such as yeast, can pack only to about 70%. The resulting high porosity offers low hydraulic resistance, and thus a cake of substantial thickness must build up in order to provide the requisite hydraulic resistance (29).

The transient behavior (i.e., rate of flux decrease following an increase in pressure) is dependent on the mechanical properties of the retained species. In ultrafiltration of macrosolutes and microfiltration of highly deformable solids, the flux may initially decrease relatively rapidly and then become quasi-steady over a long period with a low or negligible flux decline. In microfiltration of rigid particles, the flux may decrease more slowly, but the flux decline continues over a long period. For example, several studies (35,44) demonstrated that for crossflow of a suspension of red blood cells (with a volume fraction of 40%), the flux decreased rapidly and stabilized within 30 to 60 s while for crossflow of a dilute (e.g., 1 to 5%) suspension of yeast cells, the flux continued to decrease for an hour or more. The yeast cells are much less deformable than red cells, and a bed of yeast has much less hydraulic resistance to filtration than does a bed of red cells. A longer time period is required to form a thick cake from the dilute yeast suspension in order to reduce the filtrate flux to the point where an equilibrium between cake buildup and cake removal is established. In addition, the thick yeast cake may undergo gradual compaction and consolidation in which cells are rearranged to form a more densely packed bed, while the highly deformable red cells may reach their final packing arrangement very rapidly. Cake buildup may also lead to clogging of hollow fiber devices, causing complete blockage of flow, if the steady-state cake thickness is larger than the fiber radius. The transient period of flux decline associated with cake buildup is sometimes confused with membrane fouling.

Sometimes concentration polarization, transient cake formation, and membrane fouling can interact in complex ways. For example, it was observed that the thickness of cake formation in crossflow filtration of 1% yeast suspension (in 6% bovine serum albumin solution) initially increased with time and then began to decrease at a slower rate, even though the filtrate flux was still decreasing (29). The observations indicated that the filtration resistance was largely determined by concentration polarization and transient buildup of the cake layer at the beginning, whereas membrane fouling became progressively more important at longer times.

Concentration polarization also influences the observed rejection coefficient. The true membrane rejection coefficient r is defined by

$$r = 1 - \frac{C_f}{C_w} \tag{6}$$

Because C_w is greater than C_b as a result of concentration polarization, R is always less than r. In the context of the equivalent stagnant film theory, Eqs. (2), (3), and (6) may be combined (49) to yield the relationship between R and r.

$$r = \frac{R \exp\left(\frac{J}{k}\right)}{(1-R) + R \exp\left(\frac{J}{k}\right)} \tag{7}$$

B. Membrane Fouling

The flux decline associated with fouling of membranes refers to the plugging or narrowing of membrane pores by one or more substances present in the fluid to be filtered.

It may be difficult to distinguish between flux decline associated with transient concentration polarization phenomena and that caused by membrane fouling (50). Fouling is differentiated from concentration polarization in that the fouled membrane becomes the limiting hydraulic resistance. Thus changes in flux due to fouling are generally not sensitive to an increase in crossflow velocity but are sensitive to changes in TMP. It is difficult to restore the original filtrate flux simply by changing operating conditions. Usually fouled membranes must be cleaned by use of appropriate cleaning agent(s), such as detergents, enzymes, extremes of pH, and/or oxidizing agents (e.g., hypochlorite, peroxide).

Fouling is influenced by surface chemical properties and physical morphology of membranes. Adsorption of proteins (in their native, denatured, and/or aggregated form) has been recognized as a major cause of membrane fouling in crossflow filtration. For example (51), the hydraulic permeabilities of membranes can be greatly reduced after their immersion in a protein solution for several minutes. Generally speaking, hydrophobic membranes, such as polysulfones, have more tendency to adsorb proteins due to hydrophobic interactions and the hydrophobic effect (52) than do hydrophilic membranes, such as cellulose, which may be less adsorptive to proteins and more resistant to fouling.

The irregular, interconnected pore structures of most polymeric MF membranes renders them easily blocked internally (i.e., like a depth filter). Relatively isotropic UF membranes, such as those developed during the first half of the 20th century, are quickly fouled. The anisotropic UF membranes developed in the past 25 years have a very thin retentive skin and therefore exhibit less propensity for trapping of solutes or particles internally. Although some microporous MF membranes with moderate anisotropy have appeared (22,23), most MF membranes are relatively isotropic in structure and hence suffer more from fouling problems. When using microporous MF membranes for filtration of cell suspensions or homogenates, problems often occur if deformable cells, cell debris, or protein aggregates can enter the pores and remain there due to adsorption and/or physical entrapment, thereby decreasing the filtrate flux. Backflushing (possible only with hollow fiber designs) can help to improve the flux but may not be able to restore it completely. Several reports (28,53) showed that using UF membranes for MF purposes gave less flux decline and higher overall filtration rates than did microporous MF membranes, suggesting that anisotropic UF membranes with smaller surface pores are more resistant to fouling than MF membranes.

Some studies have shown that fouling may be related to concentration polarization (54–56). Proteins may have a greater tendency to aggregate in the concentration polarization boundary layer adjacent to the membrane surface. In one study at a low crossflow velocity that resulted in a thicker concentration polarization boundary layer, the initial rate of filtration flux decline was greater than at a higher crossflow velocity. High shear crossflow filters (30) also showed fewer problems of fouling.

The presence of antifoaming agents in fermentation broths can cause serious fouling of membranes during cell separation (57,58). These materials are hydrophobic, and even at very low concentration they can foul membranes easily. Although some antifoams were found to be better than others, mechanical foam breakers should be used to facilitate downstream processing by avoiding the rapid filtrate flux decline caused by antifoam fouling of membranes.

A recent study (59) revealed that use of a laboratory peristaltic pump with a bovine serum albumin solution generated protein aggregates that fouled microporous MF membranes. The rate of flux decline increased with the number of recycles of the feed stream. These findings suggest that extensive pumping, especially with occlusive peristaltic pumps, may be deleterious to membrane filtration systems.

Fouled membranes can usually be cleaned using the agents mentioned above. However, frequent cleaning may shorten the lifetime of the membranes and disrupt filtration operations. Methods proposed for minimization of fouling include (1) selection of a hydrophilic, anisotropic membrane to avoid protein adsorption and species entrapment (6); (2) use of a high shear rate to minimize concentration polarization (60,61); (3) periodic backflush from the reverse side of the membrane to remove trapped species (56,62); (4) adjustment of pH and ionic strength (19); and (5) avoidance of antifoam use in fermentation (16).

C. Influence of Operating Conditions

It is desirable to maximize productivity and minimize the effects of concentration polarization and membrane fouling on flux and rejection properties. Filtration of streams containing labile cells and proteins puts limits on increases in temperature. The practical adjustable operating parameters are usually the transmembrane pressure, crossflow velocity, pH, and ionic strength.

1. Transmembrane Pressure

It is usually advantageous to operate at a TMP sufficiently high that the maximum flux is obtained, at least for the case when the filtrate is not drawn off at a fixed rate by a pump. If the filtrate is pumped, then operation in the pressure-dependent region is safer.

Solute rejection is often influenced by TMP, especially when a stream with components of widely different size is filtered. Studies of microfiltration of cell homogenate containing cell debris showed that increased TMP would substantially increase the rejection of proteins that were not expected to be retained (63). Utilization of TMP as low as possible has therefore been suggested as a means to increase filtration selectivity. Recently a novel process of negative transmembrane pressure pulsing has been examined for improving flux and selectivity in ultrafiltration (64).

2. Crossflow Wall Shear Rate

Equations (3) and (4) show that the ultrafiltrate flux is directly proportional to the mass transfer coefficient. The Leveque solution for laminar flow in a conduit gives

$$k \propto \left[\frac{D^2 \gamma_w}{L}\right]^{1/3} \tag{8}$$

where D is the diffusion coefficient of the rejected species, γ_w is the wall shear rate, and L is the length of the flow path.

The wall shear rate is given by

$$\gamma_w = 8 \, \frac{U_b}{d} \quad \text{for tubular channel}$$

$$\tag{9}$$

$$\gamma_w = 6 \, \frac{U_b}{h} \quad \text{for rectangular channel}$$

where U_b is the average velocity of the bulk feed stream, d is the diameter of a tube, and h is the height of a channel. Wall shear rate can be enhanced by increasing the average bulk velocity (or flow rate) and decreasing the channel dimension. Thin channel designs are based on this concept (37,60), and they generally give a high filtration flux, although the pressure drop in such channels may be high. The increase in shear rate can also be realized through rapid rotation of the rotary membrane filter described above. A high value for the mass transfer coefficient, and therefore for the ultrafiltrate flux, can also be achieved using a wide-bore tubular channel and a high bulk velocity in order to attain turbulent flow in the channel, in which case $k \propto U_b^{0.8}$, and there is a stronger dependence of mass transfer coefficient on velocity.

When a particulate solution is filtered, the shear-enhanced diffusivity of the particles is itself dependent upon shear rate:

$$D \propto a^2 \gamma f(c) \tag{10}$$

where a is the particle diameter and $f(c)$ is a function of the particle concentration. Under these circumstances,

$$k \propto \left[\frac{a^4}{L}\right]^{1/3} \gamma_w \tag{11}$$

Thus the mass transfer coefficient is predicted to increase with the first power of the wall shear rate, and microfiltration of particulate suspensions is expected to benefit even more from increased shear rate than is ultrafiltration of dissolved species. This is especially noteworthy for microfiltration of cell suspensions with a rotary membrane filter (61), because very high shear rates can be obtained with that device.

A number of experimental studies have confirmed that the filtrate flux may be represented as a power function of the feed stream flow rate. UF data are usually consistent with an exponential dependence of 0.33 (laminar) or 0.8 (turbulent). The value of the power dependence varies more in MF. For example, the power dependence on velocity for several suspensions in one study varied between 0.25 and 0.97 (65). The power for a mineral suspension was 0.6 (50). A power of 1.0 was obtained for filtration of blood cell suspensions (66) and for a bacterial suspension (19). The degree of fouling will influence the relationship between J and U_b, and it is sometimes difficult to separate out fouling effects in a practical experiment.

The use of high flow velocities is generally beneficial for obtaining high filtration rates and may help to reduce unexpected retention of solutes. However, increasing shear rate increases energy consumption and increases pumping costs. If the flux is limited by membrane fouling, increasing the shear rate may not have a large influence. In biological fluids, macromolecules such as proteins may be denatured faster at high shear rates. Protein denaturation may not be caused by shear alone. Some evidence suggests that protein denaturation most likely takes place at the gas-liquid or liquid-solid interface, and shear serves mainly to increase the transport of proteins to and from the interface (67).

3. Concentration, pH, and Ionic Strength

Most UF data are consistent with a flux decrease that is linear in the logarithm of the feed concentration, in agreement with Eqs. (3) and (4). In MF, the decrease of flux with increasing concentration is more complicated (68–70) because of the concentration dependence of the shear-induced particle diffusivity.

In a batch concentration process where the concentration of retained species increases with time as fluid is removed by filtration, flux decline is caused by the concerted effects of concentration polarization, the increase in bulk concentration, and the possibility of membrane fouling. In a membrane module, the concentration of retained species increases along the fluid path. At the feed stream outlet, the concentration may be so high that, in the case of nondeformable particulates (e.g., yeast), the retained species can block the channel completely (29).

The pH and ionic strength also affect the performance of crossflow filtration, especially with biological components (40,71). The surface charge of cells and proteins changes with pH. At the isoelectric point of a solute, precipitation may occur, which can result in an increase in retention of the solute and fouling of the membrane. High salt concentration may precipitate proteins, whereas low salt concentration may improve the solubility of some proteins.

IV. APPLICATIONS

Crossflow membrane filtration has become increasingly used in downstream processing of biological products. Ultrafiltration of solutions of various proteins was practiced as early as the 1960s (24). Microfiltration of suspensions of microbial cells appeared at the beginning of the 1970s (9). Today, UF and MF have been used for separation of a variety of bioproducts, such as proteins, viruses, microbial cells, mammalian cells, plant cells, cell homogenates, inclusion bodies, and so on. UF has proven to be an effective tool for concentrating macrosolutes. A number of reviews (7,28,72,73) have appeared on the application of UF in biotechnology. MF has moved rapidly over the last few years. However, reviews on the application of MF in biotechnology are few and not comprehensive. Therefore this section will concentrate primarily on the applications of MF.

A. Cell Separation and Cell Recycling

Cell separation is usually the first step immediately after cell cultivation in the sequence of downstream processing. The traditional biotechnology industry deals mainly with microbial cells, and cell separation has been routinely performed by centrifugation or dead-end filtration, with or without filteraid. More recently, mammalian cells and plant cells have also become of interest. Separations involving these different cell types with crossflow microfiltration have begun to receive increased attention (70).

The potential advantages of crossflow microfiltration over centrifugation and dead-end filtration with filteraid include the following. (1) It offers the possibility of efficient separation at a low cost. The density difference between cells and culture medium is usually small, thereby rendering centrifugation difficult and uneconomical. Dead-end filtration with filteraid consumes a large quantity of filteraid, and its disposal after use is an environmental problem. (2) It provides for an enclosed, contamination-free system. Centrifugation is known to produce aerosols as well as heavy noise. Filteraid contaminates products. Most traditional cell separation processes involve exposure to the open air, thereby contaminating both the environment and the products. (3) It provides a system suitable for continuous washing and recycling of cells. Cell washing is necessary to remove impurities in the culture medium if the cells themselves are products or the cells need to be disintegrated to release intracellular proteins. Crossflow microfiltration permits continuous removal of culture medium and continuous addition of washing buffers. Such an operation is difficult to realize in centrifugation and dead-end filtration. Recycling of cells is used to increase productivity of some fermentation processes. In such a process, the cell suspension is pumped through the membrane module and the filtrate containing inhibitory substances is removed. The concentrated cell suspension is recycled back to the fermentor where fresh medium is added to keep the culture conditions optimal.

Although crossflow membrane filtration offers an attractive alternative to conventional cell separation techniques, remarkably little public information is available on the nature and extent of process-scale membrane filtration systems being used in the biotechnology industry; most of the information is proprietary. It was estimated in 1984 (74) that centrifugation might be cheaper than membrane filtration for large-volume processing of cells, while membrane filtration might be better for processing small volumes of cell suspensions where the size of the cells and the density difference between cells and liquid are small. A comparison of centrifugation and membrane filtration for bacteria and yeast separations (75) showed that membrane filtration with a hollow fiber module gives a higher processing rate, lower capital cost, and lower operating cost for bacteria separations. However, for yeast separation, the total capital and operating cost for centrifugation is lower than for membrane filtration.

While there are few descriptions of actual industrial processes, numerous reports have appeared on laboratory- or pilot-scale experiments with crossflow filtration of different cell suspensions. These have dealt primarily with separations of bacteria and yeasts, less with mycelia and animal cells.

1. Bacteria

Bacteria have been used industrially to produce numerous biochemical products, such as enzymes, organic solvents, and amino acids. Over the past few years, *E. coli* has become a host for expressing recombinant proteins. The separation of products from bacteria has therefore attracted considerable research interest. The diameter of most bacteria is in the neighborhood of 1 μm, and the density difference between bacteria and culture media is very small. Therefore conventional filtration and centrifugation are difficult.

Crossflow membrane filtration for removal of bacteria (*Micrococcus bacterium*) was first reported in 1972 (12). A thin channel system and a spiral wound system, originally designed for ultrafiltration purposes, were used with both UF and MF membranes. An anisotropic UF membrane produced a higher flux than a relatively isotropic MF membrane. The influences of pressure, crossflow shear rate, and concentration on filtrate flux were investigated. The flux increased with pressure up to 40 psi, and the flux was proportional to the 1.5 power of shear rate in the thin channel system and 0.8 in the spiral wound system. Other early studies (76–79) with different membranes used to filter a variety of bacteria indicated that crossflow filtration was an efficient technique for removal of bacteria from liquid media.

More recently, *E. coli* and *Salmonella typhimurium* were concentrated using pleated crossflow modules with 0.2 μm and 1.2 μm acrylic-copolymer microporous membranes. A bacterial suspension was concentrated from

140 L to about 1 L in 160 minutes using 0.3 m^2 of 0.2 μm membrane. Membrane fouling was observed, and the membrane was effectively cleaned with an ethanol solution (60,80). In a study with a number of bacterial suspensions filtered with different membranes and modules (68), a plot of the flux versus the log of the feed concentration was a sigmoidal curve rather than a straight line. This observation was attributed to concentration polarization and an increase in suspension viscosity at high bacteria concentrations. Backflushing was also used and shown to improve the filtrate flux.

In order to operate crossflow filtration at a shear rate as high as possible, an axially rotating crossflow filter was used under conditions in which Taylor vortices formed between the rotating inner cylinder and the stationary outer cylinder (61). High values of flux ranging from 80 to 155 $L/m^2 \cdot h$ were obtained with *E. coli* suspensions and a 0.2 μm Teflon membrane at rotational speeds of 2000 to 3000 rpm. The rotating membrane filter was judged superior to conventional pumped crossflow filters because the former could provide very high shear rates without significant increase of pressure drop, thereby increasing the flux and decreasing fouling.

A number of bacterial recycling fermentations have been reported including the production of organic solvents such as ethanol (81), acetone-butanol (82), acetic acid (83), and lactic acid (84,85). In these applications, crossflow filters were coupled to the fermentors for continuous removal of the solvents that had an inhibitory effect on the fermentation at high concentrations. Several fermentation studies were carried out with *Zymomonas mobilis*, a bacterial strain that produces ethanol at a much higher rate than yeasts but suffers inhibition by the presence of excess ethanol (86–88).

2. Yeasts and Mycelia

Yeasts have traditionally been used in brewery fermentations to produce ethanol, as well as in bakeries. They are also used as a host for expressing recombinant proteins. Separation of yeast from a liquid can be accomplished by centrifugation because the size of most yeasts is larger, and the density difference between the cells and aqueous culture media is larger, in comparison to bacterial cells. Nevertheless, a number of studies on crossflow filtration of yeasts have been reported, primarily for recycling cells back to the fermentor during ethanol production (69,81,87).

The performance in crossflow filtration of yeast cells has been similar to that of bacterial cells. Membrane materials were found to have an important influence on fouling. A 20,000 NMWC polysulfone membrane was less resistant to fouling than was a sulfonic acid membrane for filtering beer stillage (89). The use of antifoaming agents caused significant filtrate flux decline during crossflow filtration of yeast; the fouled membranes could be regenerated using sodium hydroxide and ethanol as washing agents (90). A microporous stainless steel tube (2 μm NPD) that could withstand back pressure, heat sterilization, and chemical cleaning was used for filtration of yeast suspensions (91). Filtrate flux declined rapidly due to fouling. Periodic backflushing partially restored the flux. Backflushing was also used in the filtration of yeast suspensions with 0.22 μm cellulose triacetate MF membranes (92). A 20- to 50-fold reduction of filtrate flux was observed over time, presumably caused by membrane fouling.

The separation of fungal mycelia is normally done by rotary vacuum filtration in industry because of the size of the filamentary fungi. For example, *Penicillium* and *Aspergillus* are much larger than other microorganisms. Little research has been reported on crossflow filtration of filamentary fungi. In one study (62), the fungal microorganism *Trichoderma reesei* was filtered with a sterilizable crossflow microfilter of porous stainless steel. A high filtrate rate was obtained using periodic backflushing with the filtrate. Backflush frequency was also optimized to increase filtrate productivity.

Another group of filamentary microorganisms is the actinomycetes bacteria, which are widely used in the pharmaceutical industry for producing antibodies. Separation of these cells from fermentation broth is traditionally done by rotary vacuum filtration. The filtration rate is low compared with that of fungi because of the smaller size of actinomycetes. Several reports have appeared on the use of crossflow filtration to separate actinomycetes (16,93). A potential problem with mycelium microorganisms is the possible breakdown of the filamentary cells by the fluid shear stress. The broken cells release intracellular components and may be destroyed in recycling fermentation (94).

Few reports have appeared on recycling cells in mycelial fermentation. A stirred cell filter was used in connection with a fermenter to recover citric acid from *Aspergillus nigar* culture (95). In another study (96), a 40 μm nylon filter was inserted into a culture vessel for production of cellulase by *Trichoderma reesei QM9414*. Shear was created by stirring the culture suspension to minimize accumulation of the fungus on the filter, and continuous production of cellulase was realized.

3. Mammalian Cells

The recovery of products from mammalian cell cultures has become industrially important for diagnostic and therapeutic applications. Large-scale cultivation of hybridoma cells has made it possible to produce monoclonal antibodies for diagnostic and therapeutic applications. In addition, the successful cloning and expression of genes in mammalian cells for production of high-value therapeutic proteins provides another application of large scale mammalian cell cultures.

Mammalian cells lack a rigid cell wall for protection. They are easily deformed and are sensitive to damage by bulk shear stress. Filtration in the dead-end mode is difficult due to the formation of a very compressible cell bed. Crossflow filtration has been studied as a means to separate mammalian cells from culture media.

Cell lysis in crossflow MF of mammalian cells was studied with red blood cells as a model system (44,48,97). The results were consistent with the hypothesis that hemolysis (i.e., lysis of a red blood cell) occurred by rupture of the erythrocyte membrane after its deformation into the membrane pores. The strain causing rupture of the deformed red cell membrane was influenced by the transmembrane pressure drop, which forced the cell membrane into the pores, and by the residence time of the deformed cells in the pores (which was taken to be inversely proportional to the wall shear rate). Subsequently, these findings were found applicable to cell damage in crossflow microfiltration of other cell lines including myeloma, hybridoma, trioma, and insect cell lines (98).

Cell damage was also examined in a recent study in which a suspension of MCSF CHO cells in serum-free media underwent crossflow MF with a modified polysulfone hollow fiber membrane cartridge (99). The experiment was run with a constant pumped filtration rate. The transmembrane pressure increased with time, presumably as a result of membrane fouling. When transmembrane pressure increased to 80 mm Hg, the filtration was automatically stopped, and a backflush was performed to regenerate the filter and to wash the suspension with buffers. Forty-five liters of the suspension was concentrated to 3.5 liters in about 200 minutes. An average flux of about 0.1 cm/min was achieved with a membrane area of 0.21 m^2 and a shear rate of about 5000 s^{-1}. Cell lysis was checked by measuring the concentration of lactate dehydrogenase (LDH) in the filtrate. The concentration of LDH increased with time, indicating occurrence of cell lysis attributable to the increase in transmembrane pressure and consequent deformation of cell membranes into the membrane pores but not to bulk shear damage by pumping the suspension in crossflow mode.

Cell damage was not explicitly reported in other studies. No loss in cell viability was found in 80 min of crossflow filtration of basophilic leukemia cells from tissue culture media using 0.2 μm polysulfone hollow fibers and 0.45 μm polyvinylidene fluoride membranes in a thin channel MF filter (100). The linear flux decrease with time was attributed to membrane fouling and to an increase in the viscosity of the cell suspension. A few other examples of crossflow filtration for separation of different mammalian cells have been reported, including hybridoma cells (93), leukemia cells (101), and BHK 21 cells (102).

B. Removal of Cell Debris

Many valuable proteins are located inside microbial cells and cannot be secreted into the culture medium. Recovery of these products requires disintegration of the cells by mechanical or chemical methods. After cell disintegration, the suspension (cell homogenate) contains cell fragments and some unbroken cells (cell debris). Further purification of the released products requires removal of the cell debris.

The size of cell debris varies widely, ranging from cytoplasmic proteins and small cellular organelles up to membrane fragments larger than 0.1 μm. Consequently, the specific cake resistance of the debris is very high (103). Separation of the debris by centrifugation requires an ultra-high-speed centrifuge, and it is difficult to obtain a clear supernatant. Therefore crossflow MF has been investigated as a possible solution to the problem by retaining the debris within the membrane while allowing the soluble proteins to pass through in the filtrate.

Several studies indicated that MF membranes performed better than UF membranes for the separation. For example, cell debris was removed from the homogenate of *Pseudomonas* sp. with 0.45 μm cellulosic and 0.5 μm PVDF membranes. These membranes gave clearer filtrate and higher enzyme yield than ultrafiltration membranes of 10^5 and 10^6 NMWC (22). In another study, a higher flux and higher enzyme yield were obtained with MF membranes than with UF hollow fiber membranes when filtering *E. coli* homogenate (104). The quality of separation was dependent on the operating conditions. In one study, crossflow filtration of disrupted *E. coli* under turbulent flow resulted in less enzyme retention than under laminar flow (105). Use of a rotating membrane filter to obtain high shear rates resulted in a filtrate flux about three times that obtained with a pumped system, and the enzyme recovery in the filtrate was also greatly improved (61). Other studies (23,106–108) of the influence of operating conditions and filter membranes concluded that crossflow membrane filtration is a better choice for cell debris removal than centrifugation.

C. Separation of Inclusion Bodies

Many recombinant proteins produced by *E. coli* form insoluble aggregates known as inclusion bodies inside the cell (109). Purification of product from inclusion bodies involves protein refolding, a necessary but difficult step which often results in significant loss of product. However, the insoluble nature of these inclusion bodies facilitates their separation from other soluble proteins by a simple solid-liquid separation step. A recent study on separation of inclusion bodies with crossflow membrane filtration used a flat sheet module with 0.6, 0.45, and 0.22 μm hydrophilic polyvinylidene fluoride MF membranes having 120 cm^2 surface area (110). The sizes of the inclusion bodies were not measured, but the use of a 0.6 μm membrane resulted in partial leaking of the inclusion bodies. Therefore 0.45 and 0.22 μm membranes were used that could retain the inclusion bodies and allow passage of the soluble proteins. The filtration rate was about 8 L/m^2•h for the 0.45 μm membrane at 100 g/L concentration. The main problem encountered was retention of soluble proteins during filtration. Increasing crossflow shear rate could not reduce the retention because the transmembrane pressure, which might counteract the effect of increasing shear rate, was simultaneously increased in this system. With use of buffer exchange, i.e., addition of buffer to the feed during filtration, 87% of soluble proteins was removed from the suspension of inclusion bodies after three volumes exchange of buffer.

Inclusion bodies containing recombinant porcine somatotropin produced by *E. coli* and having a mean diameter of 0.4 μm and a density about 1.26 g/cm^3 underwent crossflow filtration using a hollow fiber membrane cartridge of 500K NMWC (111). The flux decreased from 46 to less than 10 L/m^2•h when the concentration was increased 1.8-fold. The final inclusion body concentration was about 228 g/L (dry weight) with a recovery yield >99.9%.

D. Concentration and Removal of Viruses

Large-scale separation of viruses from protein solutions is required in two processes. The first is in vaccine production, where viruses are produced in tissue culture. The second is in the modern biotechnology industry, where viruses are removed from therapeutic protein preparations as possible pathogenic contaminants and to meet the regulatory standards on product safety. The diameters of viruses range between about 0.01 and 0.1 μm, larger than those of most proteins. Therefore UF membranes have been used to concentrate and remove viruses in processes designed to allow soluble proteins to pass through and to retain viruses by membranes of appropriate pore size.

UF membranes have been used to concentrate viruses in preparation for biological studies and in vaccine production. The advantages of this method are contamination-free operations and high efficiencies. For example, arenavirus in 3–6 L of cell culture supernatant was concentrated about 30–100-fold by ultrafiltration in less than 90 min without significant loss of particle infectivity (112). This process proved superior to the conventional concentration method using PEG precipitation, which is cumbersome, time-consuming, and unsafe. The influence of membrane type, virus concentration, and operating conditions on virus concentration using hollow fiber membranes was investigated in a study in which polio I virus was successfully retained by polysulfone hollow fibers (113). The large-scale concentration of baboon endogenous virus (BaEV) with hollow fiber ultrafiltration has been described (114). About 40 L of cell culture supernatant were concentrated with three cartridges of hollow fibers having 50,000 NMWC. The separation rate was about 27 L/h, and the BaEV recovery was as high as 98%. However, proteins were also concentrated together with the virus. Other reports of concentration include rubella (115), influenza (116), lymphoma (93), and enteric viruses (117) with membranes ranging from 30K to 1000K NMWC.

The potential virus contamination in products derived from mammalian cell culture is of major concern for product safety. UF membranes have a skewed pore size distribution, and large pores in the tail of the distribution can allow passage of viruses. Recently, a membrane having a unique structure was developed based on size exclusion that could separate viruses from protein solution with high selectivity and reproducibility (118). The membrane displayed protein rejection properties nearly equivalent to that of a 100,000 NMWC UF membrane. By truncating the pore size distribution at a certain point, the same membrane displayed particle and virus retention characteristics that increased monotonically from 3 to 8 logs as a function of particle diameter in the range of 28 to 93 nm.

E. A New Application—Affinity Membrane Adsorption

Affinity adsorption and ion exchange are increasingly used for purification of biological products. However, the hydrophilic gels traditionally used in packed beds for adsorption of proteins have disadvantages of diffusional limitations and deformation under high pressure, resulting in low flow rates and consequently long residence times that limit their large-scale commercial utilization.

The concept of using membranes as supporting materials for affinity and ion exchange separation was proposed several years ago (4). A membrane based affinity adsorption processes for purification of proteins was first reported in 1988 (119). Affinity ligands were coupled to microporous membranes. Affinity adsorption took place between a specific protein and the ligand when protein solution flowed through the membrane pores. Other proteins that did not specifically bind to the ligand passed through in the filtrate. The membrane was washed and the adsorbed protein was eluted with an agent that disassociated the protein from the ligand. Purifications of fibronectin and IgG were demonstrated using such affinity membranes. The purity and yield were comparable to those obtained using affinity gels. The throughput rate, however, was much higher for the membranes than for the gels. Recently, a system of stacked, flat sheet affinity membranes was described and analyzed experimentally and theoretically (120).

Microporous membranes have potential advantages over packed beds of particles for affinity and ion exchange separations. A configuration in which the feed solution flows through the membrane approaches the limit of a very short, wide bed. High superficial velocities are attainable with modest transmembrane pressure drop, thereby providing the possibility of very short residence times. Furthermore, pore size on the order of 1 μm or less brings the ligate and ligand into close proximity, essentially abolishing diffusional limitations. Lastly, the denaturation of product or ligand in conventional chromatographic columns, arising from long time exposure to harsh elution conditions (121), could be minimized in adsorption membranes because of very short residence times.

The advantageous characteristics of affinity adsorption membranes suggest that they may be able to play an important role in downstream processing of high-molecular-weight therapeutic proteins. In particular, their ability to handle high throughput with high selectivity may be especially valuable at the initial stages of bioprocessing, i.e., isolation and purification of products present in very dilute concentration from complicated mixtures typical of fermentation and cell culture broth, a difficult problem still in need of innovative separation methods. In this application, a combination of crossflow filtration and direct adsorption can, in principle, be carried out simultaneously in one device, so long as irreversible fouling and capacity loss are not a significant problem. It is likely that adsorption membranes will receive increasing research attention and find more applications in biotechnology.

ACKNOWLEDGMENT

Preparation of this chapter was supported in part by NSF Grant No. BCS 9012574.

REFERENCES

1. Gregor, H. P., and Gregor, C. D. (1978). Synthetic membrane technology, *Sci. Am.*, *239*: 88.
2. Londsdale, H. K. (1982). The growth of membrane technology, *J. Memb. Sci.*, *10*: 81.
3. Michaels, A. S., and Matson, S. L. (1980). Membrane technology and biotechnology, *Desalination*, *35*: 329.
4. Michaels, A. S. (1985). Membranes in biotechnology: State of the art, *Desalination*, *53*: 231.
5. Strathmann, H. (1985). Membrane and membrane processes in biotechnology, *Trends in Biotechnol.*, *3*: 112.
6. Gabler, F. R. (1985). Cell processing using tangential flow filtration, *Comprehensive Biotechnology*, vol. 2 (C. L. Cooney and A. E. Humphrey, eds.), Pergamon Press, Oxford, p. 351.
7. O'Sullivan, T. J., Epstein, A. C., Korchin, S. R., and Beaton, N. C., (1984). Application of ultrafiltration in biotechnology, *Chem. Eng. Prog.*, *80*: 68.
8. Podall, H. E. (1972). Reverse osmosis, *Recent Developments in Separation Science*, vol. 2 (N. N. Li, ed.), CRC Press, Boca Raton, Florida, p. 171.
9. Henry, J. D. (1972). Cross flow filtration, *Recent Developments in Separation Science*, vol. 2 (N. N. Li, ed.), CRC Press, Boca Raton, Florida, p. 205.
10. Vadia, P. H., Kraus, K. A., Shor, A. J., and Dresuer, L. (1971). Preliminary economic analysis of cross-flow filtration, Oak Ridge National Lab., USA, Report ORNL-4729.
11. Lukaszewicz, R. C., Korin, A., Hank, D., and Chrai, S. (1981). Functionality and economics of tangential flow microfiltration, *J. Parent. Sci. Tech.*, *35*: 231.
12. Henry, J. D., and Allred, R. C. (1972). Concentration of bacterial cells by cross-flow filtration, *Dev. Ind. Microbial.*, *13*: 177.
13. Dahlheimer, J. A., Thomas, D. G., and Kraus, K. A. (1970). Application of woven fiber hoses to hyperfiltration of salts and cross-flow filtration of suspended solids, *Ind. Eng. Chem. Proc. Des. Dev.*, *9*: 566.
14. Tobler, W. (1979). Dynamic filtration—The engineering concept of the Escher Wyss pressure filter, *Filtr. Sep.*, *16*: 630.

15. Tobler, W. (1982). Dynamic filtration: Principle and application of shear filtration in an annular gap, *Filtr. Sep.*, *19*: 329.

16. Zahka, J., and Leahy, T. J. (1985). Practical aspects of tangential flow filtration in cell separations, *Purification of Fermentation Products*, ACS Symposium Series 271, p. 51.

17. Tiller, F. M., and Cheng, K. S. (1977). Delayed cake filtration, *Filtr. Sep.*, *14*: 13.

18. Nielson, W. K., and Kristensen, S. (1983). The application of membrane filtration to the concentration of fermentation broths, *Process Biochem.*, *18*: 8.

19. Fane, A. G., and Radovich, J. M. (1990). Membrane systems, *Separation Processes in Biotechnology* (J. A. Asenjo, ed.), Marcel Dekker, New York, p. 209.

20. Brock T. D. (1983). *Membrane Filtration*, Science Tech, Madison, Wisconsin.

21. Belfort, G. (1987). Membrane separation technology: An overview, *Advanced Biochemical Engineering* (H. R. Bungay and G. Belfort, eds.), John Wiley, New York, p. 239.

22. Quirk, A. V., and Woodrow, J. R. (1984). Investigation of the parameters affecting the separation of bacterial enzymes from cell debris by tangential flow filtration, *Enzyme Microb. Technol.*, *6*: 201.

23. Le, M. S., Spark, L. B., and Ward, P. S. (1984). The separation of acryl acrylamidase by cross-flow microfiltration and the significance of enzyme/cell debris interaction, *J. Memb. Sci.*, *21*: 219.

24. Blatt, W. F., David, A., Michael, A. S., and Nelson, L. (1970). Solute polarization and cake formation in membrane ultrafiltration, *Membrane Science and Technology* (J. E. Flinn, ed.), Plenum Press, New York, p. 47.

25. Colton, C. K., Henderson, L. W., Ford, C. A., and Lysaght, M. J. (1975). Kinetics of hemodiafiltration. I. In vitro transport characteristics of a hollow-fiber blood ultrafilter, *J. Lab. Clin. Med.*, *85*: 355.

26. Olsen, O. J. (1987). Membrane filtration as a tool in biotechnical down-stream processing, *Desalination*, *62*: 329.

27. Cheryan, M. (1986). *Ultrafiltration Handbook* (1986). Technomic, Lancaster, Pennsylvania.

28. Tutunjian, R. S. (1983). Ultrafiltration processes in biotechnology, *Ann. N.Y. Acad. Sci.*, *413*: 238.

29. Ofsthun, N. J. (1989). Cross-flow membrane filtration of cell suspensions, Ph.D. Thesis, Massachusetts Institute of Technology, Cambridge, Massachusetts.

30. Murkes, J., and Carlsson, C.-G. (1988). *Crossflow Filtration*, John Wiley, Chichester.

31. Kraus, K. A. (1974). Cross-flow filtration and axial filtration, *Eng. Bull.*, *Purdue University*, *145*: 1059.

32. Morton, C. D. (1927). Method of filtration, US Patent No. 1762560.

33. Kasper, J., Soudek, J., and Gutwirth, K. (1967). Improvements in or relating to a method and apparatus for dynamic filtration of slurries, British Patent No. 1057015.

34. Vilker, V. L., Colton, C. K., Smith, K. A. (1981). The osmotic pressure of concentrated protein solutions: Effect of concentration and pH in saline solutions of bovine serum albumin, *J. Colloid Interface Sci.*, *79*: 548.

35. Ofsthun, N. J., and Colton, C. K. (1987). Visual evidence of concentration polarization in cross-flow membrane plasmapheresis, *Trans. Am. Soc. Artif. Intern. Organs, 33*: 510.
36. Goldsmith, R. L., deFilipi, R. P., Nossain, S., and Timmins, R. S. (1971). Industrial ultrafiltration, *Membrane Processes in Industry and Biomedicine* (M. Bier, ed.), Plenum Press, New York, p. 267.
37. Porter, M. C. (1972). Concentration polarization with membrane ultrafiltration, *Ind. Eng. Chem. Prod. Res. Dev., 11*: 234.
38. Leveque, M. A. (1928). Les lois de la transmission de chaleur par convection, *Ann. Mines, 13*: 201.
39. Nakao, S.-I., Nomura, T., and Kimura, S. (1979). Characteristics of macromolecular gel layer formed on ultrafiltration tubular membrane, *AIChE J., 25*: 615.
40. Vilker, V. L., Colton, C. K., Smith, K. A., and Green, D. L. (1984). The osmotic pressure of concentrated protein and lipoprotein solutions and its significance to ultrafiltration, *J. Memb. Sci., 20*: 63.
41. Vilker, V. L., Colton, C. K., and Smith, K. A. (1981). Theoretical and experimental study of albumin ultrafiltered in an unstirred cell, *AIChE J., 27*: 637.
42. Jonsson, G. (1984). Boundary layer phenomena during ultrafiltration of dextran and whey protein solutions, *Desalination, 51*: 61.
43. Wijmans, J. G., Nakao, S., and Smolders, C. a. (1984). Flux limitation in ultrafiltration: Osmotic pressure model and gel layer model, *J. Memb. Sci., 20*: 115.
44. Zydney, A. L., and Colton, C. K. (1982). Continuous flow membrane plasmapheresis: Theoretical models for flux and hemolysis prediction, *Trans. Am. Soc. Artif. Intern. Organs, 28*: 408.
45. Zydney, A. L., and Colton, C. K. (1986). A concentration polarization model for the filtrate flux in cross-flow microfiltration of particulate suspensions, *Chem. Eng. Commun., 47*: 1.
46. Zydney, A. L., and Colton, C. K. (1988). Augmented solute transport in the shear flow of a concentrated suspension, *PhysicoChemical Hydrodynamics, 10*: 77.
47. Zydney, a. L., Saltzman, W. M., and Colton, C. K. (1989). Hydraulic resistance of red cell beds in an unstirred filtration cell, *Chem. Eng. Sci., 44*: 147.
48. Zydney, A. L., and Colton, C. K. (1987). Fundamental studies and design analyses for cross-flow membrane plasmapheresis, *Artificial Organs*, Proceedings International Symposium on Artificial Organs, Biomedical Engineering and Transplantation, Salt Lake City, Jan. 20–23, 1986 (J. D. Andrade et al., eds.), VCH, New York, pp. 641–655.
49. Colton, C. K., Friedman, S., Wilson, D. E., and Lees, R. S. (1972). Ultrafiltration of lipoproteins through a synthetic membrane, *J. Clin. Invest., 51*: 2472.
50. Baker, R. J., Fane, A. G., Fell, C. J. D., and Yoo, B. H. (1985). Factors affecting flux in crossflow filtration, *Desalination, 53*: 81.
51. Reihanian, H., Robertson, C. R., and Michaels, A. S. (1983). Mechanisms of polarization and fouling of ultrafiltration membrane by proteins, *J. Memb. Sci., 16*: 237.

52. Israelachvili, J. N. (1985). *Intermolecular and Surface Forces*, Academic Press, New York, p. 102.

53. Gravatt, D. P., and Molnar, T. E. (1986). Recovery of an extracellular antibiotic by ultrafiltration, *Membrane Separations in Biotechnology* (W. C. McGregor, ed.), Marcel Dekker, New York, p. 89.

54. Howell, J. A., and Velicangil, O. (1982). Theoretical considerations of membrane fouling and its treatment with immobilized enzymes for protein ultrafiltration, *J. Appl. Polym. Sci.*, *27*: 21.

55. Suki, A., Fane, A. G., and Fell, C. J. D. (1984). Flux decline in protein ultrafiltration, *J. Memb. Sci.*, *21*: 269.

56. Fane, A. G., and Fell, C. J. D. (1987). A review of fouling and fouling control in ultrafiltration, *Deslination*, *62*: 117.

57. Kroner, K. H., Hummel, W., Volkel, J., and Kula, M.-R. (1986). Effects of antifoams on cross-flow filtration of microbial suspensions, *Membranes and Membrane Processes* (E. Drioli and M. Nakagaki, eds.), Plenum, p. 223.

58. McGregor, W. C., Weaver, J. F., and Tansey, S. P. (1988). Antifoam effects on ultrafiltration, *Biotechnol. Bioeng.*, *31*: 385.

59. Chandavarkar, A. S. (1990). Dynamics of fouling of microporous membranes by proteins, Ph.D. thesis, Massachusetts Institute of Technology, Cambridge, Massachusetts.

60. Tanny, G. B., Hauk, D., and Merin, U. (1982). Biotechnical applications of a pleated crossflow microfiltration module, *Desalination*, *41*:299.

61. Kroner, K. H., and Nissinen, V. (1988). Dynamic filtration of microbial suspensions using an axial rotating filter, *J. Memb. Sci.*, *36*: 85.

62. Su, A. G., and Brown, D. E. (1990). Cross-flow filtration of fungal suspension with reversed-flow cleaning, *J. Chem. Ind. Eng.*., *5*: 144.

63. Kroner, K. H., Schütte, H., Hustedt, H., and Kula, M.-R. (1984). Problems and improvements of cross-flow filtration in enzyme recovery processes, *Proc. 3rd Eur. Congr. Biotechnol.*, *3*: 549.

64. Rodgers, V. G. J., and Sparks, R. E. (1991). Reduction of membrane fouling in the ultrafiltration of binary protein mixtures, *AIChE J.*, *37*: 1517.

65. Belfort, G., and Altena, F. W. (1983). Toward an inductive understanding of membrane fouling, Proceedings 1983 Membrane Technology/Planning Conference, Business Communications, Stamford, Connecticut, pp. 45–67.

66. Zydney, A. (1985). Cross-flow membrane plasmapheresis: An analysis of flux and hemolysis, Ph.D. thesis, Massachusetts Institute of Technology, Cambridge, Massachusetts.

67. Thomas, C. R., and Dunnill, P. (1978). The action of shear on enzymic proteins, Proceedings of International Workshop on Technology for Protein Separation and Improvement of Blood Plasma Fractionation (H. E. Sandberg, ed.), DHEW Publication No. (NIH) 78-1422, pp. 40–43.

68. Kroner, K. H., Schütte, H., Hustedt, H., and Kula, M.-R. (1984). Cross-flow filtration in the downstream processing of enzymes, *Process Biochem.*, *19*: 67.

69. Hoffmann, H., Kuhlmann, W., Meyer, H.-D., and Schugerl, K. (1985). High productivity ethanol fermentations with cross-flow membrane separation techniques for continuous cell recycling, *J. Memb. Sci.*, *22*: 235.

70. Hanisch, W. (1986). Cell harvesting, *Membrane Separations in Biotechnology* (W. C. McGregor, ed.), Marcel Dekker, New York, p. 61.

71. Fane, A. G., and Fell, C. J. D. (1983). Ultrafiltration of protein solution through partially permeable membrane—The effects of adsorption and solution environment, *J. Memb. Sci.*, *16*: 211.

72. Beaton, N. C., and Steadley, H. (1982). Industrial ultrafiltration, *Recent Developments in Separations Sciences* vol. 7 (N. Li, ed.), p. 2.

73. Popp, D. M. (1983). Crossflow microfiltration of medical solutions, *Filtr. Sep.*, *20*: 118.

74. Datar, R. (1984). Centrifugal and membrane filtration methods in biochemical separation, *Filtr. Sep.*, *21*: 402.

75. Tutunjian, R. S. (1985). Cell separation with hollow fiber membranes, *Comprehensive Biotechnology*, vol. 2 (C. L. Cooney and A. E. Humphrey, eds.), Pergamon Press, Oxford, p. 367.

76. Reid, D. E., and Adlam, C. (1974). Large-scale harvesting and concentration of bacteria by tangential flow filtration, *J. Appl. Bacteriol.*, *41*: 321.

77. Cox, J. C. (1975). New method for large-scale preparation of diphtheria toxoid: Purification of toxin, *Appl. Microbial.*, *29*: 464.

78. Goto, S., Kuwajima, T., Okamoto, R., and Inui, T. (1979). Separation of biomass by membrane filtration and continuous culture with filtrate recycling, *J. Ferment. Technol.*, *57*: 47.

79. Valeri, A., Gazzei, G., and Genna, G. (1979). Tangential flow filtration of Bordetella pertussis submerged cultures, *Experientia*, *35*: 1535.

80. Tanny, G. B., Mirelman, D., and Pistole, T. (1980). Improved filtration technique for concentrating and harvesting bacteria, *J. Envir. Microbiol.*, *40*: 269.

81. Cheryan, M., and Mehaia, M. A. (1984). Ethanol production in a membrane recycle reactor. Conversion of glucose using Saccharomyces cerevisiae, *Process Biochem.*, *19*: 204.

82. Pierrot, P., Fick, M., and Engasser, J. M. (1986). Continuous acetonebutanol fermentation with high productivity by cell ultrafiltration and recycling, *Biotechnol. Lett.*, *8*: 253.

83. Reed, W. M., and Bogdan, M. E. (1986). Application of cell recycle to continuous fermentative acetic acid production, *Biotechnol. Bioeng. Symp.*, *15*:641.

84. Ohleyer, E., Blanch, H. W., and Wilke, C. R. (1985). Continuous production of lactic acid in a cell recycle reactor, *Appl. Biochem. Biotechnol.*, *11*: 317.

85. Taniguchi, M., Kotani, N., and Kobayashi, T. (1987). High-concentration cultivation of lactic acid bacteria in fermentor with cross-flow filtration, *J. Ferm. Technol.*, *65*: 179.

86. Lee, K. J., Lefebvre, M., Tribe, D. E., and Rogers, P. L. (1980). High productivity ethanol fermentations with Zymomonas mobilis using continuous cell recycle, *Biotechnol. Lett.*, *2*: 487.

87. Dostalek, M., and Haggstrom, M. (1982). A filter fermenter-apparatus and control equipment, *Biotechnol. Bioeng.*, *24*: 2077.

88. Charley, R. C., Fein, J. E., Lavers, B. H., Lawford, H. G., and Lawford, G. R. (1983). Optimization of process design for continuous ethanol production by Zymomonas mobilis ATCC 29291, *Biotechnol. Lett.*, *5*: 169.

89. Lee, T. S., Omstead, D., Lu, N.-H., and Gregor, H. P. (1981). Membrane separations in alcohol production, *Ann. N.Y. Acad. Sci.*, *100*: 367.

90. Cabral, J. M. S., Casale, B., and Cooney, C. L. (1985). Effect of antifoam and efficiency of cleaning procedures on the cross-flow filtration of microbial suspensions, *Biotechnol. Lett.*, 7: 749.
91. Kavanaph, P. R., and Brown, D. E. (1987). Cross-flow separation of yeast cell suspensions using a sintered stainless steel filter tube, *J. Chem. Tech. Biotechnol.*, 38: 187.
92. Matsumoto, K., Katsuyama, S., and Ohya, H. (1987). Separation of yeast by cross-flow filtration with backwashing, *J. Ferment. Technol.*, 65: 77.
93. Ricketts, R. T., Lebherz, W. W., III, Klein, F., Gustafson, M. E., and Flickinger, M. C. (1985). Application, sterilization, and decontamination of ultrafiltration systems for large-scale production of biologicals, *ACS Symposium Series, 271*: 21.
94. Abdul-Salam, F. R. (1984). Cross-flow filtration and re-suspension of fungal cells, Ph.D. thesis, University of Manchester Institute of Science and Technology, U.K.
95. Al-Obaidi, Z. S., and Berry, D. R. (1979). Extended production of citric acid using an exchange filtration technique, *Biotechnol. Lett.*, 1: 221.
96. Taniguchi, M., Kato, T., Matsuno, R., and Kamikubo, T. (1983). Continuous cellulase production by cell-holding culture, *Eur. J. Appl. Microbiol. Biotechnol.*, 18: 218.
97. Zydney, A. L., and Colton, C. K. (1984). A red cell deformation model for hemolysis in cross flow membrane plasmapheresis, *Chem. Eng. Commun.*, 30: 191.
98. Maiorella, B., Dorin, G., Carion, A., and Harano, D. (1991). Crossflow microfiltration of animal cells, *Biotech. Bioeng.*, 37: 121.
99. Sterman, M. D. (1990). Personal communication, April 4, 1990.
100. Shiloach, J., Kaufman, J. B., and Kelly, R. M. (1986). Hollow fiber microfiltration methods for recovery of rat basophilic leukemia cells (RBL-2H3) from tissue culture media, *Biotechnol. Prog.*, 2: 230.
101. Maizel, A. L., Mehta, S. R., Hauft, S., Franzini, D., Lachman, B., and Ford, R. J. (1981). Human T lymphocyte/monocyte interaction in response to lectin: Kinetics of entry into the S-phase, *J. Immun.*, 127: 1058.
102. Radlett, P. J. (1972). The concentration of mammalian cells in a tangential flow filtration unit, *J. Appl. Chem. Biotech.*, 22: 494.
103. Su, Z. G., Kleizen, H. H., van Brakel, J., and Wesselingh, J. A. (1987). Influence of cell disruption on filtration of yeast homogenate, *Proceeding 4th European Congress Biotechnology*, vol. 2 (O. M. Neijssel et al., eds.), Elsevier, pp. 554–557.
104. Eriksson, A. (1985). Some examples of the use of crossflow filtration in the downstream processing in a biochemical industry, *Desalination*, 53: 259.
105. Datar, R. (1985). Studies on the separation of intracellular soluble enzymes from bacterial cell debris by tangential flow membrane filtration, *Biotechnol. Lett.*, 7: 471.
106. Gabler, R., and Ryan, M. (1985). Processing cell lysate with tangential flow filtration, *Purification of Fermentation Products*, ACS Symposium Series 271, pp. 1–20.
107. Le, M. S., Spark, L. B., Ward, P. S., and Ladwa, N. (1984). Microbial asparaginase recovery by membrane processes, *J. Memb. Sci.*, 21: 307.

108. Thompson, J. S., and Humphries, M. (1986). Bacterial cell wall isolation by filtration, *Enzyme Microb. Technol.*, *8*: 93.

109. Kane, J. f., and Hartley, D. L. (1988). Formation of recombinant protein inclusion bodies in Escherichia coli, *Trends in Biotechnol.*, *6*: 95.

110. Forman, S. M., DeBernardez, E. R., Feldberg, R. S., and Swartz, R. W. (1990). Crossflow filtration for the separation of inclusion bodies from soluble proteins in recombinant Escherichia coli cell lysate, *J. Memb. Sci.*, *48*: 263.

111. Hamel, J.-F. P., Breslau, B. r., Holeschovsky, U. B., Snoswell, M., and Cooney, C. L. (1990). Ultrafiltration studies of recombinant porcine somatotropin producing Escherichia coli and of inclusion bodies, presented at Engineering Foundation Conference on Recovery of Biological Products V, St. Petersburg, Florida, May 13–18, 1990.

112. Gangemi, J. D., Connel, E. V., Mahlandt, B. G., and Eddy, G. A. (1977). Arenavirus concentration by molecular filtration, *Appl. Environ. Microbiol.*, *34*: 330.

113. Belfort, G., Rotem, Y., and Katzenelson, E. (1976). Virus concentration using hollow fiber membranes II, *Water Res.*, *10*: 279.

114. Weiss, S. A. (1980). Concentration of baboon endogenous virus in large-scale production by use of hollow-fiber ultrafiltration technology, *Biotech. Bioeng.*, *22*: 19.

115. Trudel, M., and Payment, P. (1980). Concentration and purification of rubella virus hemagglutinin by hollow fiber ultrafiltration and sucrose density centrifugation, *Can. J. Microbiol.*, *26*: 1334.

116. Valeri, A., Gazzei, G., Morandi, M., Pende, B., and Neri, P. (1977). Large-scale purification of inactivated influenza vaccine using membrane molecular filtration, *Experientia*, *33*: 1402.

117. Sekla, L., Stackiw, W., Kay, C., and VanBuckenhout, L. (1983). Enteric viruses in renovated water in Manitoba, *Can. J. Microbiol.*, *26*: 518.

118. DiLeo, A. J., Allegrezza, A. E., Jr., and Builder, S. E. (1992). High resolution removal of virus from protein solutions using a membrane of unique structure, *Bio/Technology* (in press).

119. Brandt, S., Goffe, R. A., Kessler, S. B., O'Conner, J. L., and Zale, S. E. (1988). Membrane-based affinity technology for commercial scale purifications, *Bio/Technology*, *6*: 779.

120. Briefs, K.-G., and Kula, M.-R. (1992). Fast protein chromatography on analytical and preparative scale using modified microporous membranes, *Chem. Eng. Sci.*, *47*: 141.

121. Antonsen, K. P., Colton, C. K., and Yarmush, M. L. (1991). elution conditions and degradation mechanisms in long term immunoadsorbent use, *Biotechnol. Prog.*, *7*: 159.

5

Liquid-Liquid Extraction

Dennis J. Kubek

Merck Sharp & Dohme Research Laboratories, West Point, Pennsylvania

I. OVERVIEW

Liquid-liquid extraction is of great importance in the isolation of chemical and biological products. It is interesting that many of the systems being investigated today are rewrapped packages of old principles. Due to the interest in biologicals for human use and consumption around the world, many more novel separation schemes are yet to be implemented. Furthermore, existing technology is ripe for optimization for these purposes. Proteins and peptides are areas of high interest as a result of the rapid advancement of molecular biology and genetics. The isolation and purification of these molecules is a natural and logical requirement in order to allow their prescribed use. However, the resulting protein or peptide is, in the eyes of regulatory agencies, usually a product of its isolation. In industry one often has preconceived notions of what the molecules' structure should be like, the degree of cross-linking, and the existence or absence of side groups, etc. Protein isolation thus becomes an interesting combination of science, engineering, art, and politics.

This chapter will address liquid-liquid extraction pertaining to protein isolation and purification. The majority of the discussion will be in the area of two-phase extraction with a lesser emphasis on alternative liquid-liquid extraction techniques.

It is particularly disappointing that the use of two-phase aqueous extraction has not found greater use other than for enzymes at the industrial scale. The method is particularly useful in that it is gentle to biological molecules, which aids in preserving activity. Most of the large-scale enzyme work with this liquid-liquid extraction technique has come from our European counterparts (1). Process development and scale-up will be addressed as required.

The area of liquid-liquid extraction for protein isolation on a large scale encompasses, for the most part, aqueous two-phase extraction. Although liquid emulsion membranes and reversed micelles have been investigated for protein isolation, more work is necessary to apply this type of separation on a large scale. Supercritical fluid extraction (2–6) is used when conventional distillation cannot be applied and is of increasing importance to the chemical industry. Unfortunately few examples of supercritical fluid extraction used in conjunction with proteins (enzymes) are available in the literature (7–9). This method will not be discussed further.

The practical considerations associated with liquid-liquid extraction will be developed with examples given to emphasize both beneficial and problem areas. Isolation of biomolecules is a matter of choice that relies on final product purity, yield, and economics as well as the characteristics of the product itself and any implied or explicit federal regulatory constraints.

II. INTRODUCTION

Liquid-liquid extraction is the transfer of certain components from one phase to another when immiscible or partially soluble liquid phases are brought into contact with each other (4). The transfer can be of a strictly physical nature only or one in which a chemical reaction can result, depending on phase makeup. Early applications of liquid-liquid extraction used two organic phases or an organic and an aqueous phase. In recent years, the isolation of biological compounds has been achieved through the use of aqueous-aqueous interactions. This type of transfer is extremely useful when proteins and peptides are involved because of their more labile nature in organic solvents.

To maximize extraction efficiency, the contact between phases should be as intimate as possible. This maximization of mass transfer can then be used to effect separations and increase yields. After contacting the liquid phases and equilibrium is established, separating the phase that contains the product of interest becomes the next important unit operation. Centrifuges, settlers, columns, etc. (10–13), have all been used to separate liquid phases for a limited number of products at the commercial scale for many years. Developing settling g forces and times is simply a matter of doing small-scale studies to verify the separation parameters and scaling up in the equipment designed for the various solvents being used (e.g., two-phase extraction) (14). Settling times are also determined by small-scale experiments. Large-scale isolations, e.g., enzymes, by two-phase aqueous extraction (14), have been accomplished. Therefore scale-up of liquid-liquid extraction separation systems is not at issue regarding the problems of isolation in general.

Since proteins are the biomolecules of interest, distillation, evaporation, etc., are typically ruled out because most solvents have a denaturing effect on certain proteins and require harsh techniques for removal. The biochemical engineer involved in the isolation of proteins is faced with the task of selecting the proper solvents (most often aqueous) and the exact conditions to effect the highest degree of purification prior to final chromatographic polishing steps (15–17). Most of the following comments will be applicable to the pharmaceutical industry and in particular biologicals, where purity and activity are of paramount importance.

Phase diagrams are routinely used to predict two-phase formation in extraction systems. However, when dealing with cell extracts it is not essential to keep to the two-phase region of a particular diagram. In certain situations, solvent concentrations below the boundary on a two-phase diagram, where only a single phase results using pure components, may be used. Using a protein solution instead of the buffer in the extract free system may give the desired two-phase separation (e.g., 18). In addition to the importance of two-phase formation, the ease with which the separation of the phases occurs aids in selecting the appropriate solvents. Organic-aqueous phase systems and PEG (polyethyleneglycol)-salt phase systems typically can give rise to a large interfacial tension between phases, while PEG-dextran interfacial tension is quite small by comparison (10,19,20). Product activity during isolation plays an important part in selecting the mode of separation. For large-scale extraction, short separation times are desirable so that simple static settlers can be used. For high-value products, the added expense of centrifuges (batch or continuous) may be justified. It is difficult to provide a rule of thumb for such separations since the wide variety of protein products leads to a large range of unit operation design parameters and system economics.

Single contact/mixing of phases on the laboratory scale and their subsequent separation is least effective in terms of yield and purity unless the proper parameters have been optimized. The degree of mixing and contact time are important in developing an isolation procedure. Continuous countercurrent extractors have maximum efficiency but are unnecessary if single-stage extractors give maximum partitioning of the product of interest (10,21). The rate of extraction and contact efficiency, of course, actually control the results in either case. Classical column separators as well as the standby centrifugal separators provide a variety of unit operations to separate phases successfully (11–13,22–24). Columns or differential extractors are not commonly used for the isolation of biologically important molecules (21).

The chemical properties of certain solvents have been exploited for years in organic-organic extraction systems. Computer methods to derive or predict liquid phase activity coefficients (25) are in place to select the proper solvents for separation processes, or at least narrow the field of choice. Calculations can be performed to determine when equilibrium is reached. Unfortunately, the results can rarely be directly applied. Problems such as emulsion formation, which may interfere with phase separation, are not readily predictable. The models in the literature serve to better explain the fundamentals of extraction.

The same modeling will need to be applied to aqueous-aqueous systems in the future. The system of choice still needs to be piloted in the lab in order to answer the majority of questions. A robust process is the desired final result of the laboratory activity. While separation predictions obtained from existing/future theory are certainly desirable, the bottom line is that good experimental work is necessary to aid in the design of a liquid extraction process in the limited time frame of industrial development.

In addition to the time needed to develop a process, often the time of the liquid extraction itself is of extreme importance in minimizing the degradation of the product protein due to the presence of proteases in the cell extracts. Protease inhibitors are useful. Most are toxic or carcinogenic in nature and may irreversibly bind to the product protein. Their use may result in a request for costly clearance studies by federal regulatory agencies. The separation process should be designed to eliminate the need for inhibitors as well as other toxic/carcinogenic chemicals. Of course if a separation can be accomplished by no other means in the time frame available (i.e., prior to clinical trials), then the removal of inhibitors is left as a future process development goal.

Finally, the practice of scale-up and design has evolved over the years in essentially the following manner (11):

1. Small-scale tests are carried out in the lab on a test system that is leased from a vendor.
2. The scale-up is more or less direct, since only a larger-sized unit is necessary.

For the most part, this strategy is followed today. The last several years have seen more theoretical input to model separation processes. Various classes of proteins will benefit by enabling the elimination of improper solvents. The models used to predict performance are both proprietary and nonproprietary (26). The proprietary models, however, could increase the existing data base and aid in future separations.

III. TWO-PHASE EXTRACTION

A. Theoretical

The use of two-phase aqueous extraction was initially investigated and popularized for protein extraction by Albertsson et al. (18,19). There are several excellent references that trace the development and current interest in this method of protein isolation (27,28). Albertsson (18) defined a partition coefficient K as

$$K = \frac{C_t}{C_b} \tag{1}$$

where C_t is the concentration of the molecule of interest in the top phase and C_b is the concentration of the molecule of interest in the bottom phase.

Maximizing or minimizing K, depending on which phase is to receive the bulk of the product, as well as maximizing specific activity, are the ultimate goals of early process research. Two aqueous phases are typically used to avoid the harsh action of organic solvents on chemically labile proteins. However, some proteins may or may not be affected by the use of solvents and may be refolded after solvent removal if necessary. This latter procedure is typically not used in an isolation scheme simply because the mechanism and conditions for refolding are generally unknown. Also, in a partially purified state, impurities may become trapped within the refolded product. Although some examples of organic solvent use will be mentioned in this summary on two-phase extraction, the bulk of the discussion will concern aqueous partitioning of proteins.

The mechanism of partitioning is largely unknown, although various models have been described in the literature with good results for the systems studied. Usually the various strong interactions (hydrogen bonding, ionic and hydrophobic interactions) as well as additional weaker forces are integrated or summarized with the net effect likely to be different in the two phases (18). Bronsted (29) defined partitioning as follows:

$$K = \frac{C_1}{C_2} = \exp\left(\frac{LM}{kT}\right) \tag{2}$$

where C_1, C_2 represent the concentrations of the molecule of interest in the two phases, L is a factor that depends on properties of the molecule of interest other than molecular weight, M is the molecular weight, T is the absolute temperature, and k is the Boltzmann constant.

There are other effects, which in turn lead to defining the partition coefficient based on size, hydrophobic surface charge, and conformational effects (18,30). The known theory states that any small changes in the above-mentioned effects can give rise to a high degree of selectivity during partitioning. This is the advantage of using aqueous two-phase partitioning for protein isolation. Not only are there a great number of parameters available for adjustment within a given system (e.g., salt, pH, temperature), but there are in addition a large number of solvents available that can give rise to two-phase systems (18,31). Single-stage extractions can give high recovery of products; however, to increase yield in systems that cannot be resolved in a single step, multistage centrifugal partition chromatography or countercurrent distribution may be required.

Multiple two-phase systems to partition a protein back and forth between hydrophobic and hydrophilic phases can be used in order to increase the degree of selectivity. Also, affinity ligands bound to the polymers used during extraction, as well as extractive reactions in the phases themselves to provide high yield and increased specificity, only increase the potential of this method of isolation. In other words, the possibilities for isolation are virtually unlimited. The problem, however, is finding the correct solvent, pH, salt distribution, etc., to effect the desired separation. This daunting task typically involves a lot of work at the bench scale. Certain systems may be eliminated due to the type of molecule to be isolated. However, even though training and experience may dictate that certain solvents or conditions are not suitable for a particular protein, these solvents and conditions may still prove effective. Although this situation may not occur often, it may represent the ideal set of conditions for an effective separation. For example, a protein may become unstable when heated; however, coupling heat with a properly formulated chemical environment may effect the desired separation while maintaining product activity.

B. Example 1: Hepatitis B Surface Antigen from S. cerevisiae

1. General Description

The best way to discuss in a more practical manner how to approach a separation problem is to use specific examples. The following example will address the isolation of hepatitis B surface antigen (HBsAg) and some pertinent aspects of the isolation of Pre S2+S hepatitis B antigen (32). Both are hydrophobic lipoproteins with several disulfide bonds and a molecular weight of approximately one to two million daltons. The aggregated proteins are approximately twenty nanometers in diameter and form particles similar to the HBsAg isolated from blood. The only major difference between the Pre S2+S and HBsAg particles is the Pre S2 sequence of approximately fifty amino acids. The antigens are expressed in recombinant yeast cells and have specific activities in the clarified broken yeast cell extracts between 0.5 and 2%. Because fermentation broths may vary from batch to batch, the isolation procedure must be able to adjust to changes in extract composition without affecting overall recovery of product.

Two-phase aqueous partitioning is one procedure that is able to maintain product activity quite well and give reproducible yields from batch to batch under controlled conditions. Antigen isolated by two-phase aqueous extraction with subsequent purification by additional chromatographic methods has been used in clinical trials with excellent results. The antigen was virtually indistinguishable from an immuno-affinity purified product as well as being free from contaminating antibodies due to column bleed-off. This leads to one of the first considerations in isolation after product properties, namely intended use. Since in this example the antigen is injected, the protein must be as pure as possible while exhibiting minimal side effects. Two-phase partitioning may or may not be able to provide truly "clean" products on its own merit; however, the use of other separation methods coupled with two-phase partitioning can result in a pure product. In certain cases, high purity may be unnecessary (e.g., enzymes). Another point to consider is the intent of this phase of the isolation. In other words, what is really required? The recombinant HBsAg was to replace the existing product isolated from human blood plasma collected and frozen at donor centers. The recombinant HBsAg project was originally initiated due to the fear that donors might become more scarce at some future time.

2. Immuno-Affinity and Two-Phase Isolations

To begin preliminary animal studies or preliminary clinical trials, a small amount of purified antigen is necessary. Initially, antibodies to the HBsAg were obtained by immunizing goats with antigen isolated from human plasma. Therefore immuno-affinity columns could be prepared using the purified antibody and recombinant HBsAg isolated from broken yeast cell extracts. For HBsAg a feed stream free of cell debris and as much waste proteins, etc., as possible was necessary prior to contacting the antibody in the immune affinity column. The expensive antibody could then be protected from a majority of waste cell products. The resulting top phase of a centrifuged PEG/dextran two-phase system that could be filter sterilized prior to use was deemed the preferred starting material. Column chromatography benefited from the cleaner filtered PEG feed stream. Since unbroken cells were removed by the two-phase system and sterile filtration of the top phase was used to ensure their complete removal, live organisms were not introduced into the column. No dissolved gas production indicating anaerobic microbial growth was evident. Such treatment eliminates the direct use of centrifuged broken cell slurry extracts (typically unfilterable due to high contaminating waste concentrations of proteins, lipids, etc., as well as membrane fragments).

The development of a two-phase system for HBsAg was investigated as a possible replacement for an existing tangential flow microporous membrane system in addition to a batch adsorption/desorption unit operation already in place in production. After two-phase extraction of the antigen and phase separation, the top PEG phase was diluted and sterile filtered to remove any living yeast cells. PEG was removed from the diluted top phase by diafiltration using 100,000 MW hollow fiber cartridges. The diafiltrate was discarded. The recoveries or yields from this use of two-phase aqueous extraction resulted in as good as or better yields than the existing process (10–20% improvement) and a product with a higher specific activity (by as much as 20–30%) for use in subsequent purification. Although this procedure is not used in the current manufacturing process, it allowed for investigation of a useful isolation technique. The membrane system and adsorption/desorption unit operation performed well, and the two-phase system therefore became a model system by which extraction could be followed using variable conditions. This isolation method could then be applied to second-generation products during the process research and development stages.

3. Experimental Analysis and Results

Table 1 shows a small-scale test (10 ml) where 6% PEG and 4% dextran were used with a broken yeast cell slurry to develop a two-phase system. The molecular weight of the PEG was varied in order to discover the effect on recombinant HBsAg partitioning. PEG 3350 (average molecular weight = 3350) and dextran T500 (molecular weight = 500,000) gave the best product recovery (100% yield) with adjustment of additional experimental parameters. Using a lower-molecular-weight PEG often aids in partitioning larger molecules into the PEG phase to effect the greatest yield. It was desired that the top, more hydrophobic, PEG phase should contain essentially all the antigen, that the phase should be clear to facilitate sterile (0.2μ) filtration, and that the antigen should be stable during the two-phase process. The yield and phase clarity criteria were easily met with this choice of system components. Stability of the antigen was found to vary after separation of the phases. On standing at 4°C the top phase became cloudy; low speed centrifugation would reclarify the phase. The antigen activity, however, decreased by as much as 50%. The 8–9% concentration of PEG in the top phase appeared to be just great enough to aid in precipitating the protein. Therefore to avoid precipitation, the top phase was diluted twofold with buffer following separation of the two phases, to reduce the overall PEG concentration and maintain activity of the antigen. If a nonactive antigen (by radioimmune assay, RIA) is acceptable, then precipitation of antigen would be one method of separating PEG from antigen. Criteria for this product, however, required the specific activity of the final purified product to be approximately unity (the same as the antigen isolated from blood plasma).

Other parameters were investigated to discover their effect on isolation. These tests were by no means an in-depth study; however, the data generated proved adequate in preparing sufficient quantities of product for further characterization studies as well as for clinical trials. Figure 1 shows the

Table 1   Recovery of HBsAg in the Top PEG Phase of a 6% PEG/4% Dextran Two-Phase System at Various PEG Molecular Weights; Dextran = 500,000 MW

PEG MV (av.)	% Yield of HBsAg in top PEG phase	Description of phase system
1500	100	Large pellet + turbid liquid phase
3350	100	Two liquid phases; clear upper phase
8000	3	Two liquid phases; clear upper phase
20,000	32	Two liquid phases; turbid upper phase

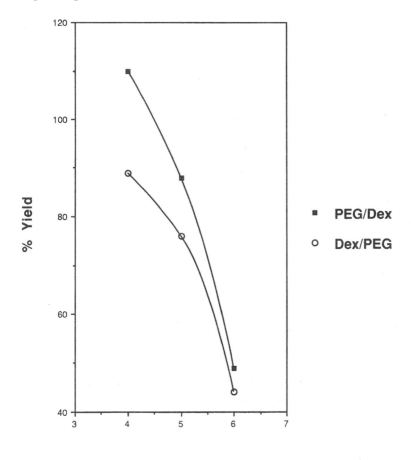

% Dextran T500

Figure 1 Recovery of HBsAg in the top PEG (6%) phase of a PEG 3350/dextran T500 two-phase system at various concentrations of dextran.

effect on yield in a PEG/dextran two-phase system when the dextran T500 concentration is varied while maintaining the PEG 3350 concentration at 6%. Variation in the RIA assay is responsible for yields greater than 100% (when compared to standards). The 4% dextran concentration proved optimal under these experimental conditions. Order of addition of the polymers showed higher titers, and therefore yield, if PEG is added prior to the dextran. This may have been due to incomplete experimental equilibrium conditions as a result of limited PEG contact time with the antigen; error in the RIA assay is another possible reason for these differences. Since the rel-

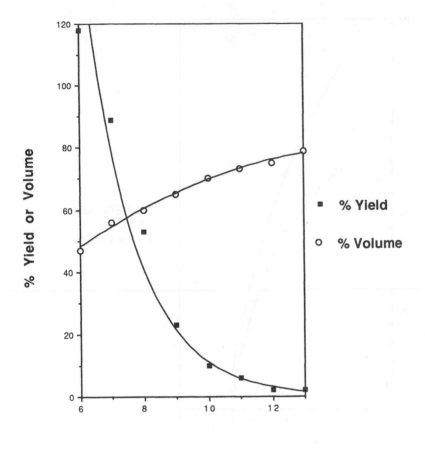

% PEG 3350

Figure 2   Recovery of HBsAg in the top PEG phase of a PEG 3350/dextran T500 (4%) two-phase system and % PEG phase volume to total system volume at various concentrations of PEG.

atively pure dextran is more expensive, minimizing its use is definitely necessary even for high-value, low-volume products. Figure 2 shows the effect of varying the concentration of PEG 3350 while maintaining dextran T500 concentration at 4%. Again the 6% concentration is the more effective in terms of higher product recovery. The above tests were performed in the presence of 0.2% Triton X-100, a nonionic surfactant. Figure 3 shows that without adding Triton the membrane antigen prefers the more hydrophilic dextran phase under the experimental conditions used. Using Triton aids in partitioning hydrophobic proteins into the PEG phase. An additional aim is to minimize the use of raw materials as much as possible and reduce volumes

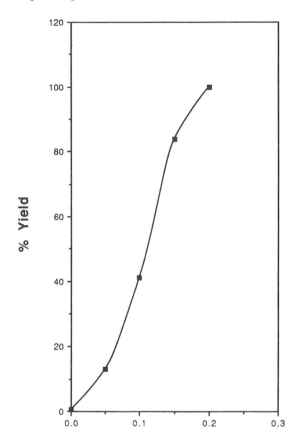

% Triton in broken cell slurry

Figure 3 Recovery of HBsAg in the top PEG phase of a PEG 3350 (6%)/dextran T500 (4%) two-phase system at various concentrations of Triton X-100.

to effect higher concentrations. Cells were broken at 50% wet weight per volume in order to minimize overall two-phase system volume with no apparent adverse effect due to protein concentration on yield.

The removal of PEG now becomes important so that the protein can be further processed. One method is to use a PEG-salt (e.g., dibasic potassium phosphate) two-phase system and have the antigen partition into the bottom phosphate phase. Figure 4 shows that taking a 6% PEG/4% dextran with Triton top phase (after separation of the phases) and adding solid dibasic potassium phosphate to achieve 0.6 molarity resulted in a complete recovery

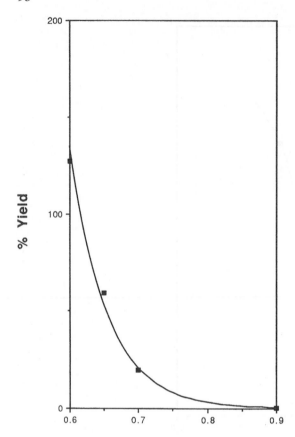

Phosphate   Molarity

Figure 4   Recovery of HBsAg in the bottom PO_4 phase of a PEG 3350/PO_4 two-phase system at various phosphate molarities [first phase system: PEG 3350 (6%)/dextran T500 (4%)].

of antigen in the bottom phosphate phase. The phosphate phase was then diafiltered to change the buffer for subsequent chromatographic purification and removal of residual protein, etc., contaminants as well as equilibrium concentrations of PEG. A direct PEG-phosphate system did not effect as clean a separation as the above-described two-step system.

4.   Pre S2+S Batch Extraction
The Pre S2+S antigen is quite similar in structure to the HBsAg, and therefore two-phase system parameters should be approximately the same. While avoiding a lengthy discussion of this system (to be published else-

where), it can be stated that at the same PEG and dextran concentrations used for HBsAg (100%) and at the same Triton level, approximately 70% of the antigen would partition into the upper phase. Increasing salt concentration (phosphate and NaCl) aided in recovery of most of the antigen in the PEG phase along with additional contaminating protein. This clear, filterable stream was able to be used as a feed to the immuno-affinity column in order to prepare purified material for characterization, animal studies, etc. (32). This method was also useful for evaluating several cell candidates from experimental fermentations (different modes of product induction). Antigen isolated using two-phase aqueous extraction followed by final chromatographic purification has been used in clinical trials with the expected immune response.

Scaling up to one kilogram of yeast cells was accomplished by simple batch mode using a bottle centrifuge. The top phase was drawn off under vacuum and diluted as described earlier (to prevent product precipitation). The resultant product was then processed further to remove a greater degree of waste contaminants than seen in the HBsAg example.

5. Countercurrent Partition Chromatography

Pre S2+S antigen was also isolated from broken yeast cell slurry clarified extracts using a continuous countercurrent centrifugal partition chromatography system (33–35). This method gives high recovery, scalability, versatility (change of mobile phase alters the two-phase system), biocompatibility, and rapidity. Sutherland et al. (22,24) and other investigators (23) report using a similar apparatus (a toroidal coil planet centrifuge) with aqueous two-phase systems. Since the single-stage extraction worked well, the continuous partition chromatography system proved unnecessary for this particular isolation. However, the method has proved extremely useful for other products and test systems during evaluation experiments in this laboratory. Dahuron and Cussler (36) used hollow fibers to separate two-phase systems and extract protein on a continuous basis. This method with pressure control works well with organic-aqueous two-phase systems that have a large surface tension between the phases (in contrast to PEG/dextran, which has a surface tension approximately 100-fold less). The hollow fibers provide the large surface area needed to optimize mass transfer of the product from one phase to the other.

6. Other Considerations

The efficient separation of a protein as large as HBsAg or Pre S2+S is predicted by Bronsted's equation (29). Since the antigen is a hydrophobic membrane protein, using Triton X-100 aids in driving the product into the upper phase (37,38). Reducing the molecular weight of the polymer (PEG) should enhance the separation as well (18,31). This in fact was verified by experimentation. The two-phase system can also be used to measure the hydrophobicity of proteins (18,30). Selecting phase compositions to minimize raw materials without compromising yield was accelerated due to the presence of existing phase diagrams (40). These diagrams and their important correlations can be predicted by the statistical mechanical theory of two incompatible polymers in solution as derived by Flory and Huggins (30,41,42). King et al. (43) have used low-angle laser light scattering to determine osmotic second virial coefficients to predict polymer-polymer-water phase diagrams and protein partition coefficients from a thermodynamic model to optimize system performance. More work is necessary (e.g., including buffer salt contribution into the model) for a better correlation between system fundamentals and actual performance. Grossman and Gainer (44) have used changes in free volume to correlate aqueous two-phase partitioning of proteins. Their model is based on salt and pH effects. Other work in this area has also broadened our understanding of protein partitioning behavior (45–47). In the future, models may be more advanced and indicate areas to investigate for various classes of molecules. At present, additional research is needed to explain, for example, interactive events when proteins differ slightly in structure but behave quite differently in two-phase systems.

C. Example 2: Beta-Galactosidase from *E. coli*

Frej et al. (48) report an example of two-phase aqueous extraction of an enzyme from a cell homogenate coupled with adsorption. This use of two separation techniques illustrates the potential of liquid-liquid extraction to aid in product recovery by minimizing protein degradation.

An *E. coli* cell slurry was homogenized in a Dyno Mill to release the product, beta-galactosidase. Phenyl-sepharose CL-4B was added to the broken cell slurry along with potassium phosphate and allowed to stand for an hour. PEG 4000, potassium phosphate, and water were added and the mixture centrifuged at low speed to separate the phases. While the top PEG phase contains the phenyl-sepharose adsorbed product, the bottom salt phase contains the cells, cell debris, waste proteins, etc. The carrier adsorbent was then prewashed in a high-salt buffer. The enzyme was eluted using a salt gradient and purified further using ion exchange chromatography and gel filtration (desalting). Complete recovery of the enzyme from the broken cell homogenate, as measured by activity, was reported with final product close to homogeneity.

Coupling two-phase aqueous extraction with adsorption, therefore, may allow for enhanced separation. In the cited example, the adsorbent appeared responsible for the purification aspect of the isolation. Separation of the adsorbent from cell debris was facilitated by using liquid-liquid extraction.

D. Example 3: Fumarase from *Brevibacterium ammoniagenes*

Hustedt et al. (14,19) discuss an example of two-phase aqueous extraction using a continuous cross-current extraction technique on a large scale for the isolation of the enzyme fumarase from *Brevibacterium ammoniagenes*. PEG and salts were added to the broken cell slurry, mixed, and the resultant two-phase mixture was separated using a centrifugal separator. Equilibrium was achieved by the use of a residence loop after the first mixer. The lower phase, which contains cell debris, protein waste, etc., was discarded. The upper PEG phase with product was sent to a holding vessel. Salts were added to the upper phase prior to the second mixer. Again the two phases were separated; however, this time the bottom salt phase contained the product. The use of such large-scale equipment can generate approximately the same yield and degree of purity as the small scale (10 ml) laboratory experiments as long as no undue separation problems arise. One such separation used 100 kg of cells from a 4000-L fermentor and a process time of 10 h (14,19). Therefore with the proper definition of process parameters, a truly large-scale isolation using two-phase aqueous extraction is possible.

E. Equipment

Belter et al. (21) provide a summary of the theory, equipment description, and examples useful for liquid-liquid extraction. The descriptions give adequate preparation for calculations involving number of stages, etc., and will not be repeated here. Some of the points discussed as well as other considerations bear emphasizing. Essentially, extraction equipment was designed and used in antibiotic isolations and, as such, many variations now exist. However, the underlying principles make use of the fact that two immiscible or partially miscible fluids are able to partition solutes selectively based on conditions set in the laboratory. It is interesting to note that all but one example used by Belter et al. (21) involves organic-aqueous two-phase systems. The aqueous-aqueous PEG-PO_4 system is used in separate batch extractor unit operations. This phase system separates more rapidly than a PEG-dextran two-phase mixture. If time is an important constraint due to product breakdown, then centrifugal separations (continuous single stage or continuous multistage) are necessary (49). The equipment being used for protein extraction normally is of simple batch, single or multiple extractor-settler combinations, or centrifugal single- or multistage systems (19). The problems with these devices are usually the same. Contact between the phases must be efficient enough in order to facilitate mass transfer. The separation of the phases, whether by gravity or by centrifugation, must be effective within time, product, and raw material constraints. The rate of settling, which is dependent on density differences between the phases and the interfacial tension and the viscosities of the phases, did not really enter into the discussion due to the use of a centrifuge to speed up the separation process. All, however, are important if settlers are to be used on a large scale.

The equipment used for separation is basically at the discretion of the investigator. Centrifugal countercurrent multistage systems allow separation of phases as well as intimate contact between the phases to effect maximum mass transfer. It is possible to use the same multistage countercurrent centrifugal extractor to separate a protein from a clarified broken cell extract into a stationary surfactant phase, then back-extract into a salt phase by varying physical parameters (e.g., pH). Whether or not staged, differential or fractional (with one or two moving phases) extraction in columns or in centrifuges (where density differences and interfacial tension determine the method of choice) are used, the underlying concept is still the separation of the phases. Determining the maximum contacting time for mass transfer based on product considerations will aid in making this choice. In addition, cost of equipment, toxicity of chemicals, phase makeup, and ease of operation within production limitations all have to be considered.

Transferring the process to production after sufficient piloting should hopefully be a painless operation. When proteins are the product of interest, care must be taken to define the conditions of separation as closely as possible. Often feeds from fermentation are of variable consistency; process control, however, can minimize any differences that occur from batch to batch. There can still be problems due to degradation of fermentation seed with time as well as loss of product-specific activity prior to isolation. Fortunately, liquid-liquid extraction is unaffected by this type of problem; however, other downstream isolation unit operations may have to be adjusted in order to better cope with the changing feed composition

F. General Considerations

Some general remarks concerning how to proceed with a two-phase system are in order. Several polymer-polymer or polymer-salt systems should be selected to investigate the partitioning characteristics of interest. Small-scale experiments should be carried out, the results evaluated, and changes in phase system components made in a systematic manner to determine their effect on separation. In addition, positions on the phase diagram should be selected that tend to give more stable systems (away from the two-phase boundary) and along tie-lines for adequate volumes of the phase of interest. Temperature may enhance separation; however, the maximum effect occurs at the critical or plait point on the phase diagram. Since this would lead to greater control problems, as well as phase stability problems, processing conditions are chosen to minimize temperature effects (18). The two-phase system temperature is usually selected as a result of product stability requirements. The pH of a system can greatly affect the partition coefficient for certain products. For the case of the Pre S2+S protein, using dibasic phosphate aided in achieving higher antigen concentration in the top phase of a PEG/dextran two-phase system. Higher pH's than those experienced with phosphate present did not increase the partition coefficient of the antigen. Other ways to increase partition coefficients are by using charged polymers (which typically are better at partitioning charged proteins than salt), PEG with bound hydrophobic groups, and selective ligands bound to the desired polymer. The use of selective ligands (50–53) approaches affinity isolation but should avoid the problem of antibody bleed-off.

Johansson (54) gives an excellent summary of the use of two-phase extraction for the isolation of proteins including blood proteins, histones, interferon, and enzymes. Hustedt et al. (14,19) discuss methods of phase separation on a larger scale as well as large-scale two-phase systems in general. Westfalia, Podbelniak, and Alfa Laval are some of the centrifuge manufacturers whose equipment is reported to be useful in separating two liquid phases on a larger scale (Ref. 19, as well as individual product manuals). Belter et al. (21) present equations for extractors (as does Perry's, Ref. 10) with examples for bioseparations. The design of existing extractors often must be modified in order to provide the maximum contact between the phases for the two-phase system of interest.

At present the larger-scale systems have been used primarily for enzyme isolation. In these cases, the economics of using a PEG/phosphate system or a dextran substitute (e.g., Reppel-PES, a starch-based polymer) (20,55) or PEG removal play a more important role. Other examples of protein isolation on a small scale using two-phase extraction demonstrate the versatility of the procedure (56–64). Areas of further interest include the ligand-polymer complex to increase yields (28,52,53,56,65–68) and the reactive extraction systems (69–71). For reactive extraction an enzyme would be in one of the phases of a two-phase system, substrate would be added along with a salt to the phase with the enzyme, and the product would be isolated in the phase free of enzyme and substrate. Adsorbents can also be used in a two-phase system. With proper design, the adsorbent can be made to partition into the top phase. The top phase can then be passed through a column, which retains the adsorbent. The use of surfactants to aid in partitioning and their subsequent removal in other phase systems, including multiple phase systems, has also been investigated (48,68).

One important point to consider is that in-depth research of a particular method in order to derive equations to predict behavior during isolation typically comes after the fact or, in some cases, not at all. With the advent of increasingly sophisticated analytical techniques, more data is generated for model development. At the time a novel product is being isolated, often very little is known of its compatibility with different chemicals, environments, and other constraints. The storehouse of information concerning various classes of proteins and peptides is growing and definitely provides methods of isolation to investigate as well as discard. The luxury of complete understanding of any isolation process is typically not realized in industry. Discretionary time can be and is used to understand mechanisms with information stored for future reference. Since pharmaceuticals can take years of development to produce a marketable product, one project may supersede another, and the time to define properly the reactions and phenomena involved by modeling may disappear. Understanding what is happening during isolation and knowing the limiting constraints of processing conditions aid in providing the best process. This allows making the required product to meet marketing demands at that point in time. In the future, the knowledge of the mechanisms involved during isolation may catch up to and, hopefully, precede final process development.

G. Problem Areas

One major potential problem area is the removal of PEG (65). Loading a top phase containing an adsorbent into a column, followed by washing the adsorbent free of the PEG and subsequent elution of the protein from the adsorbent, is one suggested method to solve this problem (58). Ultrafiltration, ion exchange chromatography, and hydrophobic interaction chromatography are other ways to separate the solute of interest from the PEG (32). However, build-up of PEG on ultrafiltration membranes may require additional diafiltration volumes for removal. Also, complete removal of PEG by this method may not be possible under high concentration conditions. However, repartitioning the solute into a salt phase will separate most of the PEG from the product.

Another major issue is the problem of waste solvents and biodegradability, which are important considerations when dealing with extraction systems. There have been reports of reuse of solvents (14). Reuse of solvents is of less concern at the smaller scale or where high-value products are involved. The problem area of disposal of solvents for large-scale applications will also have to be addressed if reuse of the solvents is unacceptable. The aqueous two-phase systems are nontoxic to biological systems and are also nonflammable. Integrated systems of isolation during fermentation have also been discussed in the literature (72,73). Such product removal can relieve feedback inhibition and allow further product production by the cells.

A degree of control not yet mentioned that might enhance separation potential/strategy is incorporating the geneticist and molecular biologist in the development of the purification scheme. Since industry prides itself on using interdisciplinary groups to solve problems, the geneticists can add their expertise in developing a successful purification (72). Because downstream processing is the bulk of product cost (1,28), doing everything possible to make this aspect easier and more efficient is necessary. The area of vaccines, for example, involves lower-volume higher-value products. For smaller-scale processes (on the average about 50 L of concentrated cell slurry) the process engineering may appear less demanding. However, every process will need control and reproducibility, which in turn means adequate monitoring of important parameters (temperature, flow rates, degree of mixing, etc.). If the group interested in providing the marketplace with a product to improve the overall condition of mankind can work together, the isolation/purification of a biological can be made less stressful. Logical process development goals as results of interdisciplinary cooperation are as follows: secreted products, non-growth-associated products, organisms tolerant to high product concentrations, stable products, and high specific activities (ratio of product to total protein) are desirable (40). The accomplishment of goals such as these should, in most instances, make the research and development activities of the engineer much more efficient.

H. Summary

In summary, two-phase partitioning (74) for the separation of proteins and peptides is an extremely useful method of isolation. The number of factors that can be varied and can therefore increase selectivity are almost limitless. An increasing number of two-phase systems of polymers and salts are being developed in order to increase further the degree of selectivity. Scale-up is straightforward based on systems that have been used for years for organic separations. Modeling of protein two-phase systems needs to be better delineated to increase both our understanding of the partitioning during extraction and the predictability of these extractive systems. Ligands, multiphase systems, and reactive extraction also add to the attractiveness of two-phase partitioning as a powerful separation tool. The use of two-phase aqueous extraction has great potential to perform initial isolation of product from cell debris, etc. Final purification may be accomplished using the same technique or other purification methods (e.g., chromatographic procedures). For vaccines (or other products administered by injection), final product purity is of paramount importance. Coupling two-phase technology with other separation procedures is one way in which the methodology may meet with greater acceptance.

IV. OTHER LIQUID-LIQUID EXTRACTION SYSTEMS

A. General

Other systems that may prove useful for separating proteins are emulsions, microemulsions or micellar solutions, and reversed micelles. These methods are very versatile tools for separation in general. A brief discussion of each technique follows. At present, however, no large-scale use of these methods for protein isolation is documented in the literature.

1. Emulsions and Microemulsions or Micellar Solutions

a. General Description. An emulsion is a heterogeneous system consisting of at least one immiscible liquid intimately dispersed in another in the form of droplets whose diameters, in general, exceed 0.1 μ (75). These systems are generally unstable and may separate into two distinct phases as the average drop size grows with time. Microemulsions or micellar solutions are considered to be thermodynamically stable. In many cases microemulsions are formed when a cosurfactant is titrated into a coarse emulsion (composed of a mixture of water/surfactant in sufficient quantity to obtain microdroplets/oil). The resulting system is low in viscosity, transparent, isotropic, and very stable (76). When the system is subjected to stress, it will return to the original state after removal of the disturbance. The physical state of the system is defined by specifying the concentrations of the various components, the pressure, and the temperature (77).

Liquid membrane systems are typically used for recovery of low concentrations of solutes in wastewater (metal ions) or gas separation (e.g., oxygen separation from air) (78). Some applications of this technology to biochemical separations have been documented (79). Generally speaking, such systems make use of an organic and aqueous phase plus surfactant to isolate a solute selectively. An emulsion of two immiscible phases is dispersed in a third continuous phase. The encapsulated phase never directly contacts the continuous phase. For most applications (including proteins), the encapsulated and continuous phases are aqueous in nature. The concentrated product is then recovered from the emulsion by heating, centrifugation, application of an electric field, or extraction into a separate stripping phase (80). When recovering proteins, a cosurfactant may be used to aid in solubilizing the protein over a wider pH range and increasing the efficiency of the protein extraction. Other factors influencing protein solubility are salt type and ionic strength.

Liquid membrane separation, a rate process, is accomplished by a driving force rather than equilibrium between phases (80). Proteins may suffer from low mobility and solubility. The basic modes of action in liquid membrane systems are simple diffusion (uncharged solutes), facilitated transport (which utilizes a carrier ion not soluble in the organic phase), and coupled transport (80). Use of carriers leads to higher fluxes, selective separations, and concentration of products. In coupled transport, the carrier agent couples the flow of two or more species, which allows one species to move against its concentration gradient as the concentration gradient of the other species is large. Typical areas of concern (81) in using these systems on a large scale include mechanical stability of the system as a whole (proper formulation of the system should limit this problem) (82), membrane swelling due to water transport, the degree and reproducibility of agitation to create globules of uniform size for maximum mass transport, and the efficiency of product recovery. Maintaining the activity of the product is also of paramount importance.

b. Scale-Up and Additional Uses. Models, including reversible reaction and advancing front (83–85), have been formulated that attempt to describe the extraction using liquid membrane systems. The design of extractors/separators for these systems will need to be investigated once larger-scale applications are available. Extractor/separator design can make use of developing models in order to effect the best separation (83). The existing technology of extraction, settling, and separation may be adequate as a starting point to meet the needs of liquid membrane systems. Recovery of proteins may present a problem if the solvent must be recovered and reused in order to make the system economically viable.

Phase separation using hollow fibers can aid in providing a high surface area for contact (86) and continuous extraction of solutes from one aqueous phase to another across an immobilized organic phase within the membrane itself. Enhancement of transport of large molecules across a membrane by applying a periodic pressure gradient transverse to the membrane has also been suggested (87).

2. Reversed Micelles

a. General Description. An aqueous protein solution contacted with a surfactant containing organic solvent, using controlled conditions, will result in the protein being solubilized in reversed micelles. System conditions are controlled by surfactant structure and concentration, the nature of the organic phase, and the pH and electrolyte concentration of the aqueous phase (88,89). Movement of a protein into a reversed micelle is, in general, maximized by protonating/deprotonating protein surface groups by pH control in addition to using low electrolyte concentrations. At the pH chosen for the aqueous phase, the surfactant should be oppositely charged to the protein. Reversing the movement of protein from the reversed micelle back to the aqueous phase may be performed by operating at the isoelectric point of the protein and by increasing the electrolyte concentration (88).

b. Scale-Up. Hatton (89) discusses process considerations for scaling up reversed micelle extractions. Only the mixer-settler system has been demonstrated when mechanical means are used to disperse one phase into the other (90). The use of agitation to effect contact between the two phases may cause emulsion formation. In order to overcome this process limitation, a microporous membrane system may be used (36). One phase, which preferentially wets the membrane, is used to fill the membrane pores. The nonwetting phase may then be used to maintain the interface within the membrane pores to avoid emulsion formation. Pressure distribution, whatever the operating configuration, plays an important part in the transfer of solute, emulsion formation, etc. (89).

c. Example: Alpha-Amylase. An example from the literature that demonstrated the application of modeling to system design was the reversed micellar extraction of alpha-amylase (90,91). This system was discussed in regard to optimization, enzyme inactivation, and modeling. The developed model allowed for the prediction of changes in process conditions (for example, the effect of residence times and mass transfer rate coefficients), as well as changes in composition of the aqueous and reversed micellar phases (for example, the effect of inactivation rate constants and distribution coefficients) on the extraction efficiency. This type of analysis is very useful in predicting which parameters are important not only for the processing conditions themselves but for scale-up as well. Therefore if a model predicts that a shorter residence time is beneficial, then centrifugal equipment for extraction/separation may be necessary. This will aid in providing the proper input for scale-up. Certainly, existing equipment may need modification in order to handle various reversed micelle systems.

d. Other Examples. Examples of proteins being separated in reversed micelle systems have all been on the small scale (81,92,93). Rahaman et al. (94) discuss recovery of alkaline protease from whole fermentation broth using reversed micelles. A three-stage cascade recovery scheme resulted in a 56% yield of product with a purification factor as high as six being observed. The system was not optimized as to solvent use, composition, etc.; however, the system demonstrated the potential of reversed micelles as an isolation technique. Goklen (95) used several proteins in reversed micelle systems and monitored their isolation by varying solvent compositions, surfactants, etc. Enzymes can be encapsulated in reversed micelles in order to drive various reactions (96). More work is necessary in order to understand the changes a protein undergoes after solubilization and the conditions required to maximize recovery of active proteins (97,98).

B. Summary

In summary, emulsion, microemulsion, and reversed micelle systems are not used on a large scale for protein purification at this time. In the future, it is possible that these methods of liquid-liquid extraction will be applied. Since solvents may wreak havoc with many proteins, these types of isolations may be limited to specific protein classes (e.g., enzymes) (81).

V. CONCLUSIONS

The liquid-liquid extraction of proteins and peptides on a large scale at present encompasses the area of two-phase extraction, mainly aqueous-aqueous and aqueous-organic. These extractions are generally used for enzyme recovery. Examples were presented on how two-phase aqueous extraction was useful in providing feed streams for immuno-affinity chromatography or hydrophobic interaction chromatography. The scale-up of liquid-liquid extraction systems has been considered as straightforward. Using existing equipment with various modifications appears to enable the separation and isolation of large quantities of enzymes of relatively high purity. The problem arises as to how the best separation can be effected using the least number of stages, where applicable, and the minimum number of two-phase systems. Defining optimum pH, salt concentration/distribution, polymer concentration and type, and appropriate additives still remains essentially a trial-and-error ritual. Experience and some knowledge of the product itself aids, however, in narrowing options. The great variety of conditions that can be manipulated is both a blessing and a curse. One has enough variables to effect a high degree of selectivity, but the number and combination of different chemical combinations may appear daunting. Only a systematic approach during laboratory isolation experiments will lead to optimal separation conditions. Modeling of two-phase systems has progressed significantly; however, additional work is needed to understand protein interactions in solution during separation.

The use of reversed micelle systems offers the potential for application to protein isolation. No large-scale use of reversed micelle systems with proteins has been reported in the literature as yet. Scale-up should be initially able to make use of existing liquid-liquid extraction technology. The modeling of surfactant based extraction systems will also need additional investigation in order to understand better the capabilities and limitations of this emerging technology.

Working with proteins is both interesting and frustrating, since the product obtained following isolation appears to be based on its purification unit operations. Activity, as measured by a variety of tests, can be easily lost through inappropriate use of any separation technique. Generally speaking, robust process development is based on considering a wide variety of separation techniques, rather than just deciding in advance that only one or two types of separations should be used. Liquid-liquid extraction is one versatile isolation method that provides separations in which high yield and activity, as well as increased specific activity, are realized. Two-phase aqueous extraction in particular has been shown to be very useful for large-scale protein isolation; it is hoped that this method will be considered more frequently for use in every large scale protein purification process.

REFERENCES

1. Kula, M.-R. (1987). Use of phase partitioning to scale-up protein purification, *Protein Purification Micro to Macro, Proceedings of a Cetus-UCLA Symposium*. (R. Burgess, ed.), Alan Liss, New York, p. 99.
2. Widom, B., and Sundar, G. (1986). Some theoretical aspects of critical phenomena in fluids, *Fluid Phase Equilibria*, *30*: 1.
3. Brignole, E. A. (1986). Supercritical fluid extraction, *Fluid Phase Equilibria*. *29*: 133.
4. Kumar, S. K., Suter, U. W., and Reid, R. C. (1986). Fractionation of polymers with supercritical fluids, *Fluid Phase Equilibria*, *29*: 373.
5. Mathias, P. M., Copeman, T. W., and Prausnitz, J. M. (1986). Phase equilibria for supercritical extraction of lemon flavors and palm oils with carbon dioxide, *Fluid Phase Equilibria*. *29*: 545.
6. King, M. B., Bott, T. R., and Chami, J. H. (1987). Extraction of bio-materials with compressed carbon dioxide and other solvents under near critical conditions, *Separations for Biotechnology* (M. S. Verrall and M. J. Hudson, eds.), John Wiley, New York, p. 293.
7. Hammond, D. A., Karel, M., Klibanov, A. M., and Krukonis, V. J. (1985). Enzymatic reactions in supercritical gases, *Appl. Biochem. Biotech.*, *11*: 393.
8. Randolph, T. W., Blanch, H. W., and Prausnitz, J. M. (1985). Enzymatic catalysis in a supercritical fluid, *Biotech. Lett.*, 7: 325.
9. Nakamura, K., Chi, Y., Yamada, Y., and Yano, T. (1986). Lipase activity and stability in supercritical carbon dioxide, *Chem Eng. Commun.*, *45*: 207.
10. Perry, R. H., Chilton, C. H., and Kirkpatrick, S. D., eds. (1963). *Perry's Chemical Engineers' Handbook*, McGraw-Hill, New York, p. 14–40.
11. Todd, D. B. (1983). Solvent extraction, *Fermentation and Biochemical Engineering Handbook* (H. C. Vogel, ed.), Noyes, New Jersey, p. 175.

12. Reissinger, K. H., Schroeter, J., and Bayer, L. (1978). Selection criteria for liquid-liquid extractors, *Chem. Eng., 85*: 109.
13. Karr, A. E., Gebert, W. and Wang, M. (1980). Extraction of whole fermentation broth with Karr reciprocating plate extraction column, *Can. J. of Chem. Eng., 58*: 249.
14. Hustedt, H., Kroner, K. H., and Kula, M.-R. (1980). Extraction in aqueous two-phase systems—A new method for large-scale purification of enzymes, *Kontakte, 80*: 17.
15. Wheelwright, S. M. (1989). The design of downstream processes for large-scale protein purification, *J. Biotech., 11*: 89.
16. Naveh, D. (1990). Industrial-scale downstream processing of biotechnology products, *BioPharm, 2*: 28.
17. Paul, E. L., and Rosas, C. B. (1990). Challenges for chemical engineers in the pharmaceutical industry, *Chem. Eng. Prog., 86*: 17.
18. Albertsson, P. (1986). *Partition of Cell Particles and Macromolecules*, John Wiley, New York.
19. Hustedt, H., Kroner, K. H., and Kula, M.-R. (1985). Applications of phase partitioning in biotechnology, *Partitioning in Aqueous Two-Phase Systems* (H. Walter, D. E. Brooks, and D. Fisher, eds.), Academic Press, p. 529.
20. Mattiasson, B., and Ling, T. G. I. (1987). Extraction in aqueous two-phase systems for biotechnology, *Separations for Biotechnology* (M. S. Verrall and M. J. Hudson, eds.), John Wiley, New York, p. 270.
21. Belter, P. A., Cussler, E. L., and Hu, W. (1988). Extraction, *Bioseparations-Downstream Processing for Biotechnology*, John Wiley, New York, p. 99.
22. Sutherland, I. A., Heywood-Waddington D., and Peters, T. J. (1985). Counter-current chromatography using a toroidal coil planet-centrifuge: A comparative study of the separation of organelles using aqueous two-phase partition, *J. of Liquid Chromatography, 8*: 2315.
23. Ito, Y., and Bowman, R. C. (1971). Countercurrent chromatography with flow-through coil planet centrifuge, *Science, 173*: 420.
24. Sutherland, I. A., Heywood-Waddington, D., and Peters, T. J. (1984). Toroidal coil countercurrent chromatography: A fast simple alternative to countercurrent distribution using aqueous two-phase partition, *J. of Liquid Chromatography, 7*: 363.
25. Brignole, E. A., Bottini, S., and Gani, R. (1986). A strategy for the design and selection of solvents for separation processes, *Fluid Phase Equilibria, 29*: 125.
26. Fair, J. R. (1988). A half-century of progress in separations technology, *Chemical Processing*, Mid-March: 58.
27. Albertsson, P. (1985). History of aqueous polymer two-phase partition, *Partitioning in Aqueous Two-Phase Systems* (H. Walter, D. E. Brooks, and D. Fisher, eds.), Academic Press, p. 1.
28. Mattiasson, B., and Kaul, R. (1986). Use of aqueous two-phase systems for recovery and purification in biotechnology, *Separation, Recovery and Purification in Biotechnology* (J. A. Asenjo and J. Hong, eds.), ACS, Washington, D.C., p. 78.
29. Bronsted, J. N. (1931). Molecular magnitude and phase distribution, *Z. Phys. Chem. Abt. A, 157*: 257.
30. Brooks, D. E., Sharp, K. A., and Fisher, D. (1985). Theoretical aspects of partitioning, *Partitioning in Aqueous Two-Phase Systems* (H. Walter, D. E. Brooks, and D. Fisher, eds.), Academic Press, p. 11.

31. Bamberger, S., Brooks, D. E., Sharp, K. A., Van Alstine, J. M., and Webber, T. J. (1985). Preparation of phase systems and measurement of their physiochemical properties, *Partitioning in Aqueous Two-Phase Systems* (H. Walter, D. E. Brooks, and D. Fisher, eds.), Academic Press, p. 85.

32. Ellis, R. W., Kniskern, P. J., Hagopian, A., Schultz, L. D., Montgomery, D. L., Maigetter, R. Z., Wampler, D. E., Emini, E. A., Wolanski, B., McAleer, W. J., Hurni, W. M., and Miller, W. J. (1988). Preparation and testing of a recombinant-derived hepatitis B vaccine consisting of Pre-S2+5 polypeptides, *Viral Hepatitis and Liver Disease*: 1079–1086.

33. Cazes, J. (1988). Centrifugal partition Chromatography, *Biotechnology, 6*: 13988.

34. Cazes J. (1987). Separation of proteins with centrifugal partition chromatography, *Am. Lab. News, 19*: 30.

35. Cazes J., and Nunogoki, K. (1987). Centrifugal partition chromatography, *Am. Lab., 19*: 126.

36. Dahuron, L., and Cussler, E. L. (1988). Protein extraction with hollow fibers, *AIChE Journal, 34*: 130.

37. Albertsson, P. (1973). Application of the phase partition method to a hydrophobic membrane protein, phospholipase A1 from *Escherichia coli, Biochemistry, 12*: 2525.

38. Lukoyanova, M. A., and Petukhova, N. M. (1976). Use of phase partition for the fractionation of hydrophobic membrane proteins, *Biokhimiya, 41*: 1810.

39. Eiteman, M. A., and Gainer, J. L. (1990). Peptide hydrophobicity and partitioning in poly(ethylene glycol)/magnesium sulfate aqueous two-phase systems, *Biotech. Prog., 6*: 479.

40. Belfort, G. (1987). Challenges and opportunities in product recovery, *Advanced Biochemical Engineering* (H. R. Bungay and G. Belfort, eds.), John Wiley, New York, p. 187.

41. Flory, P. J. (1941). Thermodynamics of high polymer solutions, *J. Chem. Phys., 9*: 660.

42. Huggins, M. L. (1941). solutions of long-chain compounds, *J. Chem. Phys., 9*: 440.

43. King, R. S., Blanch, H. W., and Prausnitz, J. M. (1988). Molecular thermodynamics of aqueous two-phase systems for bioseparations, *AIChE Journal, 34*: 1585.

44. Grossman, P. D., and Gainer, J. L. (1988). correlation of aqueous two-phase partitioning of proteins with changes in free volume, *Biotech. Prog. 4*: 6.

45. Chen, C.-C., Zhu,, Y., and Evans, L. B. (1989). Phase partitioning of biomolecules: Solubilities of amino acids, *Biotech. Prog., 5*: 111.

46. Diamond, A. D., and Hsu, J. T. (1990). Protein partitioning in PEG/dextran aqueous two-phase systems, *AIChE J., 36*: 1017.

47. Hayes, C. A., Carson, J., Blanch, H. W., and Prausnitz, J. M. (1991). Electrostatic potentials and protein partitioning in aqueous two-phase systems, *AIChE J., 37*: 1401.

48. Frej, A. Gustafsson, J., and Hedman, P. (1986). Recovery of beta-galactosidase by adsorption from unclarified *Escherichia coli* homogenate, *Biotechnology and Bioengineering, 28*: 133.

49. Sutherland, I. A. (1985). Other types of countercurrent distribution apparatus and continuous flow chromatography techniques, *Partitioning in Aqueous Two-*

Phase Systems (H. Walter, D. E. Brooks, and D. Fisher, eds.), Academic Press, p. 149.

50. Harris, J. M., and Yalpani, M. (1985). Polymer-ligands used in affinity partitioning and their synthesis, *Partitioning in Aqueous Two-Phase Systems* (H. Walter, D. E. Brooks, and D. Fisher, eds.), Academic Press, p. 589.

51. Mustacich, R. V., and Weber, G. (1978). Ligand-promoted transfer of proteins between phases: Spontaneous and electrically helped, *Proc. Nat. Acad. Sci. USA*, *75*: 779.

52. Suh, S.-S., and Arnold, F. H. (in press). A mathematical model for metal affinity protein partitioning, *Biotechnology and Bioengineering*.

53. Wuenschelll, G. E., Naranjo, E., and Arnold, F. H. (in press). Aqueous two-phase metal affinity extraction of heme proteins, *Bioprocess Engr.*

54. Johansson, G. (1985). Partitioning of proteins, *Partitioning in Aqueous Two-Phase Systems* (H. Walter, D. E. Broks, and D. Fisher, eds.), Academic Press, p. 161.

55. Gustafsson, A., and Wennerstrom, H. (1986). Aqueous polymer two-phase systems in biotechnology, *Fluid Phase Equilibria*, *29*: 365.

56. Johansson, G., Joelsson, M., and Olde, B. (1985). Affinity partitioning of biopolymers and membranes in ficoll-dextran aqueous two-phase systems, *J. of Chromatography*, *331*: 11.

57. Gineitis, A. A., Suciliene, S. P., and Shanbhag, V. P. (1984). Dissociation and isolation of chromatin proteins in salt solutions by an aqueous two-phase system, *Analytical Biochemistry*, *139*: 400.

58. Hedman, P. O., and Gustafsson, J. G. (1984). Protein adsorbents intended for use in aqueous two-phase systems, *Analytical Biochemistry*, *138*: 411.

59. Clemetson, K., Bienz, D., Zahno, M. L., and Luscher, E. F. (1984). Distribution of platelet glycoproteins and phosphoproteins in hydrophobic and hydrophilic phases in Triton X-114 phase partition, *Biochim. Biophys. Acta*, *778*: 463.

60. Andreasen, P. A. (1983). Aqueous two-phase partition studies of glucocorticoid receptors exposed to limited trypsinization, *Mol. Cell Endocrinology*, *30*: 229.

61. Albertsson, P. A., and Andersson, B. (1981). Separation of membrane components by partition in detergent-containing polymer phase systems. Isolation of the light harvesting chlorophyll a/b protein, *J. Chromatography*, *215*: 131.

62. Fex, G., Albertsson, P. A. and Hansson, B. (1979). Interaction between prealbumin and retinol-binding protein studies by affinity chromatography, gel filtration and two-phase partition, *Eur. J. Biochem.*, *99*: 353.

63. Petersen, L. C. (1978). Measurements of cytochrome c–cytochrome aa3 complex formation by aqueous two-phase partition, *Bioochem. Soc. Trans.*, *6* 1274.

64. Vernau, J., Kula, M.-R. (1990). Extraction of proteins from biological raw material using aqueous polyethylene glycol-citrate phase systems, *Biotech. and Appl. Biochem.*, *12*: 397.

65. Scopes, R. K. (1987). *Protein Purification—Principles and Practice*, Springer-Verlag, New York.

66. Johansson, G., Kopperschlager, G., and Albertsson, P. (1983). Affinity partitioning of phosphofructokinase from baker's yeast using polymer-bound Cibacon Blue F3G-A, *Eur. J. Biochem.*, *131*: 589.

67. Birkenmeier, G., Ehrlich, U., and Kopperschlager, G. (1986). Partition of purified human thyroxine-binding globulin in aqueous two-phase systems in response to reactive dyes, *J. of Chromatography*, *360*: 193.

68. Walter, H., and Johansson, G. (1986). Partitioning in Aqueous two-phase systems: An overview, *Analytical Biochemistry, 155*: 215.
69. Likidis, Z., and Schugerl, K. (1987). Recovery of penicillin by reactive extraction in centrifugal extractors, *Biotechnology and Bioengineering, 30*: 1032.
70. Tjerneld, F., Persson, I., Albertsson, P., and Hahn-Hagerdal, B. (1985). Enzymatic hydrolysis of cellulose in aqueous two-phase systems. I. Partition of cellulases from *Trichoderma reesi, Biotechnology and Bioengineering, 27*: 1036.
71. Tjerneld, F., Persson, I., Albertsson, P., and Hahn-Hagerdal, B. (1985). Enzymatic hydrolysis of cellulose in aqueous two-phase systems. II. Semicontinuous conversion of a model substrate Solka Floc BW200, *Biotechnology and Bioengineering, 27*: 1044.
72. Riet, K. V. (1984). Research on downstream processing in the Netherlands, *Innovations in Biotechnology* (E. H. Houwink and R. R. van der Meer, eds.), Elsevier, Amsterdam, p. 351.
73. Bjurstrom, E. (1985). Biotechnology, *Chemical Engineering*, Feb. 18: 126.
74. Sutherland, I. A., and Fisher, D. (1985). Partitioning: A comprehensive bibliography, *Partitioning in Aqueous Two-Phase Systems* (H. Walter, D. E. Brooks, and D. Fisher, eds.), Academic Press, p. 627.
75. Becher, P. (1965). *Emulsions: Theory and Practice*, Reinhold, New York, p. 2.
76. Rosano, H. L., and Clausse, M. (1987). *Microemulsion Systems*, Marcel Dekker, p. xv.
77. Bourrel, M., and Schechter, R. S. (1988). *Microemulsions and Related Systems*, Marcel Dekker, New York, p. v.
78. Noble, R. D., and Way, J. D. (1987). Applications of liquid membrane technology, *Liquid Membranes—Theory and Application* (R. D. Noble and J. D. Way, eds.), ACS, Washington, D.C., p. 110.
79. Thien, M. P., Hatton, T. A., and Wang, D. I. C. (1986). Liquid emulsion membranes and their applications in biochemical separations, *Separation, Recovery, and Purification in Biotechnology* (J. A. Asenjo and J. Hong, eds.), ACS, Washington, D.C., p. 67.
80. Noble, R. D., and Way, J. D. (1987). Liquid membrane technology: An overview, *Liquid Membranes—Theory and Application* (R. D. Noble and J. D. Way, eds.), ACS, Washington, D.C., p. 1.
81. Chaudhuri, J., and Pyle, D. L. (1987). Liquid membrane extraction, *Separations for Biotechnology*(M. S. Verrall and M. J. Hudson, eds.), John Wiley, New York, p. 241.
82. Borwankar, R. P., Chan, C. C., Wasan, D. T., Kurzeja, R. M., Gu, Z. M., and Li, N. N. (1988). Analysis of the effect of internal phase leakage on liquid membrane separations, *AIChE Journal, 34*: 753.
83. Reed, D. L., Bunge, A. L., and Noble, R. D. (1987). Influence of reaction reversibility on continuous-flow extraction by emulsion liquid membranes, *Liquid Membranes—Theory and Application* (R. D. Noble and J. D. Way, eds.), ACS, Washington, D.C., p. 62.
84. Leiber, J. P., Noble, R. D., Way, J. D., and Bateman, B. R. (1985). Mathematical modeling of facilitated liquid membrane transport systems containing ionically charged species, *Separation Science and Technology, 20*: 231.
85. Bouboukas, G., Colinart, P., Renon, H., and Trouve, G. (1986). Transfer of barbiturates through emulsified liquid membranes, *CRC Recent Developments in Separation Science*, (N. Li and J. Calo, eds.), CRC Press, New York, p. 209.

86. Sengupta, A., Basu, R., and Sirkar, K. K. (1988). Separation of solutes from aqueous solutions by contained liquid membranes, *AIChE Journal, 34*: 1698.

87. Leighton, D. T., Jr., and McCready, M. J. (1988). Shear enhanced transport in oscillatory liquid membranes, *AIChE Journal, 34*: 1709.

88. Scamehorn, J. F., and Harwell, J. H. (1988). Surfactant-based treatment of aqueous process streams, *Surfactants in Chemical/Process Engineering* (D. Wasan, M. Ginn, and D. Shah, eds.), Marcel Dekker, New York, p. 77.

89. Hatton, T. A. (1989). Reversed micellar extraction of proteins, *Surfactant-Based Separation Processes* (J. F. Scamehorn and J. H. Harwell, eds.), Marcel Dekker, New York, p. 55.

90. Dekker, M., Riet, K. V., Weyers, S. R. Buthissen, J. W. A., Laane, C., and Bysterbasch, B. H. (1986). Enzyme recovery by liquid-liquid extraction using reversed micelles, *Chem. Eng. J. 33*: B27.

91. Dekker, M., Riet, K. V., Bysterbasch, B. H., Wolbert, R. I. G., and Hilhurst, R. (1989). Modeling and optimization of the reversed micellar extraction of alpha-amylase, *AIChE J., 35*:2.

92. Giovenco, S., Verheggen, F., and Laane, C. (1987). Purification of intracellular enzymes from whole bacterial cells using reversed micelles, *J. Microb. Tech.*, Aug.: 470.

93. Woll, J. M. Dillon, A. S., Rahaman, R. S., and Hatton, T. A. (1987). Protein separation using reversed micelles, *Protein Purification Micro to Macro, Proceedings of a Cetus-UCLA Symposium*, (R. Burgess, ed.), Alan Liss, p. 117.

94. Rahaman, R. S., Chee, J. Y., Cabral, J. M. S., and Hatton, T. A. (1988). Recovery of an extracellular alkaline protease from whole fermentation broth using reversed micelles, *Biotechnology Progress, 4*: 218.

95. Goklen, K. E. (1986). Liquid-liquid extraction of biopolymers: Selective solubilization of proteins in reverse micelles, Ph.D. thesis, M.I.T.

96. Hilhorst, R., Laane, C., and Veeger, C. (1984). Reversed micelles as a medium for enzyme-catalyzed synthesis of apolar compounds, *Innovations in Biotechnology* (E. H. Houwink and R. R. van der Meer, eds.), Elsevier, Amsterdam, p. 81.

97. Rao, A. M., Nguyen, H., and John, V. T. (1990). Modification of enzyme activity in reversed micelles through clathrate hydrate formation, *Biotech. Prog., 6*: 465.

98. Phillips, J. B., Nguyen, H., and John, V. T. (1991). Protein recovery from reversed micellar solutions through contact with a pressurized gas phase, *Biotech. Prog., 7*: 43.

6

Differential Precipitation of Proteins

Science and Technology

Fred Rothstein

Bio-Separations Consultants, Long Beach, California

I. INTRODUCTION

The following classification of protein separations methodologies was proposed by the author in 1976 (1):

1. Methods based on differential solubility
2. Methods based on differential interactions with solid media
3. Methods based on differential interactions with physical fields

Methods based on differential solubility can obviously be subdivided into two categories: (1) differential solubility between two immiscible liquid phases and (2) differential solubility between a liquid phase and a solid phase. It is the latter category involving the separation of one protein, or family of proteins, from other proteins by means of *reversible* differential precipitation with *chemical reagents* that is the subject of this chapter. The discussion will not address *irreversible* differential chemical precipitation (e.g., differential acid denaturation) and Class C methods, which include the low temperature, *reversible* insolubilization of a group of proteins (the cryoglobulins), as well as differential, *irreversible* precipitation caused by a physical field, e.g., differential thermal denaturation. This chapter is meant to complement and supplement the major review of protein precipitation published by Dunnill and colleagues (2). A qualitative description of the essential aspects of the science and technology of differential protein precipitation will be presented.

II. GENERAL PRINCIPLES OF SOLUBILITY

In simplistic terms, the solubility of a given solute in a given solvent is determined by the net result of solvent-solvent, solute-solute, and solute-solvent interactions (3–5). These interactions can be attractive or repulsive. A solute will be soluble in a given solvent if the free energy change due to solute-solvent interactions is sufficiently negative (attractive) that it more than counterbalances any free energy decrease occurring as a result of either or both of the other interactions. Solubility will be additionally favored when the free energy of solute-solute interactions is positive (repulsive). The strength of solute-solute interactions is modulated by the chemical nature of the solvent. On the other hand, insolubility results if the free energy decrease due to solvent-solvent and/or solute-solute interactions is greater than the free energy decrease due to solute-solvent interactions. The solute will also be insoluble if the free energy change due to its interactions with the solvent is positive and the free energy changes associated with solvent-solvent and/or solute-solute interactions are negative. Thus *a soluble molecule can be insolubilized by any perturbation that will result in a decrease in its attractive interactions with the solvent, an increase in its attractive interactions with other solute molecules, and/or an increase in attractive solvent-solvent interactions; the overall result being a net decrease in the free energy of the system.* Reference to the free energy of the interactions highlights the potentially critical role of entropic effects in solubility phenomena.

From a kinetic point of view, an essential parameter of insolubilization is the translation energy of the solute molecules responsible for their Brownian motion. In order for two molecules to adhere, the total energy of attraction between them must be greater than $1.5\ kT$, the energy of Brownian motion. As additional molecules adhere, the complex grows in size, and its mean displacement due to Brownian "bombardment," which is inversely proportional to the square root of the radius of the aggregate, becomes increasingly smaller. Ultimately a solid phase appears in the form of an amorphous precipitate or a crystal.

A. Forces of Intermolecular Interaction

The forces to be considered are noncovalent. In contrast to covalent forces, which are characterized by electron pairing and the loss of the discrete nature of the bonded atoms, noncovalent forces of interaction are not concerned with electron pairing, and the interacting entities maintain their identity (6–9). Kollman has defined noncovalent interactions "as those in which: (1) electrons stay paired in reactants and products and (2) there is no change in the type of chemical bonding in reactants and products" (10).

The basis of all interatomic and intermolecular interactions is the electromagnetic force as described by quantum mechanics. For our purposes, most of the noncovalent interactions can be approached from a classical point of view. The interacting moieties can have a fixed charge, can have a permanent dipole due to separation of charge within the molecule,* or can be totally neutral. Thus the noncovalent interaction energies between these types of entities can be grouped, in classical terms, as follows: electrostatic, polarization (induction), and dispersion. In addition there are interactions derived from quantum mechanics: exchange repulsion and charge transfer.

1. Electrostatic Interactions

Electrostatic interactions include those between (1) two ions, (2) an ion and a fixed dipole, (3) an ion and a rotating dipole, (4) two fixed dipoles, and (5) two rotating dipoles. (Multipolar interactions will not be discussed. See Ref. 11.) The Helmholtz free energy expressions for each of these are as follows (6):

1. Ion–ion

$$A = \frac{Q_1 Q_2}{4\pi D_0 D r}$$

2. Ion–fixed dipole

$$A = \frac{-Qu \cos\theta}{4\pi D_0 D r^2}$$

3. Ion–rotating dipole

$$A = \frac{-Q^2 u^2}{6(4\pi D_0 D)^2 k T r^4}$$

4. Two fixed dipoles

$$A = \frac{-u_1 u_2 f(\theta_1, \theta_2, \phi)}{4\pi D_0 D r^3}$$

5. Two rotating dipoles

$$A = \frac{-u_1^2 u_2^2}{3(4\pi D_0 D)^2 k T r^6}$$

This interaction is referred to as the *Keesom orientation* interaction. Q is the charge on the ion, D_0 is the permittivity of free space, D is the dielectric constant of the medium, u is the dipole moment, θ_1, θ_2, and ϕ are the appropriate angles between interacting dipoles, k is Boltzmann's constant, T is the Kelvin temperature, and r is the distance, in meters, between ions, between an ion and the center of a dipole, or between the centers of two interacting dipoles.

It is to be noted that the free energy of these interactions is in all cases inversely proportional to the dielectric constant of the medium *between and surrounding* the interacting charges and dipoles. This is the basis for the dif-

---

*Covalent bonds can have partial ionic character due to a difference in the electronegativity of the two bonded atoms. This is manifested by a measurable bond dipole moment. Electrons will be attracted more to one of the atoms, resulting in a fractional negative charge on the more electronegative atom and an equal positive charge on the other atom. The bond dipole moment is obviously smaller than that of a molecule, but it is of great significance in intermolecular interactions.

ference in solubility of charged and polar molecules* in diverse solvents. As described by the Born equation (12) at a given temperature, the log of the relative solubilities of a salt or charged polar molecule in different solvents is an inverse function of the difference between the dielectric constants of the solvents. The potent solubilizing power of water for ionic and polar molecules is partially based on its high dielectric constant and the resulting large reduction in the free energy of interaction between ions and between polar solutes. The existence of free ions in aqueous solution is also a reflection of the high dielectric constant of water.

An additional factor contributing to the water solubility of an ionic or polar molecule is its specific interaction with the solvent water. The strong interaction between an ion or a dipole with the dipole of water at small values of r leads to a restriction of molecular motion and the creation of a structured layer of oriented water molecules surrounding the ion: the primary *hydration shell* of the ion. The electric field of the ion influences the water dipoles beyond the first hydration layer in an exponentially decreasing manner. As one progresses from the surface of the ion, the freedom of motion of the water molecules increases until it is identical to that of bulk water. This region of modified properties of water (density, restricted translation and rotational motion, structure, etc.) is referred to as the *hydration zone*, and the phenomenon is referred to as *hydrophilic solvation*. These remarks also pertain to the interaction of water dipoles with the charged groups and bond dipoles on a molecule. The existence of hydrophilic solvation and the presence of hydration zones around protein molecules play a critical role in their solubility behavior.

An example of the effect of the solvent on ion-ion and ion-dipole interactions is the nature of the solvent composition. The latter can determine the existence or absence of a charge on a molecule as well as the interactions between charged and dipolar entities; e.g., the pH of the solvent will regulate the state of dissociation of an acidic or basic group of a molecule, and the ionic composition of the solvent will greatly influence the strength of ion-ion, ion-dipole, and dipole-dipole interactions in accordance with electrolyte solution theory. These solvent effects are of prime importance when considering the solution behavior of proteins and other zwitterions. There are molecules that have a finite net charge in addition to a dipolar structure, e.g., charged amino acids such as glutamic acid or lysine.

---

*Polar molecules are defined as those having a permanent dipole resulting from an asymmetric distribution of electrons within the structure of the molecule. In addition, there are dipolar ions (zwitterions), molecules that have charged groups of opposite sign located at different positions on the molecule. The existence of dipolar ions is a function of the solvent environment of the molecule. There are zwitterions that, due to an unequal number of oppositely charged sites, can have a net charge in addition to a dipole; e.g., glutamic acid, a nonisoelectric protein, etc.

Analysis of the interactions of such a molecule with another charged dipolar molecule will involve consideration of a composite of ion–ion, ion–dipole, and dipole–dipole interactions.

2. Electrodynamic Polarization Interactions

Electrodynamic polarization interactions occur as a result of the induced redistribution of the electrons of a molecule due to the influence of an electric field originating from a fixed charge or permanent dipole on a neighboring molecule. The resulting molecule is said to have an induced dipole. The magnitude of the induced dipole in a given electric field is a function of the ease of electron displacement, i.e., the electronic polarizability α of the molecule. It is of interest to recall that the polarizability of an atom is inversely related to its electronegativity. Thus O and N are less polarizable than C and H. There are three types of polarization interactions: (1) ion–induced dipole, (2) fixed dipole–induced dipole, and (3) rotating dipole–induced dipole. For the purposes of this discussion we shall consider dipole induction in apolar molecules. The Helmholtz free energy expressions for these interactions are as follows (6):

1. Ion–induced dipole
$$A = \frac{Q^2\alpha}{2(4\pi D_0 D)^2 r^4}$$

2. Fixed dipole–induced dipole
$$A = \frac{-u^2\alpha(1 + 3\cos^2\theta)}{2(4\pi D_0 D)^2 r^6}$$

3. Rotating dipole–induced dipole
$$A = \frac{-u^2\alpha}{(4\pi D_0 D)^2 r^6}$$

Dipole–induced dipole interactions are referred to as *Debye induction interactions*.

3. Electrodynamic Dispersion Interactions

Electrodynamic dispersion interactions derive from an ever-present electrodynamic force that acts between all atoms and molecules. Dispersion interactions are considered to be most important noncovalent interactions. They are quantum mechanical in origin, but they can be pictured as arising as follows: The time average of the fluctuations in electron distributions about the nucleus of an atom is zero. At any instant, these fluctuations yield an asymmetric electron distribution that manifests itself in an "instantaneous" finite dipole moment. The electric field of this "instantaneous" dipole polarizes the electrons of a neighboring neutral molecule and induces a dipole in it. The resulting "instantaneous" interaction between the two dipoles is attractive, and the time average of this attractive interaction is nonzero. The dispersion interaction was first described by F. London, who proposed the following expression for the free energy of the dispersion interaction between two atoms or two apolar molecules in free space:

$$A = \frac{-3\alpha_1\alpha_2 I_1 I_2}{2(4\pi D_0)^2 (I_1 + I_2)r^6}$$

where I is the first ionization potential of the respective atom or molecule. The strength of the London dispersion interaction is a function of the polarizabilities of the interacting moieties. Thus apolar atoms like aliphatic C and H have stronger dispersion interactions than polar atoms such as O and N. More complicated expressions are available for the London dispersion interaction between similar and dissimilar molecules in a given medium (6). Suffice it to say that the strength of the dispersion interactions between two molecules are significantly reduced in a solvent medium.

It should be noted that the London dispersion, the Keesom orientation, and the Debye polarization interactions are all inversely related to the sixth power of the distance between interacting entities. Collectively these three types of interactions constitute the total *van der Waals* interactions between two atoms or molecules. Whereas Keesom and Debye interactions are absent between apolar molecules, London interactions are always present and, except for highly polar molecules, they dominate the total van der Waals interaction. For apolar compounds the dispersion interactions are much stronger at nearest neighbor distances of 0.2 to 0.3 nm, and the dispersion energy falls off rapidly with distance. The r^{-6} dependence renders the London dispersion interactions very sensitive to the mutual positions and extent of close contact of the atoms in the interacting molecules. Thus complementarity of shape and mutual orientation of the interacting molecules will determine the total energy of the dispersion interaction. As molecules increase in size through macromolecules to colloidal particles, the quasi additivity of the dispersion interactions renders them considerably more important. In addition, as the size of the interacting moieties increases, the dispersion interaction takes on a long-range character.

Fowkes (13) has pointed out that intermolecular forces were initially studied in dense gases where dispersion forces, dipole-dipole interactions, and dipole–induced dipole interactions explain most of the intermolecular interactions between pairs of molecules. There has been a tendency to apply the conclusions of these gas studies to liquids and solids without the realization that the extrapolation of these equations from the two body inter-actions in gases to the multibody interactions in condensed phases might not be warranted. This is especially true for Keesom and Debye interactions. In condensed phases, equally sized uncharged molecules having dipolar character have ten or more nearest neighbors that produce opposing local dipole fields that minimize the net energy of the dipole interactions. Fowkes states that, based on available data, dipole-dipole interactions are of negligible importance in most liquids of uncharged dipolar molecules. According to Fowkes, the interactions in such systems are explained in terms of the Lewis concept of acids as electron acceptors and of bases as electron donors and the interaction of such acids and bases. Based on available data, he concludes that dipole-dipole interactions in most liquids are negligibly small compared with acid-base interactions or dispersion interactions. Studies of London dispersion interactions indicate that the extension of the relations for such interactions from gases to all types of condensed phases is valid. For molecules of low polarizabilities (high electronegativity) that possess high dipole moments, e.g., H_2O, the dipole-dependent Keesom and Debye interactions will lead to self-association of the molecules and the formation of a two- or three-dimensional structure. Such liquids are good solvents for ionic solutes. In such systems, the nearest neighbor solvent molecules will orient their dipoles toward the ionic solute, resulting in very strong ion-dipole interactions and solvation.

4. Charge Transfer Interactions

Charge transfer interactions are quantum mechanical interactions derived from the delocalization of electrons from occupied orbitals of one molecule into the unoccupied orbitals of another molecule. In classical chemistry they were referred to as coordinate bonds. The strength of such interactions, which depends on the degree of overlap of these orbitals, is roughly an exponential function of the interatomic distance. Lewis acid-base interactions may be considered to fall into this category.

5. Repulsive Interactions

It is obvious that electrostatic interactions can have a repulsive component determined by the interaction of charges of like sign. In fact, it is known that under certain circumstances the London dispersion interactions can be repulsive. Our present reference is to exchange repulsion that arises from the application of the Pauli exclusion principle to the interaction between the electron clouds of the subject molecules. Exchange repulsion interactions are of very short range and increase very sharply as two molecules approach one another. The energy of the repulsive interaction has been empirically represented as a function of the inverse 9th power or 12th power of the interatomic distances, i.e., the latter being the repulsive term in the *Leonard-Jones potential* expression for the total intermolecular pair potential. The interactions reviewed above are individually or in combination viewed as being responsible for the noncovalent interactions between atoms and molecules. In specific circumstances they give rise to what may be referred to as "derived interactions."

B. Derived Interactions

I employ the term derived interactions to refer to certain multiatomic or multimolecular interactions that have specific characteristics but result from the fundamental interactive forces described above. To this classification belong (1) the hydrogen "bond," (2) "solvation interactions," and (3) the hydrophobic interaction.

1. The Hydrogen Bond

Much has been written about the "derived" hydrogen bond interaction (14,15). The hydrogen bond is a three-atom entity in which a hydrogen atom, apparently covalently bound to an electronegative atom, interacts with another electronegative atom and confers upon the association properties similar in certain respects to those found in entities conventionally called bonds. The hydrogen bond is not a bond in the classical sense because it is a three-atom rather than a two-atom interaction. It would appear to be more appropriately named the hydrogen bridge. Because of established usage we shall employ the term hydrogen bond.

The classical explanation for the hydrogen bond is as follows: The covalent bond between a hydrogen atom and atom X, of greater electronegativity, has partial ionic character with an associated bond dipole moment. The value of the dipole moment of the bond is determined by the electronegativity difference between X and hydrogen. The bond dipole will have its positive pole at the hydrogen nucleus and the negative pole on the electronegative partner X. A hydrogen bond is said to form when this X^--H^+ dipole approaches another electronegative atom Y involved in another bond dipole and a *dipole-dipole interaction* ensues; $X^--H^+...Y^--A^+$. In addition, there is a charge transfer interaction between the lone pair electron orbital of Y and the partially or totally unoccupied orbital of the proton. The contribution of this interaction to the strength of the hydrogen bond is subject to debate, but it appears to be a function of the electronegativity of the hydrogen "donor" X.

Fowkes (16) has pointed out that the data assembled by Pimentel and McClellan (17) do not support the idea that the hydrogen bond results from a dipole-dipole interaction. The bond strengths of the hydrogen bonds reported in the literature are independent of the dipole moments of the resulting bridged entities. He emphasizes the point that hydrogen bonds are a subset of Lewis acid-base interactions in which Y is the electron donor (Lewis base) and the proton is the electron acceptor (Lewis acid). The Lewis acid-base character of the hydrogen bond can be depicted as that of a proton shared by two electron pairs.

The normal hydrogen bond can have an enthalpy value of between 3 and 6 kcal/mol, approximately 1/20th that of a typical covalent bond. The strength of the hydrogen bond increases with an increase in the electronegativity of the two bridged atoms. The bond has maximum stability when the three atoms are collinear. As a result of the small size of the proton as well as minimization of exchange repulsion by the displacement of the shared electrons toward the electronegative atom X, the hydrogen "donor" X and the hydrogen "acceptor" Y can come closer to each other than the sum of the van der Waals radii of the three atoms would otherwise allow. In almost all hydrogen bonds, the proton is closer to the "hydrogen" donor, the atom to which it would be covalently bound if no hydrogen bond were formed. Hydrogen bonds can be either inter- or intramolecular.

Normal hydrogen bonds are "two centered" with one donor and one acceptor atom. Recent studies reveal the frequent occurrence of three centered, bifurcated hydrogen bonds characterized by having one donor atom linked to two acceptor atoms. All four atoms of the complex are essentially coplanar (18).

a. Hydrogen Bonding and the Structure of Water. A single water molecule can form hydrogen bonds to four other water molecules, two with its own hydrogen atoms and two with the two lone pair orbitals interacting with the hydrogen atoms of two neighboring water molecules. In addition, water molecules have a substantial dipole moment that allows for dipole-dipole interactions between them. All the anomalous properties of water can be rationalized on the basis of hydrogen bonding and dipole-dipole interactions. There is a voluminous literature on the subject of water, its structure, physical-chemical properties, and its interactions with other molecular entities (19–22). Suffice it to say that water is a highly structured, associated liquid because of the tetrahedral structure of the water molecule and the very strong Lewis acid-base hydrogen bond interactions. There is a temperature-dependent equilibrium between an open regular tetrahedral hydrogen bonded structure in which each water molecule has four other water molecules as nearest neighbors, as found in ice, and a more compact, less ordered array in which the hydrogen bonded tetrahedral structure is no longer prominent and there is an increase in the number and close packing of nearest neighbor interacting molecules. This accounts for the relatively low viscosity for such a highly associated liquid.

2. Solvation Interactions

As previously mentioned, interaction of solute molecules with solvent molecules can introduce structural order in those solvent molecules surrounding the solute (23). When water is the solvent, the phenomenon is called hydration. The characteristics of the solvation zone, such as depth and rigidity, are determined by the strength of the solvent-solute and solvent-solvent interactions. When two solvated macromolecules approach each other, the solvation zones appear to interact in an oscillatory manner as a function of intermolecular distance; at small distances the interaction varies between attraction and repulsion. This short range oscillatory solvation force originates from the layered structure of the solvation zone and the molecular dimensions of the solvent. In water the solvation (hydration) forces differ from those in other liquids because of the enhanced ability of water molecules to self-interact. A *monotonic repulsion* between approaching hydrated hydrophilic entities is superimposed upon a modulated oscillatory behavior.   *The hydration layers act as mechanical barriers giving rise to a repulsive force that prevents the close approach of solute molecules or suspended particles,* keeping the hydrated entities separated and in solution or suspension.   In contrast, the hydration force between hydrated hydrophobic entities (hydrophobic hydration) is *monotonically attractive.*   This is a manifestation of the hydrophobic effect to be discussed below.   A detailed understanding of these solvation forces is presently not at hand.   However, they must basically arise from the net result of the interactions of solute molecules with surrounding solvent molecules, as well the interactions between solvent molecules.

3.   Hydrophobic Interactions

It is well known that apolar molecules and groups are poorly soluble in water and that water is poorly soluble in apolar solvents (24–26).   Thermodynamic analysis of such a process reveals that the increase in the Gibbs free energy of the system is due to a very large entropic decrease that more than compensates for the accompanying small decrease in enthalpy.   In some instances, e.g., benzene in water, the enthalpy change is very small and the positive free energy change is a consequence solely of the decrease in entropy.   Associated with the process is an increase in the heat capacity and a decrease in the volume of the system.   The small, negative enthalpic change indicates a slight increase in the interaction energetics in the system. This may be due to a combination of increased water-water interactions as well as water-apolar interactions.   Attractive dispersion interactions between apolar and water molecules are comparable in magnitude to those between apolar molecules with each other.   Spectroscopic data suggest that the introduction of an apolar entity into water produces an increase in the number and/or strength of the existing hydrogen bonds.   The latter events will evolve energy causing the negative enthalpy change.   The relatively large entropy decrease implies a decrease in the degrees of freedom and an increase in the order of the system.   One can depict the insertion of the apolar entity into water as restricting the motion of neighboring water molecules and impeding the bending of the hydrogen bonds between the nearby water molecules, thus stiffening the overall structure and causing the observed decrease in entropy (27).   This ordering of water molecules about an apolar entity is called *hydrophobic hydration.*   The entropy decrease accompanying the introduction of an apolar molecule into water is proportional to the surface area of the apolar molecule.   Thus the larger the surface of an apolar moiety the greater the decrease in entropy, the greater the increase in free energy, and the lower its solubility in water.   This phenomenon is referred to as the hydrophobic effect.[*]

---

[*]For recent critical discussions of the hydrophobic effect see P. L. Privalov and S. J. Gill (1989), The hydrophobic effect: A reappraisal, *Pure Appl. Chem., 61*: 1097 and N. Muller (1990), Search for a realistic view of hydrophobic effects, *Acc. Chem. Res., 23*: 23.

A direct consequence of the hydrophobic effect is the *hydrophobic interaction* or hydrophobic bond, which describes the tendency of apolar groups to withdraw from contact with water, cluster together, and in so doing remove the restrictions on H-bond bending and increase the freedom of motion of the water molecules. This results in a *net increase* of the unitary entropy* of the system. Hydrophobic bond formation may be pictured as the reverse of that for introducing apolar groups into water. The apolar entities tend to self-associate so as to reduce the extent of apolar surface accessible to water. If apolar molecules and groups did not self-associate in water, then their random distribution would be accompanied by a very large entropy decrease. When aggregation occurs, the total area of apolar surface in contact with water will decrease and, as a consequence, the hydrophobic "structuration" effect and the associated entropy decrease will be minimized. Accordingly, the aggregation of apolar moieties in water is an *entropically driven* process. This drive to self-association is responsible for the low solubility of hydrocarbons in water. It should be stressed that there is no special or unique bond associated with this essentially entropic phenomenon, and the term "hydrophobic bond" is uncalled for. As mentioned above, the interaction of apolar entities with water is not repulsive but attractive due to dispersion interactions. However, the attractive interactions between water molecules are much stronger, leading to a "passive" exclusion but not an active repulsion of apolar elements. As stated by Israelachvili (6), "Water simply loves itself too much to let other substances get in its way." One can generalize this argument to other solute-solvent systems and refer to *solvophobic interactions* characterized by an enhanced association of solute molecules in the solvent when the attractive solvent-solvent interactions are stronger than the solvent-solute interactions.

C. The Cavity Model for Solubility

Sinanoglu proposed a model to explain the effect of solvent on the solubility of a solute (28). The approach taken was to define the solvent effect in terms of the difference in the free energy of a molecule in the gas phase as compared to its free energy in a given solvent. He partitioned the process into two hypothetical steps: The first step involves the creation of a cavity in the solvent big enough to accept the solute. In the second step the solute is placed into the cavity and allowed to interact with its surroundings. The net change in free energy is determined by the work expended in creating the cavity in the solvent, ΔG_{cav}, the free energy of the interaction of the solute molecule with the solvent molecules in the wall of the cavity, ΔG_{int}, and an entropic term related to the loss of solute "free volume" in going from the gas into the solvent.

---

*The unitary entropy change of a process is equal to the total entropy change minus the ideal entropy of mixing.

The free energy of cavity formation is a function of the strength of solvent-solvent interactions, which is reflected in the value of the solvent surface tension. The greater the interactions between solvent molecules the larger the value of its surface tension and the greater the amount of work necessary to separate the solvent molecules and create a cavity. For highly associated liquids that have high surface tensions, the free energy of cavity formation will be quite high. Additionally, the larger the excluded volume of the solute molecule, the more work has to be done to form the cavity. Thus ΔG_{cav} is a function of the surface tension of the solvent and the molecular size and shape of the solute. Referring to the previous discussion of the hydrophobic effect, it becomes evident that the free energy of cavity formation in water is a reflection of the magnitude of the hydrophobic effect.

The free energy of interaction between the solute molecule and the surrounding solvent molecules will depend on the relative chemical character (apolar, polar, and ionic) of the solute and the solvent. The interaction will potentially involve all types of noncovalent interactions commensurate with the chemical natures of the solute and solvent.* Accordingly, ΔG_{int} will consist of London dispersion and electrostatic attractive and repulsive components. The electrostatic contribution can be approximated for ions from the Debye-Huckel theory (12) or for large dipoles in solution from the relations derived by Kirkwood (29) and Linderstrom-Lang (30).

The solvent effect is measured by the unitary free energy of solution ΔG^0 of a solute molecule going from a hypothetical gas phase into a solvent and is given by

$$\Delta G^0 = \Delta G_{cav} + \Delta G_{London} + \Delta G_{es} + f$$

f being the solute free volume change.

This model describes the solvent effect in terms of the following parameters: (1) the surface tension of the solvent, (2) the excluded volume of the solute and the associated surface area, (3) the relative chemical character of the solute and solvent, and (4) the effect of the presence of cosolutes and/or cosolvents. The latter two parameters determine the degree of solvation of a solute, which is a partial reflection of the solvent effect. (For a recent review of the solvent effect, see Ref. 31.) It is important to recognize that *any perturbation that will reduce the solvent effect and the degree of solvation will reduce the solubility of a solute.*

D. Surface Thermodynamic Theory of Solubility

Van Oss, Good, and colleagues treat the problem of macromolecular solubility employing the concepts of colloidal science (32,33). They posit "that

---

*It is an empirical rule that "like attracts like," i.e., an apolar solute will interact with another apolar molecule in preference to a polar or charged molecule, and polar molecules will interact more favorably with polar molecules, etc.

there is no essential difference between the molecular solution of a polymer molecule (e.g., a protein) and the stable monodisperse colloidal suspension of a small particle (e.g., a virus or a polystyrene latex particle) in an appropriate liquid. It is impossible to distinguish between the two phenomena by any physical or physicochemical method at our disposal" (34). They have extended the DLVO (Deryagin-Landau and Verwey-Overbeek) theory of hydrophobic colloidal stability (35,36) to hydrophilic systems using the methods of analytical surface thermodynamics. They base their approach on the close association of solubility and surface tension, as recorded by such workers as Hildebrand and Scott (3). Employing an extension of the Dupre equation, van Oss et al. relate the free energy of solute-solute interaction in the presence of a given solvent to the *interfacial tension* between a pure solute phase and a pure solvent phase. Their analysis relates the surface properties of condensed systems to the forces of interaction discussed above: the van der Waals electrodynamic interactions (London, Keesom, and Debye interactions), Lewis acid-base interactions (which include hydrogen bonds), and electrostatic interactions. The latter two interactions predominate in systems consisting of polar solutes and solvents (especially water.)*

III. SOLUBILITY OF PROTEINS

A. Overview of Globular Protein Structure

Globular proteins are natural high-molecular-weight heteropolymers of seemingly random sequences of some twenty amino acids linked together by the peptide bond to form a polypeptide chain. For a given protein, the length of its polypeptide chain, its amino acid composition and sequence, as well as the number of chains are genetically determined (34,37,38). A common feature of polypeptides is the coplanarity of the six atoms associated with the peptide bond. Diversity is introduced by the residues attached to the alpha-carbon of each monomeric amino acid unit. These twenty residues are commonly classified on the basis of the presence of charged polar, and/or apolar groups. Thus there are six apolar aliphatic residues (gly, ala, val, leu, ile, met), four apolar heterocyclic and aromatic residues (pro, phe, trp, tyr), five polar aliphatic residues (ser, thr, cys, asn, gln), and five ionizable residues (asp, glu, his, lys, arg). The compact conformation of a globular

---

*It should be noted that the DLVO theory was developed for hydrophobic two-phase systems consisting of particles, having charges of the same sign uniformly distributed over their surface, dispersed in an aqueous solvent. The stability of such systems is determined by the relative values of attractive van der Waals interactions and repulsive electrostatic (double layer) interactions. Hydrophobic systems are extremely sensitive to salt addition, which readily destabilizes a system, causing the coagulation and flocculation of the suspension particles. Hydrophilic systems, which are considered true solutions of polar or ionic macromolecules, are comparatively insensitive toward salt. They do not flocculate in the same sense that a hydrophobic system flocculates, but high salt concentrations will cause precipitation of the macromolecule.

protein is the result of the multiple turn folding of the polypeptide chain back on itself. Parts of the chain can assume such secondary structures as the alpha helix, the beta sheet, and beta turns, the major stabilizing forces being hydrogen bonding, van der Waals interactions, and solvophobic interactions (39–43). Kauzmann (44) enunciated a basic principle of protein structure, which claims that in an aqueous environment the folding of the polypeptide chain is entropically ("hydrophobically") driven, so that apolar residues will tend to be found in the interior of the molecule while charged and polar residues tend to be on the outside. Thus in an aqueous environment, the protein chain will assume the conformation, commensurate with its amino acid sequence, that best satisfies the requirements of minimization of the contact of hydrophobic residues with the aqueous solvent (formation of hydrophobic clusters and their internalization to form the "hydrophobic core"), maximization of intramolecular interactions (hydrogen bonds, nearest neighbor van der Waals interactions, ion pair formation, etc.), and maximization of interactions between charged and polar residues with the solvent ("polar shell" formation). Not only are hydrophobic clusters internalized but a significant number of polar entities, especially the polar components of the backbone, are also found in the interior of the globule. There they make up a skeletal network of hydrogen bonds that confers a degree of rigidity to the folded state. The compact structure resulting from the operation of these forces is characterized by the presence (or absence) of chain segments of varying lengths in helical, beta-sheet, or "random" coil configurations as well as a number of beta-turns. The native configuration of a protein is a result of the balance of enthalpic and entropic forces of interaction between the amino acid side chain residues, the peptide units of the backbone, and solvent molecules, such that a state of minimum Gibbs free energy is achieved. The net free energy favoring the native structure is of the order of only 10 to 20 kcal/mol. This small stabilization free energy is the basis for the marginal stability of the native structure and its susceptibility to denaturation by relatively small environmental perturbations (45).

Lee and Richards (46,47) were the first to attempt a quantitative analysis of the distribution of apolar, polar, and charged moieties between the surface and the interior of the protein globule. Introducing the concept of solvent accessible surface area and applying it to the x-ray data from three proteins, they reported the seemingly contradictory result that the solvent accessible areas of the three native structures were roughly evenly divided between polar and apolar *atoms*. (C and S atoms were taken as apolar and O and N atoms as polar.) They reported that in the folding of the polypeptide chain, the reduction in accessibility to the solvent was approximately the same (30–35%) for apolar and polar moieties. Charged atoms and charged groups were almost totally accessible to the solvent. Rashin and Honig (48) reported that slightly more than 95% of the ionizable groups of 36 globular proteins studied are solvent accessible. Recent work by Miller et al. (40) and Janin et al. (50) involving data obtained from 46 monomeric and 23 oligomeric proteins supports the conclusions of Lee and Richards as well as those of other workers (51,52). They report that the average solvent (water) accessible atomic surface is 57% apolar, 24% polar, and 19% charged while the average atomic surface area of the polypeptide chain buried with reduced accessibility to solvent is 58% apolar, 39% polar, and 4% charged. Note that the average percentage apolar composition of both accessible and the buried surfaces are essentially equivalent. The accessible surface is, on average, 57% apolar, varying from a low of 50% to a high of 68%; the frequency of occurrence of polar and charged groups on the accessible surface varies quite widely, e.g., 7% vs. 25% for the charged groups on the accessible surfaces of penicillopepsin and flavodoxin, respectively. Their analysis corroborates the accepted wisdom that the interior of a globular protein is predominantly composed of aliphatic and aromatic amino acids and the surface by charged amino acids. However, Miller et al. (49) point out that the atoms of few residues are totally inaccessible to the solvent; thus the larger proteins in the study have 85% of their amino acid residues, to some degree, in atomic contact with the solvent. Eisenberg and McLachlan (53) estimated the contribution of each solvent accessible protein *atom* to the solvation free energy contribution to protein stability. The author is unaware of any published analysis of the *surface distribution* of apolar, polar, and charged moieties. There are proposals that the surface of a protein consists of a patchwork of apolar, polar, and charged clusters, but a detailed analysis of the surface distribution of these groups is presently absent from the literature. Dielectric measurements indicate that the cationic and anionic groups are almost symmetrically distributed on the surface of many of the globular proteins studied (54,55).

B. Parameters of Protein Solubility

The solubility of a protein in a given solvent is determined by the effective volume it occupies and the balance between protein-protein and protein-solvent interactions. The presence of ionizable residues on the surface confers polyampholyte character on proteins and is a prime factor in the solubility of proteins in aqueous media. Solubility differences among proteins are a function of their relative size and shape and the relative concentration and distribution of charged, polar, and apolar residues on the solvent accessible surface. Thus we can identify solubility parameters as shown in Table 1.

1. Molecular Size and Shape of the Protein (Stokes Radius)
The effective volume occupied by a protein solute (excluded volume) is determined by its size and shape and described by its Stokes radius (56). Proteins with large Stokes radii (large excluded volumes) are generally less

Table 1 Parameters of Protein Solubility

1. Molecular size and shape of protein
   a. Stokes radius and excluded volume
2. Amino acid composition, sequence, and location (surface/interior)
   a. Conjugation and binding
3. Protein charge (solubility net charge)
   a. Total ionizable residues
   b. Accessibility to solvent—hydration
   c. Intrinsic dissociation constant (pK_a)
      pK_a is a function of
      1. Specific chemical composition
      2. Chemical nature of neighboring groups
      3. Temperature
      4. Chemical nature of solvent—dielectric constant
      5. Ionic strength
   d. pH of the solution
   e. Ion binding
4. Electrostatic parameters other than charge
   a. Solvent dielectric constant
   b. Dipole moment of protein
   c. Ionic strength (salting-in/salting-out)
5. Temperature

soluble than chemically similar proteins with smaller Stokes radii. This is explained by the "solvophobic" theory as resulting from the increased amount of work required to form a larger cavity in the solvent for proteins of greater excluded volume.

2. Amino Acid Composition, Sequence, and Protein Conformation

As stated above, the ratio of charged and polar to apolar residues, their distribution along the polypeptide chain (apolar and polar clusters) as well as their structural location relative to solvent accessibility will determine the solubility of the protein in a given solvent. In aqueous solutions, solute-solvent interactions will be favored by the location of charged and polar residues on the surface as well as in those areas available to the solvent. The presence of clusters of hydrophobic residues on the surface will favor protein-protein interactions and the formation of multiunit complexes. Thus in those proteins possessing quaternary structure the subunits appear to be held together by interactions between hydrophobic clusters on their surfaces. Further, the marked decrease in solubility of denatured globular proteins is a result of the exposure of hydrophobic residues that interact intermolecularly, counterbalancing the interactions of the charged and polar residues with the aqueous solvent.

Clear illustration of the importance of amino acid composition as a parameter of solubility is given by the prolamines and the histones. The prolamines, with a large predominance of apolar residues (especially proline), are insoluble in water and pure ethanol but are soluble in 70–80% ethanol. The histones, characterized by a predominance of the charged basic amino acids lysine and arginine, are soluble at and below neutrality, but are insoluble in basic solutions. It is pertinent to point out that proteins designed to exist in an apolar environment, such as membrane proteins, have a surface enriched in hydrophobic residues (57). Such proteins are soluble in apolar solvents and sparingly soluble, if at all, in aqueous environments.

a. Hydration. As discussed above, the binding of water by charged and polar groups (hydrophilic hydration) and the immobilization of water by apolar moieties (hydrophobic hydration) results in the formation of the hydration zone around the protein molecule. The problem of protein hydration was subjected to an extensive review by Kuntz and Kauzmann in 1974 (58) and to a more recent short review by Rupley et al. (59). The water bound to the protein is defined in terms of its properties that differ in value from those of bulk water. The published data show that on average 0.3 g water is bound per gram protein. In the case of lysozyme, the full hydration value is 0.38 g water per gram protein or 300 mole water per mole lysozyme. A small percentage (<10%) is tightly bound with severely restricted freedom of motion while the rest of the water molecules have properties that differ in minor ways from those of bulk water. The 0.38 g water per gram lysozyme means that the average surface area covered by a single water molecule is 20 $Å^2$ and suggest that the hydration layer is structured so as to have a minimum number of water molecules covering the maximum amount of surface. Further, the structure of the hydration layer is a subset of the structures found in bulk water and thus allows the nonperturbing melding of the protein into the bulk water structure.

In a recent paper, van Oss and Good (60) applied their "surface thermodynamic" approach to a study of the hydration of human serum albumin. They report the existence of two layers of bound water with differing structural properties. The water molecules in the primary layer are close to being totally oriented with regard to the protein surface; the hydrogen atoms are adjacent to and face the albumin surface while the oxygen atoms face away from the protein surface. In the second layer, only 30% of the water molecules are oriented.

Ben-Naim et al. (61) have reported an analysis of the energetic components of the hydration of proteins. Their results indicate that hydrogen bonds between surface groups and water molecules are the largest component of the free energy of hydration.

Mechanistically, the hydration layer(s) surrounding a protein can be viewed as promoting its solubility by serving as a physical barrier preventing the close approach of other hydrated protein molecules and their aggregation.

b. Conjugation and Binding. In addition to amino acids, other chemical entities can be part of the genetically programmed composition of a protein. They can vary from simple ions or molecules, such as iron in transferrin, copper in ceruloplasmin, etc., through more complex substances such as heme in the hemeproteins, cortisol in transcortin, etc., to very large entities such as the oligosaccharides in the glycoproteins and lipids in the lipoproteins. These moieties may be covalently linked (glycoproteins), ionically complexed (transferrin, ceruloplasmin), or hydrophobically (van der Waals) bound (lipoproteins) to the protein. The overall ionic-polar-apolar character of the protein molecule and its interactions with other protein molecules as well as with the solvent environment will be affected by the chemical nature of the entities bound; e.g., glycoproteins are very soluble in aqueous solution due to the strong hydration of the carbohydrate moieties covalently bound to asparagine, serine, or threonine residues on, or near, the protein surface.

The effect of changes in chemical composition due to binding on protein solubility can be observed with some of the transport proteins. For instance, the presence or absence of iron in transferrin has a significant effect on the solubility of this protein (62). Similarly, deoxy- and oxyhemoglobin differ in solubility, which may be a reflection of the change in structure accompanying oxygen binding.

An important technique in protein separations is the reversible differential binding of apolar or charged groups so as to achieve a differential change in the solubilities of the protein species in the mixture, e.g., the reversible ionic binding of the organic ion Rivanol contributes a large heterocyclic apolar group to the protein and reduces its interaction with the aqueous solvent (63).

3. Protein Charge

Charged molecules are substantially more soluble in water than their uncharged counterparts as a result of their greater interaction with dipolar water molecules. This enhanced solute-solvent attractive interaction is coupled to a repulsive interaction between solute molecules of like charge resulting in increased solubility.

The charged state of a simple protein is determined by (1) the total number of ionizable residues, (2) their accessibility to the solvent (ionization in the hydrophobic core is energetically prohibitive and disruptive), (3) the intrinsic dissociation constants of the different ionizable groups (pK_a values), and (4) the pH of the solution. The pK_a value of a dissociable group is a function of (1) its specific chemical makeup (carboxyl, amino, imidazole, phenolic, guanidyl groups), (2) the chemical nature of the neighboring groups (e.g., inductive effects), (3) the temperature, (4) the chemical nature of the solvent as partially reflected by its dielectric constant, and (5) the ionic strength of the solvent (12).

The charged state of a protein can be experimentally manipulated by varying the solvent properties, especially the pH. Since proteins are polyampholytes, their solution behavior is a function of the average net charge rather than the average total charge. Molecules possessing zero net charge will globally experience no net electrical repulsion and have a greater probability to aggregate and come out of solution than those species possessing a nonzero net charge of similar sign. This picture is amply supported by the pH solubility profiles of proteins reported in the literature. The characteristic profile is that of an asymmetric script U. The pH of minimum solubility is considered to be that pH where the protein has zero net charge, the isoelectric pH or isoelectric point. [Tanford (64) and Finlayson (65) have presented evidence to support the correspondence of the pH of minimum solubility with the isoelectric pH.]

As a consequence of the probabilistic nature of acid-base equilibria, there are protein molecules in solution at a given pH that have different values for their net and total charge, as well as charge distribution, and that differ from the respective mean values for all the protein molecules in the solution. Any individual molecule is constantly giving up and taking on protons so that its instantaneous net charge may be greater or less than the average net charge taken over all the molecules in solution. Furthermore, there are numerous molecules with a given net charge but having a differing distribution of total charge. All these forms of a given net charge are in dynamic equilibrium, not only with each other, but with other forms of greater or lesser net charge; at any moment in an isoelectric protein solution there are significant amounts of protein cations and anions present together with molecules of zero net charge. However, the average net charge of a given molecule, over an appreciable time interval in which many proton exchanges take place, is identical with the mean net charge (zero) of all the molecules in an isoelectric solution. A measure of the fraction of molecules whose *instantaneous* net charge differs from the *mean* net charge of all the molecules in solution is given by the difference between the *mean square value* $(\bar{Z}^2)$ and the *square of the mean value* $(\bar{Z})^2$ of the net charge. This difference is the standard deviation of the net charge and is a measure of the net charge distribution among the protein molecules in solution. In an isoelectric solution the *square of the mean value* $(\bar{Z})^2$ of the net charge is zero, but the *mean square value* $(\bar{Z}^2)$ of the net charge is nonzero. Edsall (66) has calculated that in an isoelectric solution of hemoglobin less than a quarter of the molecules are actually isoelectric at a given instant and that the root mean square value of the net charge is approximately 1.87. This means that a protein even at its isoelectric pH can behave as an ion carrying a net charge! The observed solubility of a protein in a defined solvent and given pH represents the sum total of the concentrations of the various forms (cationic, anionic, and neutral) of the protein that are all present in dynamic equilibrium in the solution.

As the concentration of a given salt (ionic strength) increases, the minimum solubility value increases (salting-in), the pH of minimum solubility decreases, and the shape of the curve becomes less flat near the minimum solubility (Fig. 1A). However, *these changes are not totally ionic strength dependent but are strong functions of the specific anion of the salts in the medium* (Fig. 1B). Leavis and Rothstein (67) as well as other workers (68) attribute these observations to differential anion binding although solvent mediated interactions of ions with the protein are to be considered.

The binding of ions will change the charged state and the solubility of a protein. The ion pair binding of a simple anion (such as Cl–, SCN–, etc.) to a positively charged site will reduce the total number of positive charges, increasing the net charge by –1, thereby reducing the isoelectric pH and the pH of minimum solubility. The extent of this reduction is determined by the number of anions bound, as well as the value of the binding constant. The

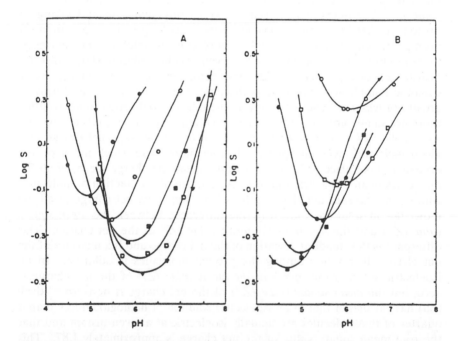

Figure 1   (A) Solubility of fibrinogen as a function of pH and concentrated NaCl, where ionic strength ($\Gamma/2$) takes the following values: 0.005 ($\blacktriangledown$), 0.01 ($\square$), 0.025 ($\blacksquare$), 0.05 (o), and 0.1 ($\bullet$). (B) Solubility of fibrinogen as a function of pH and five anions at $\Gamma/2 = 0.05$: o = F, $\bullet$ = Cl⁻, $\blacktriangledown$ = NO$_3^-$, $\square$= formate, and $\blacksquare$ = SO$_4^-$. (Adapted from Leavis and Rothstein, 1974.)

opposite behavior is observed for the binding of simple cations, i.e., higher isoelectric pH and higher pH of minimum solubility (69).

The changes in total and net charge accompanying the binding of metals depend upon the mode of binding. For instance, the ionic binding of Zn^{2+} to the nitrogen atom of imidazole increases both the total and the net positive charge by two without affecting the total number of negative charges. By contrast, the ion pair binding of Pb^{2+} to a carboxylate ion reduces the total negative charge by one and increases the total positive charge by one, but the net number of positive charges increases by two.

Charges can be added to a protein by the hydrophobic binding of organic ions such as fatty acids, anionic and cationic detergents, etc. However, the biding of such moieties is frequently accompanied by irreversible structural changes, with accompanying drastic changes in solubility.

4. Electrostatic Interaction Parameters Other Than Charge

a. Solvent Dielectric Constant. As discussed earlier, the free energy of charge interactions is inversely proportional to the first or second power of the dielectric constant of the medium in which the charges are located and through which they interact (70). In media with high dielectric constants, electrostatic interactions are minimized and the existence of charged entities is favored. As the dielectric constant of the medium decreases, the electrical free energy of the system increases and the existence of charged moieties is not favored. This results in an enhancement of electrical interactions so as to reduce the free energy of the system. For example, the pK of an uncharged acid (a carboxyl group) is increased and that of a charged acid (an amino group) is decreased upon lowering of the solution dielectric constant by addition of a miscible organic solvent (71,72). In both cases the uncharged species is favored in the lower dielectric milieu. Based on this, one could argue that the total charge on a protein will decrease and that the isoelectric point will change (increase or decrease, depending on the protein) upon lowering the dielectric constant of the solution at a fixed temperature. This reduction in overall charge on a protein would relax the hydration layer and reduce the mutual repulsion between molecules of the same species. These effects would allow for closer approach and increased attractive van der Waals electrodynamic interactions between the molecules of concern, resulting in their aggregation and insolubilization. This argument would appear to explain the precipitation of proteins by miscible organic solvents such as ethanol in terms of a reduction of the solution dielectric constant. However, as discussed below, the empirical data obtained by decreasing or increasing the *macroscopic, bulk* dielectric constant obviates its use in the analysis of electrostatic phenomena on the microscopic, molecular scale. Pertinent discussions of the concept of a dielectric on a molecular scale are given by Krishtalik (73), Rogers (74), Hopfinger (75), and Webb (9). Suffice it to say that *local* electrostatic and electrodynamic considerations involving solvent-cosolvent and specific solute-cosolvent interactions are basic to an understanding of protein stability and protein solubility in mixed solvents. One can increase the dielectric constant of a solution by addition of ionic entities, especially molecules with high dipole moments such as amino acids and peptides. According to elementary electrostatics, the solubility of proteins should be a direct function of the solution dielectric constant, which in turn is a direct function of the concentration of the added salt or dipole. However, in both cases, one observes a reduction in the solubility of the protein at sufficiently high concentrations of salt or dipolar molecules, i.e., salting-out. Specific local effects are responsible for deviations from predicted behavior; see Richards (76) and Wagner et al. (77).

One can decrease the solution dielectric constant by addition of miscible organic solvents to an aqueous solution. Exposure of proteins to such cosolvents at room temperature can result in the denaturation of the protein. However, as has been known since the work of Mellanby in 1907/1908 (78,79), irreversible denaturation can be prevented by operating at sufficiently low temperatures. Ferry et al. (80) kept egg albumin in 25% ethanol-water mixtures at -5°C for extended periods of time with no apparent denaturation. This was evidenced by the crystallization of the protein into its normal crystal lattice subsequent to the low-temperature removal of the ethanol. At +25°C, egg albumin is readily denatured in 25% ethanol-water mixtures, but it maintains its native state in water at this temperature. As reported by Wyman in 1931 (81), *the dielectric constant of a 25% ethanol-water mixture at -5°C is equal to that of water at +25°C: 78.7 vs. 78.5.* The irreversible denaturation of the egg albumin molecule in 25% ethanol at room temperature may well be a result of the lower dielectric constant value of 66.5, and the absence of denaturation at the lower temperature may be due to maintaining the "normal" dielectric constant of 78.5. Invoking bulk electrostatic effects arising from a lowering of the solution dielectric constant as a basis for the denaturation of a protein is questionable. There is strong evidence that nonbulk electrostatic factors are of far greater importance in the denaturing action of monohydric alcohols (82). These latter factors are directly related to the length of the alkyl chains of the alcohols and their effects on the hydrophobic interactions present in the system; denaturing efficiency follows the series, methanol < ethanol < propanol < butanol. Bull and Breese (83) relate the increased denaturing effectiveness of longer-chain monohydric alcohols to their being hydrophobically bound to the apolar amino acid residues of the protein and the consequent dehydration of the protein. Maurel (84) came to a similar conclusion in his study of the organic solvent effect observed with enzymes. In a calorimetric study, Velicebeli and Sturtevant (85) reported that the reduction in the denaturation temperature of lysozyme exposed to equal concentrations of methanol, ethanol and 1-propanol was correlated with the length of the alkyl chain of the alcohol. Similar results were obtained for ribonuclease and methanol by Fink (86). Arakawa and Goddette (87) presented a theoretical mechanism for the denaturation of proteins by monohydric alcohol-water mixtures. In agreement with previous workers, they concluded that the greater denaturing effect of alcohols with longer alkyl chains is a result of their enhanced hydrophobic binding to apolar groups and the consequent weakening of intraprotein hydrophobic interactions. As mentioned above, the denaturing effects of monohydric alcohols can be avoided by operating at sufficiently low temperatures. Studies by Brandts and Hunt (88) (ribonuclease/ethanol), Velicebeli and Sturtevant (85) (lysozyme/methanol, ethanol, and 1-propanol), and Fink (86) (ribonuclease/methanol) demonstrated that the free energies of alcohol denaturation of these two proteins become positive at low temperatures, i.e., the native state is stabilized by low temperature in the presence of moderate concentrations of the alcohols. However, high alcohol concentrations can cause denaturation even at low temperatures. The stabilization/denaturation temperature and alcohol concentration values are functions of the specific protein.

In the absence of ethanol, a globular protein, such as human plasma albumin or gamma globulin, is very soluble in water or dilute salt solution at its isoelectric point at 25°C. Upon controlled addition of ethanol to a concentration of 25% at -5°C, the protein precipitates in its native state. *The difference in the solubility of the protein in the two solutions cannot be attributed to a bulk dielectric constant effect since they are isodielectric* (81). An additional argument against the relationship between the solution dielectric constant and protein precipitation is based on the solubility of a protein in water and water-ethanol solutions on either side of its isoelectric point. The nonisoelectric protein molecules having a nonzero net charge will repel each other and be more soluble than at the isoelectric pH. On the basis of simple electrostatics, the mutual repulsion between similarly charged molecules and the solubility of the protein should be greater in solutions of lower dielectric constant than in water. Such is not the case; the entire pH solubility curve in ethanol-water solutions is displaced downward relative to that in water. No matter what the pH, proteins are less soluble in the presence of a miscible organic solvent than in its absence. Thus the teaching that the low-temperature precipitation of proteins by miscible organic solvents is caused by the lowering of the dielectric constant of the medium is untenable. Based on data obtained by the surface-thermodynamic approach, van Oss (89) has proposed that the precipitating action of ethanol is a result of its dehydration of the protein molecules by *competing* for the water of hydration. This allows for their close approach, enabling van der Waals interactions to cause molecular aggregation. A similar suggestion was made by Green and Hughes (90).

The salting-in of proteins by low concentrations of salt ions is enhanced in solutions of reduced dielectric constant. For instance, although the solubility of albumin decreases as the concentration of ethanol is increased, the salting-in effect increases with the ethanol concentration (70). The presence of small amounts of salt has the same solubilizing effect on water-soluble proteins in ethanol-water mixtures as does salt on the solubility of euglobulins in water at their isoelectric point. It is thought that the lowered dielectric constant of the solution enhances specific electrostatic interactions between salt ions and the charged groups of the protein molecule and thereby causes the salting-in effect to be much greater than in water alone. As discussed below, the Kirkwood theory of ion-dipole interactions appears to describe this phenomenon satisfactorily, although a mechanistic description is wanting. It should be noted that differential precipitation can be obtained by carefully balancing the solubilizing action of low concentrations of salt against the precipitating action of a miscible organic solvent at the isoelectric point of the protein of interest. This is the basis of the Cohn plasma fractionation procedure.

b. *Ionic Strength.* The global effect of ionic strength on protein solubility can be considered to be the net result of solubilizing (salting-in) and precipitating (salting-out) effects. Classically, proteins were classified on the basis of their solubility in media of differing electrolyte concentration. Those proteins insoluble in the absence of salt at their isoelectric points were named *euglobulins.* Their solubility increases upon addition of salt. They are precipitated by 33% saturated ammonium sulfate solutions. Those proteins moderately soluble in water and in moderate concentrations of aqueous salt solutions were named *pseudoglobulins* and are precipitated by 50% ammonium sulfate solutions. Proteins extremely soluble in water as well as high concentrations of salt were named *albumins.* Precipitation of albumins requires ammonium sulfate solutions whose degree of saturation is significantly greater than 50%. The difference in the solubility of globulins and albumins may be related to the marked difference in their dipole moments; globulins have a much higher dipole moment than albumins (54).

Salting-in. As a result of interactions between the ions of dissolved salts and charged groups on the protein molecule, euglobulins dissolve in the presence of small amounts of salt. This is referred to as the *salting-in effect* and was first described by Mellanby in 1905 in terms of what we now call ionic strength (91). (In order to observe the salting-in effect with solutions of pseudoglobulins and albumins, their solubilities must first be reduced, usually by addition of miscible organic solvents.)

In dilute solution, slightly soluble salts are made more soluble by the addition of another salt. The solubilizing effect of the added salt was first rationalized by the Debye-Huckel theory of dilute strong electrolyte solutions, which states that the solubility of a salt is (1) proportional to the square root of the ionic strength of the solution, (2) the product of the valences of the cation and anion of the salt, and (3) inversely related to the 3/2 power of the solution dielectric constant (28). Note that the relative solubilizing effect of the added electrolyte will be greater the lower the dielectric constant of the solution; although the solubility of a salt in a solvent of low dielectric constant is much less than in water, the increase in its solubility will be greater when other salts are added.

Kirkwood (29) has presented a theoretical treatment of the interactions between ions and dipoles that attempts to account for salting-in effects by considering the size, shape, and dipole moment of the solute, the solvent dielectric constant, the solution ionic strength, and the temperature. However, he did not consider specific solvent-solute, solvent-salt, solute-salt interactions, as well as the effect of ionic strength on the dissociation of the ionizable groups of the polyampholyte. He constructed a number of models for representing a protein as a dipole and its interaction with simple ions. The simplest model was that of a spherical dipolar ion with a point dipole moment u located at the center of the sphere. The derived relation took the form

$$\log\left(\frac{S_p}{S_o}\right) = K_i\left(\frac{\Gamma}{2}\right) - K_s\left(\frac{\Gamma}{2}\right)$$

where S_p is the solubility of the dipolar ion at the ionic strength $\Gamma/2$, S_o is the solubility of the dipolar ion in the absence of salt, K_i is the salting-in constant, and K_s is the salting-out constant. In contrast to simple ions, the relative solubility of a dipolar ion is a direct function of the first power of the ionic strength. The salting-in constant K_i is proportional to u^2 (in the other models, K_i is proportional to the first power of u) and inversely proportional to the square of the dielectric constant and the square of the temperature; i.e., $(u/DT)^2$. The salting-in term arises from the electrostatic interactions between the model dipole and the surrounding salt ions and describes the increase in solubility at low ionic strength due to perturbations in the ion atmosphere surrounding the dipole. It predicts the empirically observed strong relationship between the solubility of a dipolar ion and the size of its dipole moment as well as the greater salting-in effect observed with molecules having high dipole moments. The salting-in effect for proteins is much greater than that for amino acids, which have much smaller dipole moments. The solvent action of salts at low ionic strength is profoundly influenced by the dipole and higher electric moments of the protein that arise from the distribution of positive and negative charges on the accessible surface of the protein molecule. The electric surface configurations are highly characteristic of individual protein molecules, for some of which large changes in solubility can often be effected with small variations in ionic strength; e.g., beta-lactoglobulin with a dipole moment of 730 debye units experiences a dramatic salting-in effect as compared to horse carboxyhemoglobin, which has a smaller dipole moment of 480 debye units (54). Suffice it to say that at low ionic strength the dipole moment of the protein molecule and other characteristics determined by the number and surface distribution of the electrically charged and uncharged amino acid residues have a profound and often highly *specific* effect, varying from one protein to another. The specific interactions between proteins and electrolytes at low ionic strengths are masked in concentrated salt solutions. Consequently, separations at low ionic strength can frequently be made sharper and more specific (selective) than those carried out at high ionic strength by salting-out. In order selectively to precipitate pseudoglobulins and albumins at low ionic strength it is necessary to add a miscible organic solvent. In this regard, note should be made of the inverse relationship of K_i to the *square* of the dielectric constant, which is manifested by the greater solubilizing effect of low ionic strength on proteins in media of lower dielectric constant as compared to water. The salting-out constant K_s is inversely proportional to the first power of the dielectric constant and temperature and is a direct function of the excluded volume of the dipolar ion. The salting-out term decreases faster than the salting-in term as the solvent dielectric constant decreases. Thus the salting-out effect is greatest in aqueous solutions, in contrast to the salting-in effect, which predominates in media of lower dielectric constant. This difference is markedly demonstrated by leucine with its large aliphatic side chain. It is readily salted out from water by a small concentration of salt, but in 90% ethanol it is salted in almost to the same extent as glycine.

Dipolar ions will affect the solubility of a protein in a manner qualitatively similar to simple ions, i.e., one can observe salting-in and salting-out effects, but to a lesser extent. These dipolar effects appear to be partially related to their dielectric increment and the resultant increase in the dielectric constant of the solution. For instance, glycine-glycine has a greater dielectric increment than glycine and a greater salting-in effect. The increased solution dielectric constant will reduce generalized electrostatic interactions. However, the solubilizing action of the series of α-amino acids glycine, alanine, and valine, each possessing essentially the same dielectric increment, decreases in that order. This observation, not dealt with by the electrostatic theories of Debye or Kirkwood, is rationalized in terms of the increase in size of the apolar residue, which has the opposite effect of an increase in dipole moment. At sufficiently high concentrations of the dipolar ion, the salting-out effect will be observed.

As evidenced by the data in Fig. 1B, *specific ion effects are observed in the salting-in phenomenon.* At the same ionic strength, different anions have marked differences with regard to their effect on the salting-in of a given protein. These specific ion effects are not dealt with by the theories of Debye and Kirkwood.

Salting-out (92): The decrease in the solubility of apolar compounds from aqueous solution by addition of salts has been extensively studied (93). With minor exceptions, all the salts studied salted out apolar compounds in accordance with the Setschenow equation, $\log S/S_o = -K_sC_s$, and no salting-in effect was observed. The absence of the salting-in effect implies that even at low concentrations, neutral salts cause apolar molecules to associate and become insoluble. The introduction of polar groups into otherwise apolar compounds results in the appearance of a salting-in effect.

The solubility of most proteins at and above their isoelectric points increases upon addition of salt and reaches a maximum (salting-in), after which there is a rapid, linear decrease in solubility (salting-out). Empirically, the salting-out of proteins is described by the Cohn equation, $\log S = \beta - K_s(\Gamma/2)$ (94), where the solubility S of a given protein is related to the ionic strength $\Gamma/2$ of a concentrated salt solution. K_s is the salting-out constant, which is a characteristic function of the protein being salted out (its excluded volume as well as the polar/apolar nature of its surface) and the specific salt employed (see below). It is independent of temperature and pH at or above the isoelectric point. Recent studies by Salahuddin et al. (95) on the salting-out of nine proteins indicate that the salting-out constant K_s of a given protein is a function of its surface hydrophobicity. This is consistent with the studies on model compounds by von Hippel and colleagues (67,96,97). The term β represents the hypothetical solubility of the protein at zero ionic strength. For a given protein, it is solely dependent upon temperature and pH, with a minimum at the isoelectric point (90). Foster et al. (98) showed that β will vary depending on the salt addition technique employed. Czok and Bucher (99) pointed out that salting-out can be performed under two regimes: salting-out at constant pH and temperature and variable ionic strength (K_s-fractionation), and salting-out at constant ionic strength and variable pH and temperature (β-fractionation).

The underlying mechanism of the salting out phenomenon was first alluded to by Hofmeister in 1888 (100), who suggested that it was due to a dehydration of the protein by the added salt. Debye (101) presented a quantitative treatment of salting-out in which the salt ions attract the solvent water molecules, squeezing out other solutes such as proteins. Based on the previously discussed solvophobic theory of Sinanoglu and colleagues (28), Melander and Horvath (102) presented a theoretical treatment of protein solubility and the salting-out of proteins, as well as a proposal as to the basis of the Hofmeister series. They presented a bipartite relation for the effect of salt on the solubility of a protein, i.e., the effect of salt on the electrostatic free energy of the protein and the effect of salt on the free energy of cavity formation. The electrostatic term gives an estimate of the salt-induced free energy changes based on the classical ion (Debye) and dipole (Kirkwood) models of proteins. It is a function of the dipole moment of the protein and reflects the salting-in effect, but it is independent of the nature of the salt. The cavity term is a function of that part of the nonpolar surface area of the protein dehydrated upon precipitation and the molal surface tension increment of the specific salt employed. It is presented as reflecting an intrinsic salting-out coefficient that is a function of the area of hydrophobic contact between protein molecules in the system and the effect of the specific salt on the surface tension of the solvent. They interpret this intrinsic salting-out coefficient to be a measure of a *halophobic effect*: the enhancement of hydrophobic interactions by a salt-induced increase in solvent-solvent interactions measured by an increase in the surface tension of the solution. The theory states that the salting-out effectiveness of a series of salts is a linear function of their molal surface tension increments.

There is a body of data at variance with the conclusions drawn from the theory of Melander and Horvath. As is evident from Fig. 1B, there are significant specific ion effects manifested at low salt concentration in the salting-in of fibrinogen, an observation that cannot be dealt with by the theory. Further, the recent data reported by Przybycien and Bailey (103,104) concerned with the salting-out of alpha-chymotrypsin demonstrate a lack of correlation between the salting-out constants and the molal surface tension increments for a series of sodium and potassium salts. These authors claim that the theory of Melander and Horvath fails to describe the salting-out behavior of a conformationally labile protein due to the failure to address the interaction of the salt with the protein and the potential consequent changes in the physical properties of the protein.

Timasheff and colleagues (38,105,106) have carried out extensive studies of the interactions of solvent components with proteins and have established the general rule that chemical entities that salt out proteins at high concentration in aqueous solution are preferentially excluded from the immediate environment of the proteins resulting in the preferential hydration of the proteins. *Protein preferential hydration is a general characteristic of salting-out systems.* They posit that this nonuniform, entropically unfavorable distribution of cosolvent molecules around the protein molecule is responsible for their salting-out properties. Arakawa and Timasheff (107,108) studied the preferential interaction of a series of proteins with sodium and potassium salts and divalent cation salts. They reported that for a series of sodium salts, as well as divalent metal sulfate salts, a good correlation exists between their salting-out effectiveness, their preferential exclusion from the protein surface, and their molal surface tension increment. They asserted that for salts cosolvent exclusion was a "direct and necessary consequence of the increase by the salt of the surface free energy (surface tension) of water." Such was not the case with chloride salts of divalent cations such as $CaCl_2$, $BaCl_2$, and $MgCl_2$ at pH values near and above the isoelectric point of the protein. At these pH values, these salts tend to increase protein solubility even though they have high values for their molal surface tension increments. Below the isoelectric point of the protein, salting-out is observed with these salts. In two recent papers (109,110), Arakawa et al. postulate that the solubility of a protein in a salt solution is determined by the balance of the three different protein-salt interactions: salting-in, salting-out, and weak ion binding. Salting-in and weak ion binding are functions of the protein charge, the pH of the solution, and low salt concentration, while salting-out is a linear function of surface tension increment of the salt. At salt concentrations above which the salting-in interaction is constant, the solubility of the protein is determined by the relative magnitudes of ion binding and salting-out interactions. When ion binding is dominant, the solubility of the protein increases with salt concentration accompanied by increased ion binding due to the mass action effect. In cases of minor ion biding, preferential salt exclusion (preferential hydration), due to the increase of the surface tension of water by the salt, becomes the dominant salt-protein interaction resulting in a decrease in protein solubility. Apparent deviations from the linear relation between the molal surface tension increment of a salt and its salting-out action are accounted for by weak ion binding. A recent paper by Breslow and Guo (111) regarding the salting-in behavior of compounds with positive surface tension increments, and observations by others that precipitating agents such as polyethylene glycol and ethanol, which have negative surface tension increments, raise questions as to the generality of the concept relating solubility to surface tension increments in its present form; other factors must be involved. However, one thing is clear: the salting-out of proteins, as for simple molecules including gases, is largely dependent upon the volume of water "displaced" by the precipitating agent. Suffice it to say that a complete mechanistic description of the salting-out phenomenon is lacking.

Low ionic strength salting-out of a protein at pH values acid to its isoelectric point has been reported for serum globulin (112), casein (113), myosin (114), hemoglobin (115), and most recently fibrinogen (67). the effect is reversed as the ionic strength increases at pH values slightly acid to the isoelectric point. At more acid pH values, the solubility of the protein is a continuous inverse linear function of ionic strength and obeys the Cohn salting-out equation. The use of the Cohn equation to describe this behavior does not imply that the molecular mechanisms basic to the phenomena are the same as for the classical salting-out of proteins by concentrated salt solutions. The low ionic strength salting-out of the protein below its isoelectric point is most probably due to the formation of insoluble protein-anion complexes at low pH values.

c. Specific Ion Effects. The salting-out effectiveness of different ions having the same charge varies most dramatically. This effect is a strong function of the specific cation and anion of the salt employed, suggesting the involvement of specific nonelectrostatic factors. This was first reported by Hofmeister (100), who studied the relative effectiveness of various salts in precipitating euglobulins from aqueous solutions. In terms of molar concentration, the sequence he reported was Na_3 citrate $> Li_2SO_2 = Na_2SO_4 = K_2HPO_4 = Na_2HPO_4 > (NH_4)_2SO_4 > MgSO_4 > KAc = NaAc > NaCl > NaNO_3$. The sequences of cations and, especially, anions derived from this and many other studies are known as the Hofmeister or lyotropic series. These studies describe the apparent specific effects of simple ions on numerous phenomena, including macromolecular conformation (116). These ion-specific (lyotropic) effects appear to be related to the field strength of the ion (ion size, charge density, and polarizability), which determines the extent of ion-solvent and ion-macromolecule interactions (117).

The effectiveness of the salting-out of apolar compounds from aqueous solutions by different ions varies in conformance with the Hofmeister series (93). The absence of the salting-in effect infers that neutral salts, even at low concentrations, cause nonpolar molecules to associate and become insoluble. The interactions of neutral salts with apolar moieties is well illustrated by comparing the effect of salt on the solubility of glycine and leucine. They have the same charged groups and dipole moment but differ in the number of methylene groups as well as in their molecular size; leucine in water is insolubilized at a much lower salt concentration than glycine in water. Extrapolating to proteins, the interaction of neutral salts with hydrophobic residues would favor the folded conformation with these groups associating to form the hydrophobic core. However, proteins contain polar groups, most numerous of which are the peptide amide groups, whose effects on protein solubility in the presence of salt must be considered. The introduction of polar (amide) groups into otherwise nonpolar compounds results in the appearance of a salting-in effect that appears to be a function of ionic strength alone with no specific ion (lyotropic) effects (118,119). Schrier and Schrier (120) suggested that the presence of nonpolar groups in the solute being salted out is responsible for the Hofmeister specific ion effects and that the sign and magnitude of the salting-out constant K_s is a function of the ratio of apolar to polar groups exposed to the solvent. Recent work by von Hippel and colleagues (68) supports this idea that specific lyotropic effects arise due to the unique interactions of the ions with exposed apolar residues.

Evidence presently available indicates that high concentrations of neutral salts cause structural changes ranging from increased helix content (kosmotropes) to the unfolded "coil" state (chaotropes) in general accord with the lyotropic series (97). Chaotropic ions such as thiocyanate, perchlorate, calcium, and lithium destabilize the native structure, while kosmotropic ions on the other end of the lyotropic series (sulfate, acetate, ammonium) behave as stabilizers of macromolecular structure. Destabilizing ions increase the rate of conformational change under denaturing conditions, while the opposite is observed for stabilizing ions. Of direct interest to the fractionator are the data that demonstrate that high concentrations of ions that are conformation stabilizers decrease protein solubility (e.g., sulfate), and high concentrations of those ions that destabilize the native structure tend to increase protein solubility (e.g., thiocyanate). The relative values of the parameter that measures the molar effectiveness of a sequence of ions as conformational stabilizers closely parallel those for the salting-out constants of the ions in the sequence, i.e., the lyotropic series for salting-out parallels that for stabilization. The studies of Timasheff et al. (106,109) report that high concentrations of ions that are preferentially excluded from the protein solvation shell independent of solution conditions stabilize the native structure of proteins and act as salting-out agents. *These remarks are generalizations for which there are numerous exceptions* that appear to be related to the specific protein and ion under consideration: e.g., Fredericq and Neurath (121) reported the reversible salting-out of insulin with thiocyanate; a recent paper by Reis-Kautt and Ducruix 9122) reports that the reverse order of the Hofmeister series is observed in the precipitation and crystallization of lysozyme.

Melander and Horvath (102) proposed that the effect of a specific anion on the surface tension of water (the molal surface tension increment of the sodium or potassium salt of the anion) is linearly related to the position of the ion in the lyotropic series of Bruins (123) and Voet (117). Bull and Breese (124) presented a differing view in postulating that the lyotropic series results from the effect of the ions on the *interfacial* tension of the protein-water interface. This approach has been followed by Collins and Washabaugh (116) who relate the Hofmeister series of ions to their specific effects on the behavior of water at interfaces.

In considering the mechanism responsible for the differing interactions between ions and nonpolar moieties as well as their surface tension effects, it is necessary to account for their effects on the structure of water (18,125). The highly structured water lattice will be perturbed by the introduction of ions as a result of a number of interrelated factors: the size of the ion relative to that of the unit cell of the normal water lattice and the interactions of the ion electric field with that of the neighboring dipolar water molecules. Ions whose diameter is sufficiently small can fit into the interstices of the normal water lattice without causing a significant disturbance of the lattice. Larger ions that cannot be accommodated by the normal water lattice will cause its disruption. As the concentration of ions increases, the normal water structure will be destroyed irrespective of the ion size. The calculations of von Hippel and Schleich (96) demonstrate that in a 1 M solution of a uni-univalent salt, no two ions are separated by more than a distance equal to three times the diameter of a water molecule. This implies that in concentrated solutions of small or large ions there are no regions of normal structure and that all the molecules of water are subject to the electrostatic fields of the ions. The electrostatic interaction between an ion and the dipoles of neighboring water molecules will lead to the formation of the primary hydration layer, whose structure is totally different from that of normal water. The thickness of this layer is a direct function of the ion charge density. Between the primary hydration layer and bulk water of normal structure, there is thought to exist a region of unstructured monomeric water molecules that are under the influence of the ion electric field diminished by the shielding effect of the primary hydration layer. The reduced electric field is sufficiently strong to prevent these water molecules from entering the normal water lattice but not strong enough to draw them into the primary hydration layer. Ions of high charge density, such as PO_4^{2-} and SO_4^{2-}, have a large primary hydration layer, and their addition to water is accompanied by a decrease in the partial molal unitary entropy of solution and an increase in viscosity. Such ions are referred to as "structure makers" (kosmotropes), and their strong attraction for water, due to their high charge density, is responsible for their preeminence as salting-out agents. As the charge density of a sequence of ions decreases, so does the primary hydration layer, while the intermediate layer of unstructured water increases. Thus ions of low charge density (large ionic radii) such as Br^-, I^-, SCN^-, NO^{3-}, ClO_4^-, Rb^+, and Cs^+ reduce the overall solution structure, as evidenced by an increase in the partial molal unitary entropy of solution and viscosity decrease. They are referred to as "structure breakers" (chaotropes) and frequently behave as solubilizing agents. Taylor and Kuntz (126) have suggested that "structure makers" are poorly bound to proteins due to their large structured primary hydration layer, which is a result of their high charge density. This suggestion is supported by the extensive work of Timasheff and colleagues (38), who refer to the negative binding of ions as "preferential hydration." As stated above, the available data indicate that ions that are water "structure makers" stabilize protein conformation as well as act as salting-out agents.

The addition of nonpolar compounds to water is accompanied by a net increase in the overall solution structure due to hydrophobic hydration. the structure of this water, referred to as "icebergs," is different from the normal water lattice as well as the structure of the ion hydration layer.

If we now consider a system composed of water, ions, and nonpolar compounds, there exist three separate forces, each competing to organize the water molecules into three different types of structure. These three forces arise from the ions, the nonpolar groups, and the solvent water lattice, respectively. This suggests that specific ion effects reflect, in addition to direct differential ion pair formation, the indirect, solvent-mediated interactions between ions and nonpolar groups. The structural perturbation of water by an ion will influence the potential size of the "icebergs" surrounding exposed nonpolar entities of a protein. This in turn will determine the strength of hydrophobic interactions and the subsequent solubility of the protein. A "structure-making" ion that induces its neighboring water molecules to assume the characteristic structure of the primary hydration layer will, by some presently unrecognized mechanism, increase the number of water molecules available from the unperturbed water lattice for the formation of "icebergs" around the hydrophobic groups of protein. This will enhance hydrophobic interactions and reduce the solubility of the protein. On the other hand, "structure breakers," in some nondefined manner, reduce the number of water molecules available for "iceberg" formation around apolar entities. This will reduce the entropic driving force of hydrophobic interactions, and as a consequence the solubility of the protein will be increased. For a critique of this line of thinking, see Muller (127).

Finally, it is of interest to note the observations of Jain (128). He reported that the salt concentration needed to precipitate 90% of the gamma globulin in solution was 20% greater when the stock reagent was 6 N Na_2SO_4 + 6 N NaCl as compared to 6 N Na_2SO_4 alone. This may be a reflection of the offset of the precipitating efficiency of the sulfate ion by the solubilizing effect of the chloride ion.

5. Temperature

The aqueous solubility of a protein will be affected by the influence of temperature on (1) the structure of water and the energy needed to create a hole for the protein molecule; (2) the structure of water and its behavior as a dielectric medium; (3) the interaction between protein molecules ("crystal lattice energies"); (4) the various interactions between the protein and the solvent as well as those between salt ions and the solvent (ion hydration); (5) the pK_a of ionizable groups on the protein, of buffer molecules in the solution as well as the association constants for the binding of ionic and nonionic species present in solution; and (6) the intramolecular interactions determining the conformation of the protein. With the exception of hydrophobic interactions, the energies of all forms of noncovalent interactions (ionic, Debye, Keesom, London), including the hydrogen bond, are inversely related to the temperature. In contrast, the strength of the hydrophobic interaction increases with rising temperature up to the range of 50–60°C, after which it falls (129).

As a rule, the solubility of proteins is endothermic in salt-free solutions, low-ionic-strength solutions, and ethanol-water mixtures (positive temperature coefficient of solubility), but the absolute value of this parameter will vary with the protein. In concentrated salt solutions, the temperature coefficient of solubility may be positive or negative, depending upon the protein: e.g., myosin (114) and carboxyhemoglobin (115) have negative temperature solubility coefficients while that for lysozyme is positive (130). It is obvious that variation in temperature can be directly employed as a fractionation parameter in such instances where the proteins have opposite temperature coefficients of solubility, as well as in those instances where the parameter has the same sign but sharply differing absolute values. An excellent example of the latter situation is the separation of fibronectin from fibrinogen (131). In practice, however, temperature has been generally employed to prevent denaturation, to reduce enzymatic activity, and to restrict bacterial growth rather than as a solubility variable.

At present, published theoretical treatments of protein solubility (Kirkwood, Melander and Horvath, etc.) are inadequate. Recently, Chen et al. (132) have proposed a molecular thermodynamic model for the solubilities of amino acids and peptides. Their results are quite encouraging. They are pursuing the extension of the model to proteins.

IV. METHODS OF DIFFERENTIAL PROTEIN PRECIPITATION

As listed in Table 2, there are a number of different techniques by which one can reversibly precipitate a protein from solution (132–135). These techniques can be divided into two groups. Group A is characterized by precipitation resulting from major perturbations in the properties of the solvent caused by relatively large concentrations of the precipitant. In contrast, group B is characterized by precipitation being caused by minor perturbations in the solute protein due to direct interaction (binding) of the protein with low concentrations of the precipitant. In the former case, solute-solvent interactions are reduced by changes in the solvent and in the latter case by changes in the solute. The selective precipitation of a given protein from a mixture of proteins is a function of those unique physicochemical properties that differentiate it from the other proteins in the mixture.

A. Primary Perturbation Affects the Solvent

This class of methods is characterized by the precipitant altering the properties of the solvent so as to reduce its interactions with the solute and allow for increased solute-solute interactions. The latter are increased by adjusting the solution pH to that of the isoelectric point of the subject protein.

Table 2 Methods Based on Differential Precipitation

A. Primary perturbation affects solvent
  1. Euglobulin precipitation
  2. Salting-out
  3. Nonionic polymeric precipitation
  4. Miscible organic solvent precipitation
  5. Precipitation of a soluble affinity complex
B. Primary perturbation affects solute
  1. Isoelectric precipitation
  2. Metal ions and complex coordination compounds
  3. Cationic precipitants
      a. Organic cations (e.g., Rivanol)
      b. Natural and synthetic cationic polyelectrolytes
  4. Anionic precipitants (fatty acids, T.C.A., anionic polymers)
  5. Affinity precipitation (e.g., immunoprecipitation)

1. Euglobulin Precipitation

Euglobulins are those proteins insoluble in water but soluble in salt solutions. Maximum insolubility in water occurs at the isoelectric point of the protein. Proteins from diverse sources demonstrate such behavior. Sandor (136) has presented a valuable discussion of the euglobulins of human serum. A number of the early antitoxin preparations were euglobulins obtained by dilution of horse serum with water. The general approach to the isolation of a euglobulin is to desalt the solution and then to adjust the pH to the isoelectric point of the protein. The desalting can be accomplished by the following procedures: (1) sufficient dilution with water, (2) dialysis/diafiltration, (3) size exclusion (gel permeation) chromatography, (4) ion exchange chromatography (137,138), and (5) electrodialysis (128,139).

2. Salting-out

This technique involves the precipitation of a protein or group of proteins by the addition of high concentrations of neutral salts or amino acids under appropriate conditions of pH, total protein concentration, and temperature. It has enjoyed wide popularity and has been subjected to numerous reviews (90,92,98,99,140–143). Our previous discussion of the salting-out effect has covered the essential aspects of this procedure. The selectivity of this type of precipitation is not very great, but usually the larger proteins precipitate first, i.e., at lower salt concentrations, all other parameters being equal.

Harms (144,145) reported an interesting effect of some phenolic compounds on the salting-out of plasma proteins by ammonium sulfate. Upon addition of ammonium sulfate to plasma, the normal order of protein precipitation is fibrinogen, followed by the beta- and gamma-globulins and then albumin. However, if the procedure was conducted in the presence of 2% phenol or 1% tricresol, then the order of precipitation was reversed, albumin being precipitated first. Schilling (146) suggested that the phenolic compounds bind to albumin resulting in its reduced solubility in less concentrated salt solutions as compared to the unbound species. Michon and Arnaud (147) reported a procedure for the fractionation of plasma proteins by salting-out with ammonium sulfate in the presence of phenol.

The salting-out of proteins by amino acids was first reported by Richards in 1937 (76). She described the salting-out of egg albumin and hemoglobin by high concentrations of glycine. Salting-out by amino acids has been used in the purification of fibrinogen (148,149) and the antihemophilic factor (77).

Zahn and Stahl (150,151) reported the differential extraction of a precipitate obtained by completely salting out a mixture of proteins with ammonium sulfate. The precipitate was suspended with diatomaceous earth in the concentrated salt, poured into a column, and extracted with solutions of decreasing ammonium sulfate concentration. For additional examples of this procedure see Keil et al. (152) and King (153). A variation of this technique of *salting-in chromatography* was reported by Sargent and Graham (154). A column of a molecular sieve was equilibrated with a high concentration of ammonium sulfate. A solution of proteins was applied to the top of the column where some proteins precipitated and the rest were washed down the column. The column was then eluted with a decreasing salt gradient and the precipitated proteins were differentially extracted; see also von der Haar (155).

Porath (156) took this concept one step further by proposing *differentially to precipitate* and elute on a column in one continuous operation. He called the procedure *zone precipitation*. It is based on the difference in the flow rate of micro- and macromolecules through a column of an appropriate molecular sieve. One establishes an ammonium sulfate gradient in the column, the concentration increasing from the top to the bottom. The soluble protein mixture is applied to the top of the column. The proteins, which are totally excluded from the sieve particles, move down the column faster than the salt, which penetrates the sieve particles. When a given protein reaches the appropriate salt concentration it will precipitate and become immobile. As the decreasing salt concentration reaches the precipitated protein it dissolves and resumes movement into the gradient where it reprecipitates. The process then repeats itself until the protein is eluted from the column in the soluble state.

3. Nonionic Polymeric Precipitation

A number of water-soluble uncharged polymers of varying molecular weights have been used for the precipitation of proteins. They include (1) dextrans (151–163); (2) polyvinyl pyrrolidone (164,165); (3) polypropylene glycol (166); and (4) polyethylene glycol (PEG).

There is an extensive literature on the use of PEG for the precipitation of proteins. The initial report of the precipitation of proteins by PEG appears to be that of Stocking (167). Beginning with the work of Polson et al. (168) a vast literature has accumulated on the use of PEG in the fractionation of proteins; see especially Refs. (169–173).

Numerous papers have been written concerning the mechanism by which nonionic polymers, such as PEG, cause the precipitation of proteins. The early work of Laurent (158,159,174) demonstrated that the precipitation of proteins by the nonionic polymer dextran was a function of the size of the protein and the dextran concentration. The size of the dextran, once it exceeded a minimum value, was of little influence. He suggested that the phenomenon is a result of the steric exclusion of protein molecules from the volume of the solution occupied by the larger dextran molecules; i.e., since two masses cannot occupy the same space at the same time, addition of a nonionic polymer with a large Stokes radius and accompanying large effective volume greatly reduces the volume in the solution available to protein molecules. The volume effectively occupied by the polymer is referred to as the excluded volume, and the phenomenon is known as the "excluded volume effect." Based on Ogston's theoretical treatment of the excluded volume effect (175–178), Juckes (170), followed by Foster et al. (171), derived the following theoretical expression to describe the precipitation of proteins from *dilute* solution by nonionic polymers such as PEG:

$$\ln S = \ln S^0 - aC$$

where S is the solubility of the protein, C is the concentration of the polymer, and S^0 and a are constants. S^0 is the solubility of the protein in the polymer-free solution, and a is a virial coefficient reflecting the interaction between PEG and the protein. In agreement with an excluded volume effect, the value of a is essentially a linear function of the Stokes radius of the protein, an exponential function of the polymer molecular weight up to a limiting value of 6000 D, and a function of pH, ionic strength, and temperature (170,171,178). For concentrated protein solutions an additional term bS must be added to the left-hand side of the equation, where b is a coefficient reflecting protein-protein interactions. Critical discussions of the assumptions made in deriving this relation can be found in Refs. 179–181. Hasko et al. (182) presented an empirical equation, obtained by computer analysis of PEG-protein precipitation curves, that was in agreement with the theoretically derived relation. The experimental data reported in the cited references are in basic agreement with the theory. As indicated above, the efficiency of PEG precipitation of a given protein from *dilute* solution is a linear function of the polymer concentration and is independent of the molecular weight of the polymer as long as it is greater than 6000 daltons. Under these conditions the slope a is constant, which leads to the surprising conclusion that the excluded volumes of PEG species having molecular weights between 6000 and 20,000 are essentially the same (170,179). The displacement of proteins from solution by lower-molecular-weight PEG molecules *is* a function of the polymer molecular weight; the value of a is now an exponential function of the PEG molecular weight (168,179,183). For lower-molecular-weight PEG species, higher concentrations are needed to precipitate the same amount of a given protein, since the excluded volume of the polymer decreases as its molecular weight decreases. Honig and Kula (184) have shown that one can increase the *selectivity* of the precipitation process by using smaller-molecular-weight PEG species. However, significantly higher polymer concentrations are required. Selectivity can also be increased by decreasing the concentration of protein (169). When a given species of PEG is added to a mixture of proteins, the order of precipitation follows the decreasing value of the Stokes radii of the proteins in the mixture; the larger protein will precipitate at a lower PEG concentration than the smaller proteins. Suffice it to say that the evidence strongly supports the steric exclusion mechanism for the precipitation of proteins by nonionic polymers such as PEG.

PEGs are polymers of ethylene oxide and have the general formula $HOCH_2CH_2(OCH_2CH_2)_nOH$. These polymers are very soluble in water due to the ether oxygens spread along the length of the polymer, which are strong Lewis bases and form hydrogen bonds with water molecules. The ethylene groups contribute a degree of hydrophobic character to the molecules. Lee and Lee (185) and Arakawa and Timasheff (186) have reported that proteins are preferentially hydrated in the presence of PEG, i.e., the PEG molecule is sterically excluded from the protein domain. The extent of preferential exclusion increases almost linearly as a function of the PEG molecular weight (in the range of 400 to 1000 daltons) but decreases as the concentration of a given molecular weight PEG increases. The rate of decrease in preferential hydration (PEG exclusion) with increase in PEG concentration rises dramatically as a function of the molecular weight of the PEG species. This latter observation was explained in terms of an increase in the folding of the polymer chain as the polymer concentration increases, leading to a decrease in its excluded volume at higher PEG concentrations. Lee and Lee (187) reported that the magnitude of the preferential exclusion is a function of the normalized hydrophilicity of the proteins studied and suggested that unfavorable interactions with negatively charged groups on the protein surface may be involved in the exclusion mechanism. However, Comper and Laurent (188), based on their studies of the interaction of dextran with albumin by temperature-dependent light scattering and calorimetry, concluded that any enthalpic contributions to the interaction are minimal and that entropic phenomena (excluded volume effects) dominate the interaction.

Under normal conditions, PEG does not denature proteins. As mentioned earlier, Timasheff and coworkers (106) have found that protein structures are stabilized by substances that are preferentially excluded from the protein domain. One would expect PEG to enhance the stability of proteins. However, while not enhancing protein stability, it has no tendency to denature proteins, under normal conditions. Atha and Ingham (179) reported that PEG 400 and PEG 4000 had negligible effects on the thermal denaturation of RNase, even at concentrations up to 30%. Knoll and Hermans (189) demonstrated that PEG 6000 at a 6% concentration had a negligible effect on the thermal denaturation of RNase and the pH denaturation of sperm whale myoglobin. On the other hand, Arakawa and Timasheff (186) observed that PEG 200, 400, 600, and 1000 at concentrations of 10% in solutions of beta-lactoglobulin lowered the thermal denaturation transition temperature of this protein. Lee and Lee (187) studied the thermal stability of four proteins (lysozyme, beta-lactoglobulin, RNase A, and chymotrypsinogen) in the presence of 10 to 30% PEG 200, 400, 1000, and 4000, respectively. Except for RNase A, the presence of these polymers significantly decreases the thermal transition temperatures for the other proteins. The lowering of the transition temperature was greater as the concentration of the polymer increased. They suggested that the various PEG species lower the transition temperature by preferentially interacting, hydrophobically, with the unfolded configurations of proteins. The extent to which the transition temperature is lowered appears to be related to the average hydrophobicity of the protein (190). However, it must be recognized that protein destabilization by PEG occurs at temperatures significantly higher than room temperature (>40°C). Thus one can operate at more congenial temperatures than with miscible organic solvents and not be concerned about denaturation due to the reagent PEG. It should be noted that PEG has been shown to increase the pK_a values of both amino and carboxyl groups (189) as well as that of the phosphate system (191).

A number of studies have been done on the effect of pH, ionic strength, temperature, and protein concentration on the precipitation of proteins by PEG (171,179). One can increase the efficiency of the process by adjusting solution parameters such that the solubility of the protein of interest is at its minimum prior to the addition of PEG, e.g., solution pH equal to the pI of the protein, temperature equal to that at which the protein solubility is minimum, ionic strength at a value at which the protein of interest is minimally soluble but separated from potential complexing proteins, and a protein concentration sufficiently dilute so as to increase the selectivity of the process. Foster et al. (171) showed that the selectivity of the precipitation is improved if it is performed by a set of sequential additions of PEG (rather than continuous addition) until the desired concentration is reached. Precipitate is removed at each stage of the sequence. This type of preliminary fractionation allows for the precipitation of the desired protein from a more dilute solution.

A few final remarks about the use of PEG are in order: (1) PEG is the nonionic polymer of choice because the viscosity of concentrated solutions of PEG is comparatively low in relation to other nonionic polymers. (2) The formation and equilibration of precipitates appears to take significantly less time with PEG as the precipitating agent than with ammonium sulfate or ethanol. (3) The elimination of the polymer from protein-containing solutions can be achieved by (a) precipitation of the protein, (b) adsorption of the protein to an ion exchange or affinity medium, (c) ultrafiltration, or (d) induction of phase separation by addition of phosphate or sulfate salts and separation by differential partitioning into the two liquid phases (192,193).

4. Miscible Organic Solvent Precipitation

Alcohols, acetone, ether, and other water-miscible organic reagents have been used by analytical chemists to precipitate proteins since the early part of the last century. However, such precipitates were invariably composed of denatured protein. Mellanby in 1907 (78,79) was one of the first, if not the first, to recognize that an undenatured protein preparation can be obtained by alcohol precipitation if the procedure is conducted at low temperature. He obtained a biologically active concentrate of diphtheria antitoxin by addition of appropriate amounts of alcohol to horse serum. In 1910, Hardy and Gardiner (194) fractionated animal plasma or serum by precipitation with cold alcohol or acetone. They washed the precipitate with cold ether to extract lipids as well as residual alcohol (or acetone) and removed the ether by air drying. The resulting powder was readily soluble in water and retained biological (antitoxic) activity. This use of cold miscible organic solvents to concentrate antibody activities from plasma or serum was subsequently reported by Dean (195), Hartley (196), Felton (197), and Merrill and Fleisher (198). Liu and Wu (199), using cold methanol, were the first to attempt a systematic study of the fractionation of serum with a miscible organic solvent. They obtained three major fractions corresponding to the euglobulin, pseudoglobulin, and albumin fractions obtained by salt fractionation. In 1940, Cohn et al. (200) published the first report of the preparation of therapeutic proteins by the systematic fractionation of human plasma by use of cold ethanol. Subsequent articles (201–203) detailed the procedures known as Cohn Methods 6 and 9. Cohn methodology is based on two observations: (1) the low-temperature precipitation of a protein by an appropriate concentration of ethanol at a defined pH; and (2) the enhancement of the salting-in effect due to the presence of miscible organic cosolvents such as ethanol. The presence of the organic cosolvent is considered to cause an increase in quasi-specific electrostatic interactions between charges uniquely distributed on the surface of a given protein and the ions of a salt present at low concentration. The differences in the salting-in effect at a given ionic strength on the solubility of different proteins are magnified as the concentration of organic solvent is increased. Thus *differential precipitation is obtained by carefully balancing the enhanced solubilizing action of low ionic strength in the presence of an organic cosolvent against the precipitating action of the organic cosolvent at the isoelectric pH of the protein or family of proteins of interest.* It should be noted that whereas three of the five variables of the Cohn process are manipulated as solubility parameters (pH, ethanol, and salt concentration), such is not the case with the remaining two (temperature and protein concentration). Temperature is not employed as a solubility parameter but is kept low to reduce the potential denaturing action of the organic cosolvent. The teaching with regard to protein concentration is to keep it as low as economically feasible so as to reduce coprecipitation and occlusion.

Besides ethanol, methanol—e.g., Pillemer (204), Fasoli (205), Dubert et al. (206)—acetone, e.g., Askonas (207)—ether, Mackay (208), and dioxane—Sumner and Dounce (209), have been used in the differential precipitation of proteins. Blomback et al. (210) described the use of the polar aprotic solvent, dimethylformamide (DMFA), in the fractionation of proteins in plasma and milk. It should be recalled that such polar aprotic solvents solvate cations very well but do not solvate anions to any appreciable extent. This fits with their observation that less DMFA was required for precipitation on the acid side of the pI of the protein. They suggested an inverse correlation between the polar/nonpolar ratio of amino acids and the concentration required to precipitate a given protein.

5. Precipitation of a Soluble Affinity Complex

Schneider and colleagues (211,212) introduced the procedure of precipitating a soluble affinity complex. They employed specific ligands fixed to water-soluble polymers that bound the protein containing the target group. The soluble complex was then precipitated by a change in pH or by salting-out. They applied this concept to the isolation of trypsin from beef pancreas by copolymerizing aminobenzamidine, acrylamide, and *p*-aminobenzoic acid. The resulting water-soluble polymer bound trypsin from a pancreatic homogenate, and the soluble complex was precipitated by lowering the pH. More recent use of this procedure was reported by Taniguchi et al. (213) employing bound Protein A to isolate IgG and by Ngyuen and Luong (214), who bound *p*-aminobenzamidine to a soluble polymer for the isolation of trypsin. Senstad and Mattiasson (215,216), expanded this concept by employing a hetero bifunctional molecule, where one functionality interacts with the molecule of interest and the other functionality interacts with the precipitating molecule; e.g., lactic dehydrogenase was bound to Blue Dextran (protein-dye affinity interaction) and the resulting soluble complex was precipitated by another affinity reaction, concanavalin A binding to the saccharide portion of the Blue Dextran. Bradshaw and Sturgeon (217) coupled Protein A to a water-soluble galactomannan. The soluble conjugate forms a soluble biospecific complex with IgG, which is then insolubilized by the specific interaction of borate ions with the galactomannan.

B. Primary Perturbation Affects the Solute

1. Isoelectric Precipitation

As discussed, the solubility of a protein in aqueous solution is a minimum at the pH where it is isoelectric, the pI of the protein. Thus for many proteins titration of a low-ionic-strength solution to that pH at which the protein has a zero net charge will lead to its insolubilization. When attempting to precipitate a protein from a mixture of proteins having an array of different pI values, one should adjust the solution pH to a value above or below the highest or lowest pI of the proteins present. Under either of these conditions all proteins present will be soluble and have charges of the same sign. The solution is then gradually titrated to the nearest pI, precipitate allowed to form and then separated, followed by adjustment of the solution pH to the next lower (or higher) pI (218). If the pH of the solution is between that of the pI values of two proteins, then they will bear net charges of opposite sign and form an ion-ion interaction complex. The solubility of the complex will be at a minimum at some intermediate pH, e.g., beta-lipoprotein has a minimum solubility at pH 5.4, and gamma-globulin is minimally soluble at pH 7.3. The complex formed in mixtures of these two proteins is much less soluble between these two pH values, having a broad solubility minimum centered about pH 6.7 (219).

2. Metal Ions and Complex Coordination Compounds

It has been known since the 1905 reports of Osborne and Harris (220) and that of Mellanby (78,79,91) that low concentrations of salts of heavy metals are potent reversible protein precipitants. Divalent and trivalent metal cations form well-defined complexes with carboxyl, alpha, and epsilon amino, imidazole, and sulfhydryl groups in proteins: Ca^{2+} and Pb^{2+} combine with carboxyl groups; Zn^{2+}, Cu^{2+}, and Cd^{2+} combine with imidazole groups; and Hg^{2+} and Ag^{2+} preferentially combine with sulfhydryl groups. Metals interact with different proteins in very specific ways. The specificity resides in the location, chemical makeup, and reactivity of the protein-combining sites. Not all metal-protein complexes are insoluble. Fractionation and separations can be effected by using a metal that specifically precipitates a given protein from a mixture of proteins. It should be noted that the solubility minima of metal proteinates occur at higher pH values than the pI values of the proteins alone. This allows for fractionation to occur without extensive swings in pH (221). Detailed discussions of the solubility behavior of metal-protein complexes can be found in (222) and (223).

Two general types of metal-protein complexes can be envisioned: (1) a simple ion-ion complex in which the metal ion combines with a single binding site and (2) a coordination complex in which the metal ion combines with two or more intra- or interprotein ligand groups as described by ligand field theory. The formation of a simple complex can affect solubility by changing the pI of the protein as well as the hydration of the protein. The formation of an intermolecular coordination complex due to the multivalent character of heavy metal ions would appear to be the primary factor contributing to he formation of insoluble metal-protein complexes. It should be noted that pH and the anion of the metal salt can have significant effects on the precipitation of the protein by the metal cation. The pseudo-specificity of most metal precipitations is related to the presence of binding sites on the protein capable of being involved with the metal in the formation coordination complexes; e.g., the ring nitrogen of histidine and tryptophane.

Numerous studies concerning the fractionation of serum and plasma proteins have been reported. Astrup et al. (224) used $CdCl_2$, $CuCl_2$, and $PbCl_2$ as precipitants in the fractionation of bovine and horse serum. Uriel (225) and Aoki and colleagues (226,227) studied the differential precipitation of serum proteins by an array of heavy metals and employed different gel electrophoretic assay techniques. Steven et al. (228) and Maeda et al. (229) reported the precipitation of fibrinogen by Zn^{2+}, Cu^{2+}, Ni^{2+}, Fe^{2+}, Hg^{2+},

Co^{2+}, Cr^{3+}, and La^{3+} ions but did not observe any insolubilizing effect of Ca^{2+}, Mg^{2+}, or Mn^{2+}. Escribano (230) used Cu^{2+}, as the acetate salt, selectively to precipitate the total gamma globulin fraction from human serum under defined conditions of ionic strength and pH. Van Dam et al. (231) used bis-copper chelates in their study of the relationship between the precipitating action of the metal ion, the bis-copper chelate, and the number of accessible histidine residues on the surface of a protein. Aluminum chloride was used by Lewin (232,233), and aluminum tartrate by Rejnek and Skvaril (234–236) to isolate gamma-globulin from plasma. $ZnSO_4$ was used by Heremans et al. (237) for the purification of IgA and by Cambier and Butler (238) for the purification of IgM. Cohn Methods 10 and 12 (239,240) for the fractionation of plasma proteins employ zinc glycinate as the precipitating reagent. In so doing, the zinc ions are slowly made available to the binding sites on the protein, allowing for a greater selectivity than is obtained by the use of a fully dissociated zinc salt. Zaworski and Gill (241) used $ZnCl_2$ reversibly to precipitate recombinant proteins (porcine urokinase, a TPA analog, and human interleukin-1 beta) from tissue culture and fermentation broth supernatants. All the studies referred to above involved the sue of millimolar concentrations of the metal ion and were performed at a slightly acid pH. When working close to or above neutrality, addition of metal ions to aqueous solution results in the formation of metal-hydroxide flocs. Collingwood et al. (242,243) used Fe^{3+} and Al^{3+} to form colloidal hydroxide flocs that bound the enzymes of interest. The centrifugally separated enzyme-floc complex was dissolved by use of citrate and the active enzyme recovered at high yield.

In 1939, Michael (244) reported the use of anionic and cationic complex coordination salts of chromium for the reversible nondenaturing precipitation of such proteins as insulin, casein, and egg albumin. Brown and Rothstein (245) found potassium tetrathiocyanato-(S)mercurate to be a rather specific nondenaturing precipitant of human fibrinogen. In a continuation of this study, Mannuzza and Rothstein (246) compared the behavior of halide complexes of mercury as quasi-specific fibrinogen precipitants. They reported that the mercury bromide complex was the most efficient of the mercury halides in the isolation of fibrinogen from human plasma.

3. Cationic Precipitants

We can subdivide this category in two: (1) organic bases and (2) natural and synthetic cationic polyelectrolytes.

a. Organic Bases. Although many organic bases including cationic detergents have been used to precipitate proteins selectively, the precipitates so formed are not readily solubilized, and the precipitated proteins appear damaged. One compound that has been shown to form reversible, nondenatured protein precipitates is a yellow, bactericidal, acridine dye, 2-ethoxy-6:9-diaminoacridine lactate, which has the commercial names Rivanol and

Ethodin. The initial work on the use of this compound in the differential precipitation of proteins was pioneered by Horejsi and Smetana (247,248). They reported that all the plasma proteins with the exception of the IgG immunoglobulins were reversibly precipitated by relatively low concentrations of Rivanol, at neutral or slightly alkaline pH. The IgG molecules remaining in solution showed no evidence of denaturation. Later studies have demonstrated that the Rivanol supernatant contained other proteins in addition to IgG (249–253). Rivanol has been widely used to obtain IgG preparations as well as in the isolation and purification of numerous other proteins: transferrin (254,255), ceruloplasmin (256), haptoglobin (257), thrombin (258), plasminogen (259), alpha$_2$-macroglobulin (260,261), albumin (262), cholinesterase (263), and monoclonal antibodies (264). The staff at Behringwerke developed a commercial plasma protein fractionation process based on the use of Rivanol and ammonium sulfate (265–267).

Numerous studies of the mechanism basic to the precipitating action of Rivanol are in the literature (268–271). These studies indicate that the basic dye forms an electrostatic complex with negatively charged groups on the protein. Conditions favoring the interaction are low ionic strength and a pH above the pI of the protein. Temperature does not seem to be a variable, thus allowing room temperature operation. The latter is facilitated by the bactericidal behavior of Rivanol. The precipitate can be dissolved by decreasing the pH or increasing the ionic strength. The freed Rivanol can be removed by adsorption onto either activated charcoal (247), a cation exchange resin (258), insoluble starch (272), silica gel (273), or polyurethane foam (270). Rivanol is readily precipitated by halide ions. The preferred method is to precipitate the free Rivanol with KBr followed by adsorption onto polyurethane foam (270). It can also be separated from the proteins by size exclusion chromatography or diafiltration, as long as no halide ions are present.

A number of cationic detergents have successfully been used as reversible protein precipitants, e.g., Kurioka et al. (274) used stearyltrimethyl-ammonium chloride to precipitate and isolate fibrinogen from human plasma.

b. Natural and Synthetic Cationic Polyelectrolytes. Protamines, a group of highly basic proteins rich in arginine, have been used to precipitate selectively fibrinogen from plasma (275,276). A number of synthetic cationic polyelectrolytes have been shown to precipitate proteins, at the appropriate pH, by charge-charge interactions. Morawetz and Hughes (277) studied the precipitation of bovine albumin by polyvinylamine, as well as by the polyampholyte diethylaminoethyl (DEAE) methacrylate-methacrylic acid copolymer. Water-soluble DEAE dextran was shown to precipitate proteins under a defined set of conditions of pH, very low ionic strength and mass ratio of protein to DEAE dextran (278). Polyethyleneimines and similar cationic synthetic polymers have been used as protein precipitants in the isolation of enzymes (279–281).

4. Anionic Precipitants

We can subdivide anionic precipitants into (1) small anions and (2) anionic polymers.

a. Small Anions. Chanutin and colleagues demonstrated that low concentrations of *short chain fatty acids* (e.g., caproic, caprylic, lauric, etc.) can precipitate certain proteins from plasma at pH 4.2 (282,283). Differences were observed in the precipitation capacity of the different fatty acids; at low fatty acid concentrations albumin and the alpha- and beta-globulins are precipitated, the supernatant being rich in gamma globulin. There is no clear picture for the mechanism of the precipitating action of the short chain fatty acids. Steinbuch and colleagues, in a series of systematic studies of reversible protein precipitation by caprylic acid, developed procedures for the isolation of IgG (284,285), ceruloplasmin (286), orosomucoid (287), monoclonal IgG and IgA (288), prealbumin (289), amylase, and lactic dehydrogenase (290). They reported that the optimum conditions included a pH between 4.8 and 5.0, low protein concentration, and room temperature. The optimum concentration of caprylic acid varied with the pH and the protein(s) under study (291). Many other workers have used the caprylic acid procedures of Steinbuch et al. to purify polyclonal (292) and monoclonal IgG (293–297). Allary and Saint-Blancard (298) made the interesting observation that albumin, precipitated by caprylic acid at pH 4.8 to 5.0, is readily solubilized in a 30% ethanol, pH 6.0 solution. On the basis of this data, they developed ethanol-caprylic acid fractionation procedures for preparing albumin starting with Cohn Supernatant I+II+III and one for IgG starting with Cohn Fraction I+II+III. The procedures gave very good yields as well as purity.

A number of acids have been used in conjunction with other reagents in the fractionation of protein mixtures. *Trichloracetic acid (TCA)* has been used for the preparation of albumin from plasma or serum, based on the selective extraction of albumin by high concentrations of acetone or ethanol from the TCA precipitate of nearly all the plasma proteins (299–305). Levine (300) suggested that precipitation with TCA is due to the extensive binding of trichloromethyl groups by the albumin molecule, which becomes very hydrophobic. This increased hydrophobicity would be expected to increase the solubility of the TCA-albumin complex in organic solvents. He presented data that appeared to rule out TCA binding to free amino groups of the protein. Dirr and Farber (306) reported the results of stepwise addition of TCA to serum. All proteins except the beta-globulins and albumin are precipitated at a 0.3% TCA concentration. At a TCA concentration of 1.8%, only albumin is soluble. Albumin precipitates at higher TCA concentrations. The gamma- and alpha-globulins appear to be precipitated first, followed by the beta-globulins and finally the albumin.

Schwert (303), Kallee et al. (304), Sri Ram and Maurer (307), and Rao et al. (308) reported that TCA-treated albumin is physicochemically and immunologically indistinguishable from untreated albumin. Based on this property of albumin, the Institut Merieux developed a very large-scale process for the purification of human albumin from placental blood for therapeutic use (309).

Winzler et al. (310) were the first to employ the protein precipitating action of *perchloric acid and sulfosalicylic acid* in isolating the highly glycosylated and very soluble glycoproteins of plasma: "orosomucoid," "sero-mucoid," or "serum mucoprotein." The 0.6 N perchloric acid–soluble fraction was shown to be a heterogeneous mixture of such glycoproteins as alpha$_1$-acid glycoprotein, haptoglobin, and alpha$_1$-antitrypsin. Schultze et al. (311) reduced the concentration of perchloric acid to 0.2 N and obtained a greater number (12) and amount of the plasma glycoproteins in the soluble fraction as compared to the 0.6 N soluble fraction. Heide and Haupt (266) and Schultze et al. (311) describe the isolation of many glycoproteins from the 0.2 N perchloric acid–soluble fraction.

Astrup et al. (312) and Berry et al. (313) studied the differential precipitation of serum proteins by a series of small polyanions including *sulfosalicylate, tungstate, picrate, molybdate, phosphomolybdate, and metaphosphate.* It was suggested that these polyanions reversibly combine with accessible basic groups of the protein and change the chemical characteristics of the protein surface and its solubility. The most promising results were obtained with tungstate, sulphosalicylate, and metaphosphate. The proteins in the sulphosalicylic acid–soluble supernatant were chromato-graphically subfractioned into a number of low-molecular-weight proteins by Dolezalova et al. (314) and Pavlu (315,316). Burstein and colleagues (317–319) have successfully used sodium phosphotungstate in combination with MgCl$_2$ in the fractionation and purification of the plasma lipoproteins. Steinberg (320) purified a series of enzymes from filtrates of microbial fermentation by use of tungstophosphoric, tungstosilicic, tungstoboric, molybdophosphoric, and molybdosilicic acids. He suggested that the precipitating action of these heteropolyacids results from their combination with epsilon-amino, guanidino, and imidazole groups on the protein.

b. Natural Anionic Polymers. *Metaphosphates* were employed by Astrup et al. (312), Rane and Newhouser (321) and Etheridge et al. (322) as selective plasma protein precipitants. Nitschmann et al. (323,324) developed a plasma fractionation procedure based on the use of *linear polyphosphates.* More recently, Lee et al. (325) have used polyphosphate in the isolation of bovine plasma immunoglobulins.

It has long been known that *tannic acids*, polymers of digallic acid and glucose, will precipitate proteins. Coulthard et al. (326) employed tannic acid in the isolation of a glucose dehydrogenase from bacterial cultures. Mejbaum-Katzenellenbogen (327) has studied the interaction of tannins with proteins and the dissociation of the complexes by caffeine. In a subsequent study, she and Kubicz (328) isolated pituitary hormones using tannin as precipitant in the procedure. In a series of papers, Casillas and colleagues employed tannic acid as a quasi-specific fibrinogen precipitant in the isolation of fibrinogen (329) and in the preparation of fibrinogen-free antihemophilic factor (330). They employed polyvinyl pyrrolidone to dissociate the fibrinogen-tannin complex.

A number of natural sulfated polysaccharides such as *heparin* have been shown to precipitate proteins under a defined set of conditions. von Korff and coworkers (331,332), and Godal (333) showed that heparin will precipitate fibrinogen as well as cold-insoluble globulins. Burstein et al. (317–319) reported the precipitation of very-low- and low-density lipoproteins by heparin in the presence of $MnCl_2$. Anderson reported the precipitation of fibrinogen and beta-lipoproteins by chondroitin sulfate (334).

c. Synthetic Anionic Polyelectrolytes. There is an extensive literature on the use of synthetic anionic polyelectrolytes as protein precipitants. *Polyacrylic acids* were studied as protein precipitants by Morawetz and Hughes (275), Weiland et al. (335), Whitaker (336), Berdick and Morawetz (337), Noguchi (338), Isliker and Strauss (339), Sternberg and Hershberger (340), Sternberg (341), and Caygill et al. (342). Clark and Glatz (343) studied the precipitation of egg white proteins by *carboxymethyl cellulose.* Isliker (344) reported that *polystyrene sulfonates* can be used for the fractionation of albumin-gamma globulin mixtures.

Astrup and Piper (345) reported the apparently specific precipitation of fibrinogen from plasma by synthetic *polysaccharide polysulfuric acids.* The formation of a precipitate was observed to be a function of the composition of the solution (protein concentration, ionic strength, pH) and the specific sulfated polysaccharide employed. Precipitation occurred not only on the acid side of the pI of fibrinogen, as one would expect for multiple charge-charge interactions, but also on the near alkaline side. Walton (346) reported similar observations with *dextran sulfates* with molecular weights above a critical level. As with other anionic polyelectrolyte-protein complexes, solubility was a function of ionic strength, pH, temperature, polyelectrolyte molecular weight, and the ratio of polyelectrolyte with a given charge density to protein. The precipitates formed on either side of fibrinogen's pI behaved differently with regard to parameters of the interaction. Below the pI, precipitation is due to ordinary salt formation and was a function of the charge density of the dextran sulfate moiety employed and not its size. The amount and character of the precipitate was independent of temperature between 0 and 37°C. On the other hand, the solubility of the complex formed above the pI of fibrinogen was a function of temperature, the size of the polyelectrolyte, as well as the ratio of polyelectrolyte to protein. There was an optimum value for this ratio for maximum precipitation to occur. The complex was soluble in the excess of either component, thus resembling the specific precipitates formed in antigen-antibody systems. The character of the precipitate changed and the extent of precipitation decreased with temperature. The apparent specificity of the interaction of the appropriately sized dextran sulfates and fibrinogen may be a function of the asymmetry of the fibrinogen molecule and its consequent large excluded volume. Sasaki and Noguchi (347) confirmed the observations of Walton. Both groups reported that carboxymethyl cellulose does not form precipitates with fibrinogen above its pI.

Bernfeld et al. (34) reported that fibrinogen and beta-lipoglobulins are the only proteins precipitated from plasma by *sulfated amylopectin* in the range of pH 7.5 to 8.6. The precipitate behaved as that described by Walton. Oncley et al. (349) employed large-molecular-weight dextran sulfate in the isolation of beta-lipoproteins from human serum or defibrinated plasma. The isolation of beta-lipoproteins by precipitation with sulfated polysaccharides was reviewed by Cornwell and Kruger (350). Burstein et al. (317–319) subfractionated the lipoproteins by precipitation with different combinations of dextran sulfates and divalent cations.

5. Affinity Precipitation

The classical example of this type of precipitation is that of an *antibody-antigen* precipitate. The antigen-antibody interaction is highly specific, being a function of the structural complementarity of the interacting surfaces of the antigen and the antibody (351). It would appear that all types of noncovalent interactions are involved, with a significant contribution by dispersion forces. Maximum precipitate is formed at an optimum concentration ratio of antigen to antibody, with less precipitate being formed when either the antigen or the antibody is in excess.

The highly specific interactions of *lectins* with the glyco moieties of glycoproteins have been employed to precipitate glycoproteins (352,353). Brewer and colleagues have studied the mechanism of precipitation of a series of glycopeptides by concanavalin A (354).

A number of workers have selectively precipitated target proteins by use of modified *group-specific dyes*, such as Procion Blue (355), Reactive Red (356), and C. I. Reactive Blue 2 (357). See also Pearson (358).

Larsson and Mosbach (359) proposed to precipitate a specific protein by use of a bifunctional ligand molecule. They synthesized a soluble bifunctional molecule having a group specific moiety at each end: Bis-NAD, two NAD (nicotinamide adenine dinucleotide) moieties connected by a spacer. NAD has a strong affinity to a number of enzymes such lactic dehydrogenase (LDH). Addition of the bis-NAD to a solution of LDH led to the formation of a specific precipitate without any changes in solution parameters being required. This procedure has been discussed by Mosbach and colleagues in a number of recent papers (360,361). Hayet and Vijayalakshmi (362) employed bis compounds of the triazine dye Cibacron Blue, an affinity ligand for NAD-dependent enzymes, as well as some other proteins. The bis dye directly precipitates the target protein.

V. GENERAL PRINCIPLES OF PRECIPITATE FORMATION

Whenever particles are formed by precipitation from solution, the two processes of nucleation and growth are involved, and the fundamental concepts of crystallization are applicable (363,364). An understanding of the basic concepts of particle formation and growth is essential for successfully dealing with the technology of precipitation and subsequent liquid-solids separations problems.

Particle formation generally consists of two separate phases: an induction phase involving the formation of nuclei, followed by a growth phase during which additional solute molecules condense onto the nuclei. The particles so formed continue to grow and agglomerate until the final equilibrium state is reached. For solute molecules to come out of solution and initiate particle formation, the soluble solute concentration must be greater than the normal equilibrium solubility value; i.e., the solution must be in a metastable, *supersaturated* state with respect to that solute species. Because organized structures with defined surfaces are created from the random distribution of molecules in solution, nucleation and growth are energy-consuming processes. This energy requirement establishes the need for the solution to attain a particular level of supersaturation for nuclei to form and growth to occur. It is this excess solute concentration relative to the equilibrium solubility value that contributes the energy necessary for nucleation and growth. Thus the driving force for both processes involved in particle formation is the degree of supersaturation, but the kinetics of the two processes are affected differently by the extent of supersaturation.

Nucleation is the spontaneous generation, by noncovalent molecular association and condensation within the metastable supersaturated liquid phase, of a stable aggregate of ultramicroscopic size. Initially, clusters of molecules form and increase in size by continued addition of molecules. As their size increases, so does their chemical potential. Many of the clusters, which are indistinguishable from the mother phase, are unstable and dissociate. The more stable clusters continue to grow to a critical size to form nuclei that have a maximum chemical potential (365). The rate of nucleation is an exponential function of the degree of supersaturation and becomes "infinite" at the maximum level of supersaturation. This maximum is called the *supersolubility limit*. (See Fig. 2.) Thus fewer nuclei will be formed per unit time at low levels of supersaturation, while the maximum number of nuclei formed per unit time will occur at the supersolubility limit.

Nuclei are at the edge of the liquid/solid transition. Once formed, they act as centers for the deposition of additional solute molecules. Not all nuclei continue to grow; many disaggregate, and the freed molecules can

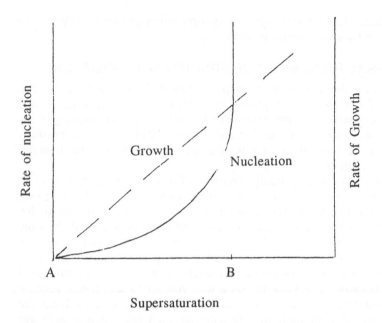

Supersaturation

Figure 2 Nucleation and growth rates as functions of the degree of supersaturation. (A) normal equilibrium solubility; (B) supersaturation limit. [(Adapted from Porter, H. F., Flood, J. E., and Rennie, F. W. (1966)]. Improving solid-liquid separations, *Chemical Engineering, June 20*: 141.)

then condense on more stable nuclei in a process referred to as "ripening." Aggregates whose size is greater than that of a nucleus form a separate phase and continue to grow and increase in size to form the size-limited primary precipitate particle. The latter collide and adhere to each other to form the precipitate aggregate particle. Particle growth continues as long as the solution remains supersaturated. The extent of supersaturation and the rate of growth are linearly related, and both decrease until reaching the saturated state, the point where no further growth occurs. As indicated, the mechanics of particle growth are described in terms of molecular as well as particle collisions resulting from their relative motion. The collisions are due to the inherent kinetic energy of the entity (diffusive transport) and bulk movement due to input of energy from external sources (convective transport). These two growth mechanisms are referred to as perikinetic and orthokinetic aggregation, respectively (366–369).

The objectives of the precipitation operation are, in order of priority:

1. Maximum separation of the solute of interest, in its native state, from other solutes (high selectivity);
2. Minimum coprecipitation;

3. Large granular particles;
4. Minimal amount of mother liquor; and
5. Maximum difference in particle density relative to that of the solution

To achieve objectives (2) through (5), the rate of nuclei formation should be minimized and the growth rate optimized. A slightly supersaturated solution will allow for the formation of larger nuclei at the expense of smaller nuclei. The solubility of small nuclei is greater than that of large nuclei as a consequence of the reduction of the total interfacial area and interfacial free energy for the large nuclei. In addition to the degree of supersaturation, the *interfacial tension* of the solid phase will greatly affect the solubility and stability of the nuclei. Materials with low interfacial tensions between the solid and liquid phases have low solubility and will favor the formation of many small, stable nuclei and the development of colloidal or highly solvated, slimy precipitates. Materials with high interfacial tensions will form fewer nuclei and larger, more dense particles.

For a particular solute, the greater the number of nuclei the more sites are available onto which a given number of solute molecules coming out of solution can adhere. This results in a large number of fine particles at the end of the growth phase. In highly supersaturated solutions nuclei appear so rapidly and in such great number that the supersaturation condition is rapidly eliminated by the formation of a colloid, a gel, or a slimy, highly solvated precipitate. For the same number of solute molecules coming out of solution, the fewer the number of nuclei, the larger the size of the final particles. However, the rate of growth is slower, and growth will take longer, than in the case of many nuclei. Suffice it to say that precipitate particles having the desired characteristics are obtained at a relatively low degree of supersaturation where the rate of nucleation and the rate of growth are *reduced*.

It follows from this discussion that for a given solute in a given solvent (fixed interfacial tension), the degree of supersaturation is a fundamental parameter in defining the physical characteristics of the precipitate. Precipitates formed under conditions of large precipitant excess, i.e., high degree of supersaturation, are voluminous, highly solvated with occluded mother liquor, very compressible, and generally have a small density difference relative to the solution and a high probability of containing coprecipitated solute molecules. Operationally, the direct addition of a precipitant to a solution results temporarily in a heterogeneity of conditions in the reactor. In the vicinity where the precipitant has been introduced, precipitant concentration varies between wide limits; there is a temporary large local concentration of precipitant in the region where the two solutions come in contact. *The major problem is the avoidance or minimization of this local excess concentration of precipitant* that produces the rapid formation of many small highly solvated particles, the coprecipitation of other more soluble solutes (overprecipitation) as well as conditions that may be conducive to damaging the solute.

The ideal situation is exemplified by the technique of "precipitation from homogeneous solution" (370–373). In this technique, the precipitant is gradually generated uniformly throughout the entire solution. This is in contrast to the conventional technique, in which a solution of the precipitant is added to a solution of the reactant accompanied by localized concentration excesses. In homogeneous precipitation, a precipitant precursor, at the appropriate concentration, is homogeneously distributed throughout the solution. The process is initiated by gradually converting the precipitant precursor to its active form. At no time is there a difference in precipitant concentration at any point in the solution. The extent of supersaturation is kept small by controlling the rate of the conversion reaction. As a result, the number of nuclei formed is relatively small, yielding a precipitate that is compact and dense, with a minimal amount of coprecipitation and occluded mother liquor. These particle characteristics can be further optimized by slowing the rate of the reaction generating the precipitate. An example of precipitation from homogeneous solution is the precipitation of thorium iodate by the generation of the iodate ion by the reduction of periodate with ethylene glycol that is slowly produced by the hydrolysis of beta-hydroxyethyl acetate. The volume of the precipitate is dramatically smaller than that of an identical amount of thorium iodate formed by direct addition of iodate (374). Precipitation from homogeneous solution yields an optimal precipitate particle because it allows for the increase of precipitant concentration uniformly throughout the solution at a nearly ideal rate without excessive supersaturation and avoids local excesses in precipitant concentration. As stated above, the primary problem in the heterogeneous precipitation process is the existence of localized regions of excess precipitant concentration and the concomitant generation of many small nuclei and coprecipitation of undesired solutes. This condition results from the rapid addition of a concentrated precipitant solution and inadequate intensity of mixing. The obvious solution is to control the precipitant concentration so that the extent of a localized excess of precipitant is minimized by changing the solubility parameters *slowly*. This can be accomplished by *gradual addition of dilute solutions of precipitating reagents accompanied by vigorous mixing* so as to approach the desired extent of supersaturation slowly as well as limit and rapidly dissipate local excess precipitant concentration. Thus the techniques employed for reagent addition and mixing are of critical importance.

In many cases, the precipitate particle initially formed is not the most stable configuration for the given set of final conditions. In such situations the precipitate, given time, will change to the stable form. This process of change is referred to as "precipitate aging" or "ripening." The "aging" process involves the gradual resolution of small, unstable particles. The resulting solute molecules deposit themselves upon the more stable particles of larger size. Imperfect precipitates obtained by rapid precipitation from concentrated solutions undergo many cycles of resolution and reprecipitation. This "aging" or "ripening" process results in the expulsion of coprecipitated impurities and in the formation of purer and larger precipitate particles. It is evident from this brief discussion that an optimized "aging" time allows for the formation of a purer precipitate in the form of large, dense particles.

In review, to obtain good precipitates the following principles should be applied:

1. Minimal degree of supersaturation that will allow for precipitation
2. Avoiding local excess concentration of precipitant by
   a. Vigorous mixing
   b. Dilute precipitant solution
   c. Slow rate of addition
3. Allowing sufficient time for resolution of fine particles and concomitant growth of larger particles

A. Protein Precipitate Formation

I will not deal with the quantitative kinetics of protein precipitation but refer the reader to the publications of Dunnill and colleagues (2,375), of Glatz and colleagues (376–380), as well as the papers of Lawson et al. (381) and Przybycien and Bailey (382).

Changes that occur during the precipitation of a protein are complex and are functions of the specific protein, the specific precipitant, and the technique of precipitant addition. Studies of protein precipitation such as those of Nelson and Glatz (378) allow one to describe the process as being made up of four stages.

Stage 1. Addition of precipitant, achievement of supersaturation, and nuclei formation. Nucleation times can range from a few seconds to several minutes depending on the specific precipitant and specific protein. During this period there occurs the diffusion-controlled agglomeration of thousands of protein molecules to form the nuclei. However, the number of nuclei formed is an inverse function of the scale of micromixing.

A number of studies of the nucleation process during protein precipitation and crystallization have been reported in the literature. Parker and Dalgleish (383) employed stopped-flow light scattering and stopped-flow turbidity to study the nucleation of the calcium-induced precipitation of alpha$_s$-casein. Their analysis was based on the theory of polyfunctional condensation: they assumed that condensing monomers have greater than two functional groups by which they associate. As the aggregate size increases so does the number of available reactive groups, as does the probability of successful collisions. A point is reached in the aggregation process when the rate of growth is no longer a function of the number of free reactive groups but rather a function of the concentration of particles and their rate of collision i.e., a diffusion-controlled process à la Smoluchow-ski. A year later, Kam et al. (384) employed quasi-elastic light scattering (QELS) to study the nucleation stage during the crystallization of lysozyme. The theory they presented allowed for the prediction from data obtained prior to and during nucleation as to whether crystallization or amorphous precipitation would result. Their approach was based on the concept that amorphous precipitation is a noncooperative irregular aggregation process, whereas crystallization is a cooperative phenomenon involving the regular, stepwise aggregation of monomers. QELS was used to study the prenuclea-tion state in protein crystallization by Baldwin et al. (385), Carter et al. (386), and Mikol et al. (387). The latter, working with lysozyme and concanavalin A, presented evidence that with certain precipitants protein aggregation occurs when the protein solutions are undersaturated. In such cases the protein is unable to crystallize and forms an amorphous precipitate when the solution becomes supersaturated. With other precipitants, the proteins remain monodisperse up to saturation and crystallize once supersaturation is attained. This raises the question as to the relationship between the nature of the protein-precipitant interaction and the formation of a crystal or amorphous precipitate. Kadima et al. (388) employed dynamic light scattering in conjunction with photon correlation spectroscopy in a study of the characteristics of the precrystallization stage of canavalin and their functional relationship to crystal or amorphous precipitate formation. Based on their experimental results they suggest that when aggregation of monomers occurs too rapidly an amorphous rather than crystalline solid phase will appear.

Stage 2. Perikinetic growth of nuclei to form microscopic, colloidal-sized entities, referred to as primary precipitate particles, which attain a limiting size.

Stage 3. Orthokinetic growth by collision and adhesion of "mature" primary precipitate particles to form macroscopic precipitate particles. Photomicrographs of isoelectric soy protein precipitates (389,390) and salted-out casein precipitates (383) clearly show the precipitate aggregates to consist of a multitude of primary precipitate particles with approximate diameters in the range of 1 micron. There have been a series of studies concerning the factors affecting particle size during the orthokinetic growth phase from Dunnill's group in the Department of Chemical and Biochemical Engineer-ing, University College, London (391–401) as well as from Glatz's group in the Department of Chemical Engineering, Iowa State University (402–407). The results of these workers highlight the fact that particles suspended in moving fluid will collide as well as being subjected to fluid shear. The collisions can lead to aggregation and growth as well as breakup of the larger aggregates. Growth of an aggregate occurs by collision with primary precipitate particles and smaller aggregates. Collisions between larger aggregates are ineffective in forming larger stable aggregates. Thus growth can be viewed as the incremental addition of small units to the growing aggregates. Fluid shear can lead to particle erosion. Precipitates formed at a high rate of shear tend to have a smaller final size distribution as a result of the greater extent of erosion at the high shear rates. The formation and average size of the final precipitate aggregate can be conceived of as resulting from a balance between orthokinetic aggregation, hydrodynamic shear-controlled breakup, and collisions between aggregates as well as with the vessel walls. Increasing the intensity of mixing (shear rate) will result in smaller-sized aggregates. Larger aggregates can be obtained at low shear rates during the growth and aging stages as well as at higher protein concentrations. Thus the particle size distribution attained at the end of the growth period is a function of the design of the reactor, the intensity of mixing, and the concentration of particles (initial protein concentration).

The physical properties of the protein precipitate particles are determined by the operating conditions employed during the peri- and orthokinetic stages as well as the subsequent aging stage. The strength of the aggregates, i.e., resistance to breakup, was shown by Bell and Dunnill (393) to be determined by the time of exposure to and the extent of the nonuniform shear fields. Aggregates of optimal resistance to breakup are gotten only with a specified exposure to shear: a Camp number, the product of the mean velocity gradient in the reactor (shear field) and the time of exposure, of 10^5. The density of the protein precipitate particle is a function of the specific precipitant as well as the operating conditions in the reactor during the various stages in the precipitation process.

Stage 4. This is the period of aging and ripening of the precipitate particles. During this stage, under appropriate conditions of shear, the aggregates continue to grow in size, strength, and density. The latter is evidenced by the decrease in hindered settling time as the time of aging increases (396,397,408). In addition, during this period the consequences of overprecipitation (coprecipitation) are partially reversed by resolution of proteins precipitated due to imperfect mixing and consequent presence of domains of local precipitant excess during the addition process. The extent of overprecipitation is a function of the rate of precipitant addition, the concentration of the stock precipitant solution, and the intensity of mixing. For example, protein x is insoluble in 20% ethanol. To attain this concentration, 95% ethanol is added to the protein solution. In the course of this addition the ethanol concentration will be progressively diluted until a 20% ethanol concentration is reached. During the addition process elements of the solution experience differing ethanol concentrations varying from say 90% to 5%. In those elements with ethanol concentrations greater than 20%, other more soluble proteins will precipitate. When the solution is homogeneously 20% in ethanol those proteins soluble at this concentration will redissolve. This occurs during the aging period.

VI. UNIT OPERATIONS EMPLOYED IN DIFFERENTIAL PRECIPITATION

Table 3 lists the important operations and variables that must be considered in designing a differential precipitation system. They have been assembled into three groups: reagent addition, mixing, and precipitate growth and aging. A qualitative, empirical discussion of these factors will be presented, the goal of which is the design of a system that will allow for an optimum separation of the protein(s) of interest from other proteins (high selectivity) and the formation of large, dense precipitate particles having a minimum amount of occluded mother liquor and coprecipitation of other species. Four techniques can be employed in determining the success of the precipitation process: (1) collect samples at intervals during the process, separate the precipitate from the supernate and determine the protein species distribution between the two; (2) record the changes of the solution turbidity during the precipitant addition and aging phases of the process; (3) measure the settling time of the suspension at appropriate intervals during the process (408); and (4) measure the particle size distribution with the appropriate equipment as a function of time during the process.

Table 3 Precipitation Parameters: Reagent Addition and Mixing

---

A. Reagent addition
    1. Processing mode (batch vs. continuous)
    2. Chemical nature of reagent
    3. Physical state of reagent (solid vs. liquid)
    4. Rate of addition
    5. Reagent concentration in stock solution
    6. Protein concentration
B. Mixing (laminar vs. turbulent flow)
    1. Batch processing in a tank
        a. Tank geometry (l/d ratio)
        b. Agitator design and placement
            1. Marine, air foil, turbine, etc.
            2. Use of baffles for center mount
        c. Sparger design and placement
    2. Continuous processing in a pipe
        a. Static mixers
    3. Dissipation of heat of mixing
        a. Jacketed tanks and piping
            1. Immersion coils
        b. Temperature of reagent
        c. Rate of reagent addition
C. Precipitate growth and aging
    1. Acoustic conditioning

A. Reagent Addition

Reagent addition involves such considerations as (1) processing mode, (2) chemical nature of the precipitant, (3) physical state of the precipitant, (4) rapid rate of addition, (5) reagent concentration of stock solution, and (6) protein concentration. These factors will dramatically affect the characteristics of the precipitate.

1. Processing Mode

Given the significance of mixing and shear in the formation of precipitates, it is not surprising that different reactor designs produce precipitate particles with distinctly different characteristics. Foster et al. (98,409) reported that reactor design—batch stirred tank reactor (BSTR) or continuous stirred tank reactor (CSTR)—can have a marked effect on the physicochemical parameters of the precipitation as well as the size of the precipitate particles. In the salting-out of a protein, the technique of salt addition to the protein solution has a marked effect on the final solubility parameters of a given protein, i.e., the salt concentration at which precipitation occurs. Compared to batch processing, operation in a CSTR required higher concentrations of precipitant to insolubilize the same amount of a given protein; i.e., an additional 25% saturation with ammonium sulfate was required to attain the same solubility of the enzyme fumarase in a CSTR as compared to a BSTR. The absolute values of the constants of the Cohn equation, β and K_s, were larger for the CSTR than for the BSTR. They also reported that residence time in the CSTR was a parameter affecting the precipitate: increased residence times in the CSTR required more salt to precipitate the same amount of protein. *The solubility of the protein was a function of the method of precipitant addition*! Other observations of note were that the particles produced in a CSTR were larger than those produced in a BSTR and that short residence times in the CSTR resulted in larger particles than obtained at longer residence times. Similar differences between a BSTR and a CSTR were also observed when PEG was the precipitant. However, less PEG was required in the CSTR than in the BSTR to achieve the same solubility of fumarase.

The isoelectric precipitation of soy proteins was studied in a BSTR (389,391,395), in a CSTR (379,390,402), and in a continuous tubular reactor (CTR) (392). The general conclusion derived from these studies was that the physical characteristics of the protein precipitate aggregate were dependent on the reactor design and its shear profile. BSTR precipitate aggregates were more compact, more regular in shape, and more resistant to shear breakup than those obtained in a CSTR and a CTR. The strength of the CTR precipitate aggregate can be increased by exposure to the variable shear field in a BSTR. The aggregates appeared to undergo a restructuring process in the high shear domain of the impeller. The mean size BSTR precipitate aggregates was half that of CTR precipitate aggregates. The differences in the physical properties of BSTR, CSTR, and CTR precipitate aggregates can be conceived to be due to the different shear profiles in the reactors and the length of time the particles are exposed to shear. (The shear field in a CTR is essentially homogeneous, whereas in a BSTR the shear field is heterogeneous, having very high shear in the region of the impeller.) Exposure to this variety of shear gradients as well as longer times of exposure to these gradients is considered to be the basis for the mechanically stronger aggregates. Virkar et al. (392) showed that the mechanical characteristics of a CTR precipitate aggregate can be improved by introducing turbulence promoters appropriately spaced along the length of the CTR or by transferring the aggregate to a BSTR. However, BSTR aggregates are stronger than the "batch" aged CTR aggregates. CTR aggregates had faster hindered settling rates than aggregates of similar size formed and aged in a BSTR. The centrifugally sedimented solids obtained from a BSTR and a CTR possessed nonlinear viscoelastic properties at low shear stresses. The CTR precipitate "pastes" were much drier and almost 120 times more cohesive and resistant to deformation than the BSTR precipitate pastes.

In the early 1970s, Watt (410,411) developed a semicontinuous version of the Cohn cold ethanol, low-ionic-strength plasma fractionation process. A description of its first iteration can be found in the article by Foster and Watt (412). Essentially it consists of a series of modules ("Watt trolleys"), each dedicated to a given step in the process. Each module is designed as a CTR, employing a static mixer and an acoustic conditioning device (see below) to conduct a specific precipitation. Foster et al. (413) observed less occlusion and coprecipitation when using the continuous mode as compared to the batch mode. Mitra and Lundblad (414) reported an increased yield, but decreased purity, of albumin isolated from plasma when conducting the Cohn process in the CTR mode ("Watt trolley") as compared to the BSTR mode. Pennell (personal communication, 1977) reported that continuous flow processing in a static mixer CTR yielded "cleaner cuts" and less coprecipitation than obtained by batch processing. Chang (415) developed a hybrid precipitation system for the Cohn process composed of a CSTR combined with a static mixer CTR. He reported less coprecipitation, denser precipitate aggregates (drier centrifuge pastes), and higher yield and purity of the final product, albumin.

These differences between the characteristics of protein precipitates obtained by batch or continuous processing modes (different reactor geometry) would appear to highlight the importance of the microscale kinetics of the interactions leading to precipitation of a protein.

2. The Chemical Nature of the Precipitant

The chemical nature of the precipitant can have dramatic effects on the precipitation process. Foster (409) reported differences in the precipitation behavior of the enzyme fumarase when comparing ammonium sulfate and

PEG as precipitants. Overprecipitation was observed with ammonium sulfate as precipitant but not with PEG, and in addition the precipitation kinetics were different. Chan et al. (375) studied the precipitation of soy proteins in a CTR in laminar flow using different precipitants: sulfuric acid (isoelectric precipitation), ethanol, Ca^{2+} ion, and ammonium sulfate. While the kinetics of precipitate growth were similar in all cases, the final mean aggregate size was strongly dependent on the type of precipitant employed (sulfuric acid > ethanol = Ca^{2+} > ammonium sulfate). Mixing intensity did not appear to affect the final mean aggregate size when sulfuric acid and Ca^{2+} were the precipitants, but it was a factor for ethanol and ammonium sulfate. Fisher and Glatz (406) observed markedly different aggregate size distributions as well as different susceptibilities to shear breakup when comparing the precipitation of egg white lysozyme by a polyelectrolyte precipitant (polyacrylic acid) and by low-molecular-weight acid precipitants. These results are a reflection of the different mechanisms of insolubilization and growth. Salt et al. (416) studied the effect of different acids in the isoelectric precipitation of soy proteins. They found that the degree of protein denaturation was a function of the acid anion. The extent of damage varied inversely with the Hofmeister series, i.e., sulfate < nitrate < phosphate < chloride. Even at low mixing intensity, sulfuric acid appeared to cause no significant damage to soy proteins. Nelson and Glatz (378) reported that the number and size of soy protein primary precipitate particles was a function of the precipitant used (vigorous mixing): HCl > H_2SO_4 > Ca^{2+}. It has been known for some time that the character of ethanol-induced plasma protein precipitates is a function of the buffer anion employed; acetate yields much drier, less "sloppy" precipitates than chloride (F. Rothstein, unpublished observations).

3. The Physical State of the Precipitant

The physical state of the precipitant is a precipitation variable. As mentioned in the discussion of salting-out, Foster et al. (98) reported a marked difference in the values of β (the hypothetical solubility of the protein at zero ionic strength) obtained when precipitating fumarase with solid ammonium sulfate and a saturated solution of this salt. The use of solid reagent yielded larger particles than the liquid form of the reagent and is accompanied by extensive coprecipitation of other proteins and occlusion of mother liquor. The resulting "nonspecific" flocculent precipitates are often highly solvated and do not settle readily due to a small density difference relative to the solvent. These observations can be rationalized in terms of the large local excess concentration of the reagent surrounding its solid phase.

4. Rapid Rate of Addition

A rapid rate of addition of precipitant often leads to gross, highly solvated, flocculent and, at times, gelatinous precipitates. The rate of precipitant addition should be reduced so as to avoid such states and possible protein denaturation due to local excess reagent concentration. Such local excesses will lead to the formation of a solid phase whose composition differs from that obtained at "equilibrium" due to extensive coprecipitation of unwanted protein species. This can significantly increase the time for equilibration. A slow rate of addition allows for the gradual increase in reagent concentration and, with good mixing, minimizes the problem of local excess precipitant concentration as well as reducing the irreversible aspects of the process. This thesis is supported by the observations of McMeekin (417), who used dialysis as the method of reagent addition, a technique introduced by Theorell in 1932 (418). The precipitant solution was contained in a rotating cellophane bag immersed in an agitated protein solution. The diffusion of the reagent into the protein solution, as well as the agitation due to rotation of the bag and a mixer, greatly reduced excess local precipitant concentration. This slow addition procedure yielded granular precipitates with reduced coprecipitation and occlusion. Separations were sharper (cleaner cuts) and much more reproducible. Vickar et al. (392) reported that relative to a slow dropwise precipitant addition to a BSTR, rapid addition of precipitant resulted in a larger mean aggregate size and a marked broadening of the size distribution curve, the effect being amplified at low mixing intensity. Fisher et al. (419) compared two extremes in the rate of precipitant addition (slow, dialytic vs. direct addition in a BSTR) in the fractional acid precipitation of the soy proteins, glycinin, and beta-conglycinin. They observed no difference in selectivity and particle microstructure, but other properties were affected. Rapid acid addition resulted in larger primary particles and larger, stronger aggregates, which, however, settled more slowly than aggregates resulting from slow acid addition. A number of years ago I attempted to perform dialytic reagent addition employing an array of hollow fibers. All went well until the precipitates occluded the intratubular space. Clark and Glatz (343) compared the effect of single vs. multiple staged addition of the precipitant, carboxymethyl cellulose, on the fractional precipitation of egg white proteins. The largest aggregates were obtained by a one-stage addition. Two-stage addition produced fewer small aggregates, but the mean aggregate diameter was smaller. Importantly, *staged addition improved the selectivity of the precipitation*. Jain (128,420) reported the use of electrodialysis (ED) for the controlled rate of addition of ionic precipitants to a protein mixture. He reported that the salt concentration required to salt out 90% of the gamma globulin was 1/3 less when added by ED than when added directly to the solution. He also compared salt addition by ED to dialysis and reported that dialytic addition required twice the concentration of salt needed to precipitate 90% of the gamma globulin as by ED. The effect of addition rate can be studied by following changes in the turbidity of the solution as the precipitant is added. Such studies were made by G. Hedenskog, D. Lanfear, and F. Rothstein (unpublished observations) by use of an immersion turbidimeter during a number of the precipitation steps in the Cohn cold-ethanol process. Rapid precipitant addition was accompanied by an ethanol process. Rapid precipitant addition was accompanied by an "overshoot" in the turbidity readings followed by a decline to a steady-state value. This phenomenon was avoided by slowing the rate of addition of the precipitant such that the turbidity follows a "gradual" sigmoidal curve to the steady-state value. (The mixing parameters were the same.) Large-scale operation requires a procedure by which the precipitant concentration in each microscopic unit volume increases at a defined slow rate, but macroscopically at a rate that allows for the total addition to occur in an economically acceptable time. Models for such a procedure are available from the field of heat transfer and will be discussed below.

5. Reagent Concentration of Stock Solution

Since the rate of reagent addition is a precipitation variable, obviously so is the *reagent concentration of the stock solution*. By employing a lower concentration of the reagent solution, the local excess concentration problem will be reduced. P. Wah and F. Rothstein (unpublished studies) observed that the settling time of an ethanol-pH-induced protein precipitate was reduced by more than 50% when the concentration of the precipitant solution was halved, all else being held constant.

6. Protein Concentration

It is well known that in many cases *protein concentration* is an inverse function of the concentration of reagent required to insolubilize a given amount of protein. On the other hand, less coprecipitation and greater selectivity are obtained with dilute protein solutions (92). Primary particle size and final aggregate size increase with protein concentration (378,392).

B. Mixing

The mixing operation serves to accelerate the blending of the precipitant with the other solution components into a homogeneous system in which the molecules are uniformly distributed. This is achieved by mechanically setting the fluids into motion, either laminar or turbulent. Turbulent mixing superimposes eddy diffusion onto molecular and bulk diffusion and is the most rapid technique to achieve the desired uniform molecular distribution. Laminar mixing involves only molecular and bulk diffusion and, as a result, is a slower process than turbulent mixing (421–423). However, the shear stresses encountered in turbulent flow are much greater than in laminar flow. This becomes a potential problem with shear-sensitive molecules as well as precipitate particles. The intensity of mixing will obviously affect precipitate formation by reducing local domains of concentrated precipitant and undesirable side reactions. The extent of denaturation of soy protein during isoelectric precipitation with HCl is inversely related to the intensity of mixing (416). While one desires sufficient mixing intensity to reduce localized high concentration of precipitant, it should not be so intense as to produce small precipitate aggregates due to shear breakup. One should strive for maximum turbulence and micromixing during precipitant addition and then significantly reduce the intensity of mixing to the laminar regime during the growth and aging phase.

Some mixing parameters to be optimized when operating in the batch processing mode are tank geometry, presence of baffles, impeller size and design (axial flow marine, axial flow air foil, radial flow turbine, axial flow pitched blade turbine, helical screw, helical ribbon, etc.), impeller placement in the tank, and sparger design and placement relative to the impeller (424–427). It is known [see, e.g., Khang and Levenspiel (428,429)] that if one injects a pulse of a "tracer" fluid into the bulk liquid in a batch-stirred tank, the initial concentration of the tracer at a given sensing point in the tank oscillates from zero to a value higher and then decreases to a value lower than the final, equilibrium value. The tracer concentration will continue to fluctuate about the final value with an exponentially decreasing amplitude (difference from the final value) until equilibrium is reached. The initial value of the amplitude is a function of the position of the sensor relative to the point of tracer addition as well as the concentration of the stock tracer solution. The frequency of the oscillation and the rate of decay of the magnitude of the concentration fluctuations are functions of the intensity of mixing (tank and impeller dimensions, rotational speed of impeller, impeller Reynolds number, etc.). The total time from injection to the final equilibrium state is referred to as the mixing or blend time. It follows that the blend time is a function of the reactor volume and the intensity of mixing. As the reactor volume is reduced, so too is the blend time. Thus blend times in a tubular reactor will be much smaller than in a tank reactor, the fluid in both cases being in the turbulent regime. In a batch stirred tank reactor, the blend time is a function of the position of the sparger relative to the impeller: the closer the sparger is to the impeller, the shorter the blend time. This is because turbulence is at a maximum at the impeller: just below an axial flow impeller and in the annulus surrounding a radial flow impeller. Even in a fully baffled tank with the accompanying turbulence behind the baffles, addition of reagent at the surface of the fluid is nonoptimal with regard to short blend times. Keep in mind that the shorter the blend time, the shorter the life of a local concentration excess. The discussion above was with reference to a pulse of reagent. In the case of continuous addition, the life of a local concentration excess is prolonged, especially at the point of addition. This can readily be visualized by adding a drop of precipitant to the surface of an agitated protein solution. When the precipitant contacts the protein solution, a white streak appears decreasing in density as the flow carries the solution away from the point of addition, until it redissolves and disappears. If one now adds additional drops of precipitant at an increasing frequency, the life of the streak increases to the point where at a given frequency of drop addition it remains continuously in view. This indicates that the local excess concentration of precipitant in the region of the addition point is being maintained and not dissipated. The observed effect of local overprecipitation can be attenuated by vigorous mixing, slow addition of precipitant in a pulsed rather than continuous manner into domains of maximum turbulence, and use of a dilute precipitant stock solution. These problems can be alleviated by operating in a continuous, tubular mode employing static mixers to ensure very short blend times and a more uniform history for each unit volume of the product.

C. Aging and Growth

As mentioned above, following nuclei formation there is a period during which the nuclei grow by diffusion and attachment of molecules coming out of solution forming macroscopic particles (perikinetic growth). Subsequently, as a result of hydrodynamic forces, the particles grow by particle-particle collision and agglomeration (orthokinetic growth). The final aggregate size represents a balance between orthokinetically controlled growth and shear controlled breakup. During the aging period, the precipitate aggregates undergo physical as well as compositional changes. The influence of reactor design, mixing intensity, and the Camp number (the product of shear rate and incubation time) on the size and strength of precipitate aggregates has been discussed above. Suffice it to say that long mean residence times and low intensity of mixing yield the largest and most resistant-to-shear precipitate aggregates.

Simultaneously, the particles can undergo the phenomenon referred to as aging, during which the precipitate proceeds to the equilibrium condition by readjusting its composition by allowing coprecipitated species to resolubilize. This was clearly demonstrated by Watt (410), who reported aging studies on precipitates obtained by the cold ethanol method of Cohn performed in the batch mode. In the case of the Fr.IV precipitate, the amount of coprecipitated albumin was 50% less, after 45 h of aging, than the amount found after 1 h of aging. Chang (415) reported the effect of aging in the precipitation of Cohn fractions Fr.IV$_1$ and Fr.IV$_4$. Significant coprecipitation of albumin was observed during the early part of the precipitation. Aging of the precipitate for 6 to 8 h resulted in the resolubiliz- ation of most of the coprecipitated albumin. There was a cursory reference by Steinbuch (430) to the effect of the time of incubation of the suspension on the concentration of precipitant necessary to insolubilize the target protein: i.e., the Rivanol concentration necessary to precipitate a specific amount of the enzyme, serum cholinesterase, was greater for extended incubation times than for very short times. Regretfully, no data were given as to the specificity of the precipitations. Suffice it to say that the final equilibrium distribution of a given protein will be a function of the various aspects of the technique of precipitant addition and the time following the completion of the addition allotted for the attainment of the equilibrium condition.

1. Acoustic Conditioning

Aging a protein precipitate by gentle agitation for an extended period of time improves its physicochemical characteristics with regard to liquid/solids separations. However, it is good manufacturing practice to reduce processing time as much as possible. Thus we would seek to accelerate the aging processes. Exposure of a suspension of particles to low-frequency acoustic waves has been used to improve particle characteristics so as to facilitate liquid/solids separation operations. Acoustic conditioning of protein precipitates was first reported by Jewett (431). In the initial design, opposing periodic mechanical vibrations at two slightly different frequencies are introduced into the suspension parallel to its flow path as it passes between two vibrating paddles (409). [In the second iteration, the acoustic vibrations were imparted perpendicular to the suspension flow path (432).] As a result, the suspension is subjected to low-frequency (5–10 Hz) traveling beat waves that impart an acceleration to the suspension and cause a transition from the laminar to the turbulent regime at low rates of flow in the chamber. This increase in micromixing is thought to promote particle-particle collisions and aggregation as a function of the time of exposure to the beat waves and the acoustical power input. At the optimum residence time and power input, the number of larger particles was hardly affected, but the number of the smallest particles was greatly reduced due to their "catalyzed" aggregation (433). A third iteration of the design of the acoustic conditioner has a rectangular chamber with a moveable wall that acts as a *single* source of acoustic energy perpendicular to the flow path (434–436). According to these authors, the low-frequency conditioning process is based on the periodic expansion and compression of the volume of the chamber by the action of the oscillating wall. The geometry of the chamber is such that its cross-sectional area is considerably larger than the inlet and outlet pipes. Thus fluid is alternately driven forward into the outlet pipe and sucked back into the chamber from the outlet pipe as a function of the frequency and amplitude of the oscillating wall and the accompanying compression and expansion of the chamber volume. During the expansion phase, the fluid flows back into the chamber as a high-velocity fluid jet in a direction counter-current to that of the suspension flow. This counter-current jet generates turbulent back mixing in the slowly forward moving suspension in the chamber. During the expansion-contraction cycle, the flow in the outlet pipe is pulsatile while the flow in the inlet pipe is constant.

With regard to particle size, there would appear to be two opposing processes consequent to the jet-mixing: (1) particle growth due to enhancement of orthokinetic aggregation by the increased frequency of particle collisions, leading to the elimination of fine particles by successful collisions with larger particles and (2) restriction of the maximum particle size as a result of the erosion of larger particles due to the shear forces existing in the zones of turbulence. The result of these two competing processes will determine the maximum steady-state particle size, which is a function of the balance between the cohesiveness of the aggregate and the destructiveness of the shear forces generated by the mixing jet. Thus there is a narrowing of the particle size distribution. In addition, they report that with appropriate values of frequency and amplitude, larger aggregates had a denser, more compact structure as well as an increased resistance to shear breakup. McIntosh et al. (437) have designed an in-line furrowed channel device for pulsatile flow that mimics the jet mixing behavior of the acoustic conditioning unit.

It should be mentioned that the use of high- and low-frequency acoustic and electroacoustic energy has been proposed for the dewatering and drying of heat-sensitive materials such as food additives and pharmaceuticals as well as sewage sludge. The reader is directed to (438–442).

D. Some Novel Precipitation System Designs

The BSTR and CSTR configurations are the most commonly used industrial protein precipitation reactor designs. As indicated above, a BSTR is optimized by having the appropriate ratio of tank height to diameter, proper impeller type, dimensions and placement relative to the tank bottom, baffles properly placed and sized, and an appropriately designed sparger, properly positioned relative to the impeller. A variation in the CSTR design is centered around the use of a very small-sized tank and the inclusion of "residence time" lengths of tubing downstream of the tank for precipitate growth and aging (443). Another CSTR design variation has the precipitating reagents added into the "mouth" of a recirculating centrifugal pump so as to get very rapid micromixing as well as a length of downstream residence time tubing (444). A CTR is in use at the Protein Fractionation Centre of the Scottish National Blood Transfusion Service in Edinburgh. The design employs a static mixer for dispersion of precipitant reagents and acoustic conditioning for the stages of growth and aging. The total amount of precipitant required is added in "one shot" into the static mixer, and the unit volume of solution passing through the static mixer is very rapidly brought to the desired final precipitant concentration (412). In the BSTR and many of the CSTR designs, the precipitant is continuously or intermittently added to the protein solution so as to reach the desired concentration of precipitant at a defined rate, slow or fast.

Chang (415,445) proposed a CSTR precipitation reactor design, Fig. 3, in which the precipitant reagents were added as a fine spray dispersed in a cone-shaped pattern onto the surface of the protein solution in a small stirred tank. The novel aspect of this design is the continuous addition, through a static mixer, of fresh protein solution to a recirculating suspension of precipitated protein having the final set of conditions, such as pH and the concentration of precipitant. The desired precipitate characteristics were obtained after a minimum residence time in the CSTR. Chang postulated

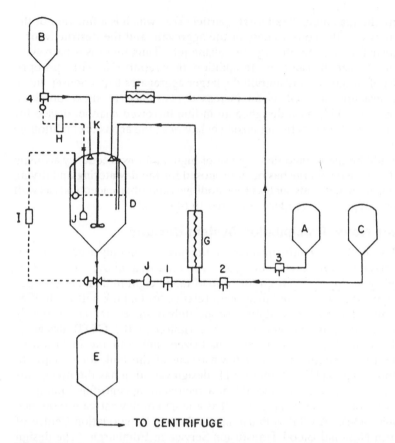

Figure 3 Process flow diagram for continuous plasma fractionation system. (A) alcohol tank; (B) buffer tank; (C) plasma tank; (D) suspension tank; (E) product receiving tank; (F) tubular coller; (G) tubular in-line static mixer; (H) pH analyzer/recorder/controller; (I) liquid level controller with gravity discharge valve; (J) pH probes; (K) agitator; (1) metering pump for precipitated suspension recirculation; (2) metering pump for feed plasma; (3) metering pump for alcohol; (4) metering pump and pneumatic control for buffer. (Taken from Chang, Ref. 415.)

that the protein in the fresh stream would preferentially condense on nuclei already present in the recirculating stream, rather than form additional nuclei. He reported supporting data, such as increased clarity of centrifugate and denser, drier pastes from the centrifuge.

Based on the general principles of crystallization and the empirical observations regarding precipitate formation, I have sought a precipitation reactor design that would eliminate or reduce the occurrence of local precipitant excess and control the number of nuclei formed during the nucleation period. The design would allow for the controlled, gradual increase in precipitant concentration in each microscopic unit volume of solution to the lower levels of supersaturation, while allowing the total addition to occur in an economically acceptable time. In 1975 (unpublished work), I proposed the system shown in Fig. 4. It consists of a residence tank connected to a recirculation line in which are found a recirculation pump, a number of static mixers, and appropriate sensors such as a turbidimeter. The precipitant is metered into the static mixers by a metering pump connected to a correctly designed manifold. Thus if one wishes to achieve a final precipitant concentration of, say, 12%, sufficient precipitant solution is injected into each static mixer so that its concentration in the product solution is increased by 1% at the exit of each static mixer, and the desired 12% precipitant concentration would be reached in three circulations. The essential characteristics of the system are the very rapid homogenization that occurs with a low viscosity solution in a static mixer, drastically reducing local precipitant excess, and the defined gradual increase of the precipitant concentration in each unit volume of the solution. After the addition is

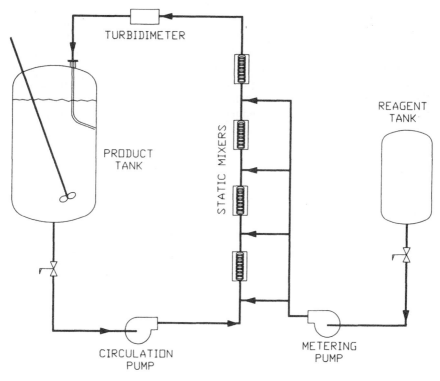

Figure 4 Reagent addition procedure proposed by the author.

complete, the recirculation rate would be greatly reduced, allowing for growth and aging to occur in the recirculation loop. Obviously, one can eliminate the recirculation loop by introducing a larger number of static mixers and have the suspension exit into a tank or an extended length of "residence time" tubing. The system has been implemented at the pilot scale, and the argument for its design was supported by the nature of the precipitates obtained. Not only were the cuts cleaner but the precipitate cake obtained in a tubular bowl centrifuge was drier and more highly organized. The latter was evidenced by the appearance of Newton colors when the paste surface was illuminated with white light.

As a result of mutual discussions concerning the problem of precipitation reactor design, a colleague, D. Severy, suggested the design shown in Fig. 5. The system is configured so that a given protein in solution never sees a precipitant concentration greater than the value required to insolubilize that protein. In addition, it allows for the gradual approach to the supersaturation condition. The central feature of the proposed design is the use of an ultrafiltration module to separate the solvent containing precipitant from the solute to be precipitated, and *using this ultrafiltrate to dilute the precipitant concentrate*. On its return to the product tank, a metered amount of concentrated precipitant reagent is added, by means of a static mixer, to the ultrafiltrate, so that it becomes a dilute solution of precipitant. In the product tank, this dilute precipitant solution is mixed with the concentrated protein in the UF retentate and the original protein solution. As the process proceeds, the concentration of precipitant in the ultrafiltrate increases, and the amount of precipitant concentrate required to be metered into the returning ultrafiltrate must be reduced. Note that the protein of interest will never see a precipitant concentration greater than that required for its insol-

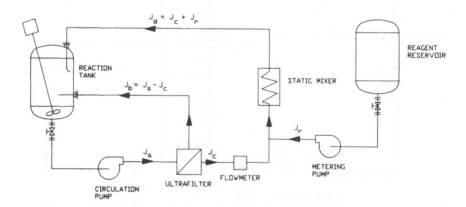

Figure 5   Reagent addition concept in precipitation reactions as proposed by D. Severy.

ubilization. Thus the problem of local excess of precipitant is eliminated. Further, the speed of approach to the final state conditions can be readily controlled by adjusting the flow through the UF module and/or the flow out of the metering pump.

REFERENCES

1. Rothstein, F. (1976). Some principles of plasma protein fractionation, *Hormones in Human Blood* (H. N. Antoniades, ed.), Harvard University Press, Cambridge, Mass., p. 3.
2. Bell, D. J., Hoare, M., and Dunnill, P. (1983). The formation of protein precipitates and their centrifugal recovery, *Advances in Biochemical Engineering/Biotechnology* (A. Fiechter, ed.), *26*: 1. Springer-Verlag, Berlin.
3. Hildebrand, J. H., and Scott, R. L. (1950). *The Solubility of Nonelectrolytes*, 3d ed., Reinhold, New York.
4. Hildebrand, J. H., Prausnitz, J. M., and Scott, R. L. (1970). *Regular and Related Solutions*, Van Nostrand Reinhold, New York.
5. Shinoda, K. (1978). *Principles of Solution and Solubility*, Marcel Dekker, New York.
6. Israelachvili, J. N. (1985). *Intermolecular and Surface Forces*, Academic Press, New York.
7. Burley, S. K., and Petsko, G. A. (1988). Weakly polar interactions in proteins, *Adv. Protein Chem.*, *39*: 125.
8. Gabler, R. (1978). *Electrical Interactions in Molecular Biophysics, An Introduction*, Academic Press, New York.
9. Webb, J. L. (1963). *Enzyme and Metabolic Inhibitors*, vol. 1 Academic Press, New York, p. 204.
10. Kollman, P. A. (1977). Noncovalent interactions, *Acc. Chem. Res.*, *10*: 365.
11. Dykstra, C. E. (1988). Intermolecular electrical interaction, *Acc. Chem. Res.*, *21*: 355.
12. Edsall, J. T., and Wyman, J. (1958). *Biophysical Chemistry*, Academic Press, New York.
13. Fowkes, F. M. (1985). Interface acid-base/charge-transfer properties, *Surface and Interfacial Aspects of Biomedical Polymers* (J. D. Andrade, ed.), Plenum Press, New York, p. 337.
14. Joesten, M. D., and Schaad, L. J. (1974). *Hydrogen Bonding*, Marcel Dekker, New York.
15. Schuster, P., Zundel, G., and Sandorfy, C. (1976). *The Hydrogen Bond*, vols. 1–3, North-Holland, Amsterdam.
16. Fowkes, F. M. (1987). Role of acid-base interfacial bonding in adhesion, *J. Adhesion Sci. Tech.*, *1*: 7.
17. Pimentel, G. C., and McClellan, A. L. (1960). *The Hydrogen Bond*, W. H. Freeman, San Francisco, Calif.
18. Saenger, W. (1987). Structure and dynamics of water surrounding biomolecules, *Ann. Rev. Biophys. Biophys. Chem.*, *16*: 93.
19. Franks, F. (ed.) (1972–1982). *Water: A Comprehensive Treatise*, vols. 1–7, Plenum Press, New York.

20. Edsall, J. T., and McKenzie, H. A. (1978). Water and proteins. I. The significance and structure of water; its interaction with electrolytes and non-electrolytes, *Adv. Biophys.* (Tokyo), *10*: 137.

21. Edsall, J. T., and McKenzie, H. A. (1983). Water and proteins. II. The location and dynamics of water in protein systems and its relation to their stability and properties, *Adv. Biophys.* (Tokyo), *16*: 53.

22. Finney, J. L. (1982). Towards a molecular picture of liquid water, *Biophysics of Water* (F. Franks, ed.), John Wiley, New York, p. 73.

23. Israelachvili, J. N., and McGuiggan, P. M. (1988). Forces between surfaces in liquids, *Science*, *241*: 795.

24. Tanford, C. (1980). *The Hydrophobic Effect*, 2nd ed., Wiley-Interscience, New York.

25. Franks, F. (1975). The hydrophobic interaction, *Water: A Comprehensive Treatise*, vol. 4 (F. Franks, ed.), Plenum Press, New York, p. 1.

26. Jencks, W. P. (1969). *Catalysis in Chemistry and Enzymology*, ch. 8, McGraw-Hill, New York.

27. Dandliker, W. B., and de Saussure, V. A. (1971). Stabilization of macromolecules by hydrophobic bonding: Role of water structure and of chaotropic ions, *The Chemistry of Biosurfaces*, vol. 1 (M. L. Hair, ed.), Marcel Dekker, New York, p. 1.

28. Sinanoglu, O. (1968). Solvent effects on molecular association, *Molecular Associations in Biology* (B. Pullman, ed.), Academic Press, New York, p. 427.

29. Kirkwood, J. G. (1943). The theoretical interpretation of the properties of solutions of dipolar ions, *Proteins, Amino Acids and Peptides* (E. J. Cohn and J. T. Edsall, eds.), Reinhold, New York, ch. 12.

30. Linderstom-Lang, K. (1953). The activity coefficient of large multipolar ions, *C. R. Trav. Carlsberg Ser. Chim.*, *28*: 281.

31. Richards. W. G., King, P. M., and Reynolds, C. A. (1989). Solvation effects, *Protein Eng.*, *2*: 319.

32. van Oss, C. J., and Good, R. J. (1989). Surface tension and the solubility of polymers and biopolymers: The role of polar and apolar interfacial free energies, *J. Macromol. Sci.-Chem.*, *A26*: 1183.

33. van Oss, C. J. Chaudhury, M. K., and Good, R. J. (1988). Interfacial Lifshitz–van der Waals and polar interactions in macroscopic systems, *Chem. Rev.*, *88*: 927.

34. van Oss, C. J., Good, R. J., and Chaudhury, M. K. (1986). Solubility of proteins, *J. Protein Chem.*, *5*: 385.

35. Shaw, D. J. (1980). *Introduction to Colloid and Surface Chemistry* (3d. ed.), Butterworths, London.

36. Verwey, E. J. W., and Overbeek, J. Th. G. (1948). *The Theory of the Stability of Lyophobic Colloids*, Elsevier, Amsterdam.

37. Cohn, E. J. (1943). The solubility of proteins, *Proteins, Amino Acids and Peptides* (E. J. Cohn and J. T. Edsall, eds.), Reinhold, New York, ch. 23.

38. Arakawa, T., and Timasheff, S. N. (1985). Theory of protein solubility, *Meth. Enzymol.*, *114*: 49.

39. Robson, B., and Garnier, J. (1988). *Introduction to Proteins and Protein Engineering*, Elsevier, Amsterdam.

40. Oxender, D. L., and Fox, C. F. (1987). *Protein Engineering*, Alan R. Liss, New York.
41. Creighton, T. E. (1983). *Proteins: Structures and Molecular Principles*, W. H. Freeman, New York.
42. Fasman, G. D. (1989). *Prediction of Protein Structure and the Principles of Protein Conformation*, Plenum Press, New York.
43. Schulz, G. E., and Schirmer, R. H. (1979). *Principles of Protein Structure*, Springer-Verlag, New York.
44. Kauzmann, W. (1959). Some factors in the interpretation of protein denaturation, *Adv. Protein Chem.*, *14*: 1.
45. Privalov, P. L. (1989). Thermodynamic problems of protein structure, *Ann. Rev. Biophys. Biophys. Chem.*, *18*: 47.
46. Lee, B., and Richards, F. M. (1971). The interpretation of protein structures: Estimation of static accessibility, *J. Mol. Biol.*, *55*: 379.
47. Richards, F. M. (1977). Areas, volumes, packing and protein structure, *Ann. Rev. Biophys. Bioeng.*, *6*: 151.
48. Rashin, A., and Honig, B. (1984). On the environment of ionizable groups in globular proteins, *J. Mol. Biol.*, *173*: 515.
49. Miller, S., Janin, J., Lesk, A. M., and Chothia, C. (1987). Interior and surface of monomeric proteins, *J. Mol. Biol.*, *196*: 641.
50. Janin, J., Miller, S., and Chothia, C. (1988). Surface, subunit interfaces and interior of oligomeric proteins, *J. Mol. Biol.*, *204*: 155.
51. Shrake, A., and Rupley, J. A. (1973). Environment and exposure to solvent of protein atoms. Lysozyme and insulin, *J. Mol. Biol.*, *79*: 351.
52. Finney, J. L. (1975). Volume occupation environment and accessibility in proteins. The problem of the protein surface, *J. Mol. Biol.*, *96*: 721.
53. Eisenberg, D., and McLachlan, A. D. (1986). Solvation energy in protein folding and binding, *Nature*, *319*: 199.
54. Oncley, J. L. (1943). The electric moments and the relaxation times of proteins as measured from their influence upon the dielectric constants of solutions, *Proteins, Amino Acids and Peptides* (E. J. Cohn and J. T. Edsall, eds.), Reinhold, New York, ch. 22.
55. Kirkwood, J. G., and Shumaker, J. B. (1952). The influence of dipole moment fluctuations on the dielectric increment of proteins in solution, *Proc. Nat. Acad. Sci. U.S.A.*, *38*: 855.
56. Tanford, C. (1970). *Physical Chemistry of Macromolecules*, John Wiley, New York, p. 196.
57. Rees, D. C., DeAntinio, L., and Eisenberg, D. (1989). Hydrophobic organization of membrane proteins, *Science*, *245*: 510.
58. Kuntz, I. D., and Kauzmann, W. (1974). Hydration of proteins and polypeptides, *Adv. Protein Chem.*, *28*: 239.
59. Rupley, J. A., Gratton, E., and Careri, G. (1983). Water and globular proteins, *TIBS, January*: 18.
60. van Oss, C. J., and Good, R. J. (1988). Orientation of the water molecules of hydration of human serum albumin, *J. Protein Chem.*, *7*: 179.
61. Ben-Naim, A., Ting, K. L., and Jernigan, R. L. (1989). Solvation thermodynamics of biopolymers. I. Separation of the volume and surface interactions with estimates for proteins, *Biopolymers*, *28*: 1309.

62. Inman, J. K., Coryell, F. C., McCall, K. B., Sgouris, J. T., and Anderson, H. D. (1961). A large scale method for the purification of human transferrin, *Vox Sang.*, *6*: 34.

63. Kaldor, G., Saifer, A., and Vecsler, F. (1961). The interaction of Rivanol with bovine serum albumin, *Arch. Biochem. Biophys.*, *94*: 207.

64. Tanford, C. (1961). *Physical Chemistry of Macromolecules*, John Wiley, New York, p. 242.

65. Finlayson, J. S. (1975). Physical and biochemical properties of human albumin, *Proceedings of the Workshop on Albumin* (J. T. Sgouris and A. Rene eds.), DHEW Publication No. (NIH) 76-925, p. 31.

66. Edsall, J. T. (1943). Proteins as acids and bases, *Proteins, Amino Acids and Peptides* (E. J. Cohn and J. T. Edsall, eds.), Reinhold, New York, ch. 20.

67. Leavis, P. C., and Rothstein, F. (1974). the solubility of fibrinogen in dilute salt solutions, *Arch. Biochem. Biophys.*, *161*: 671.

68. von Hippel, Ph. H. (1975). Neutral salt effects on the conformational stability of biological macromolecules, *Protein-Ligand Interactions* (H. Sund and G. Blauer, eds.), Walter de Gruyter, Berlin, p. 452.

69. Cohn, E. J. (1953). The formed and the fluid parts of human blood. Their discovery, characterization and separation by virtue of their physical properties and chemical interactions, *Blood Cells and Plasma Proteins: Their State in Nature* (J. L. Tullis, ed.), Academic Press, New york, p. 18.

70. Cohn, E. J. (1936). Influence of the dielectric constant in biochemical systems, *Chem. Rev.*, *19*: 241.

71. Bacarella, A. L., Grunwald, E., Marshall, H. P., and Purlee, E. L. (1955). The potentiometric measurement of acid dissociation constants and pH in the system methanol-water. pK_A values for carboxylic acids and anilinium ions, *J. Org. Chem.*, *20*: 747.

72. Bates, R. G., Bennetto, H. P., and Sankar, M. (1980). Dissociation constants of acetic acid and primary phosphate ion and standards for pH in 10, 20 and 40 wt % ethanol/water solvents at 25, 0, -5 and -10°C, *Anal. Chem.*, *52*: 1598.

73. Krishtalik, L. I. (1989). Dielectric constant in calculations of the electrostatics of biopolymers, *J. Theor. Biol.*, *139*: 143.

74. Rogers, N. K. (1986). The modelling of electrostatic interactions in the function of globular proteins, *Prog. Biophys. Molec. Biol.*, *38*: 37.

75. Hopfinger, A. J. (1973). *Conformational Properties of Macromolecules*, Academic Press, New York.

76. Richards, M. M. (1937). The effect of glycine upon the activity coefficient of glycine, egg albumin and carboxyhemoglobin, *J. Biol. Chem.*, *122*: 727.

77. Wagner, R. H., McLester, W. D., Smith, M., and Brinkhouse, K. M. (1964). Purification of antihemophilic factor (Factor VIII) by amino acid precipitation, *Thrombos. Diathes. haemorrh.* (Stuttg), *11*: 64.

78. Mellanby, J. (1907). The precipitation of the proteins of horse serum, *J. Physiol.*, *36*: 288.

79. Mellanby, J. (1908). Diphtheria antitoxin, *Proc. Roy. Soc.* (London), *B80*: 399.

80. Ferry, R. M., Cohn, E. J., and Newman, E. S. (1936). Studies in the physical chemistry of the proteins. XIII. The solvent action of sodium chloride on egg albumin in 25% ethanol at -5°, *J. Amer. Chem. Soc.*, *58*: 2370.

81. Wyman, J. (1931). The dielectric constant of mixtures of ethyl alcohol and water from -5 to 40°, *J. Amer. Chem. Soc.*, *58*: 2370.
82. Franks, F., and Eagland, D. (1975). The role of solvent interactions in protein conformation, *CRC Critical Reviews of Biochemistry* (G. Fasman, ed.), *3*: 165. CRC Press, Cleveland, Ohio.
83. Bull, H. B., and Breese, K. (1978). Interaction of alcohols with proteins, *Biopolymers*, *17*: 2121.
84. Maurel, P. (1978). Relevance of dielectric constant and solvent hydrophobicity to the organic solvent effect in enzymology, *J. Biol. Chem.*, *253*: 1677.
85. Velicelebi, G., and Sturtevant, J. M. (1979). Thermodynamics of the denaturation of lysozyme in alcohol-water mixtures, *Biochemistry*, *18*: 1180.
86. Fink, A. L. (1986). Effects of cryoprotectants on enzyme structure, *Cryobiology*, *23*: 28.
87. Arakawa, T., and Goddette, D. (1985). The mechanism of helical transition of proteins by organic solvents, *Arch. Biochem. Biophys.*, *240*: 21.
88. Brandts, J. F., and Hunt, L. (1967). The thermodynamics of protein denaturation. III. The denaturation of ribonuclease in water and in aqueous urea and aqueous ethanol mixtures, *J. Amer. Chem. Soc.*, *89*: 4826.
89. van Oss, C. J. (1989). On the mechanism of the cold ethanol precipitation method of plasma protein fractionation, *J. Prot. Chem.*, *8*: 661.
90. Green, A. A., and Hughes, W. L., Jr., (1955). Protein fractionation on the basis of solubility in aqueous solutions of salts and organic solvents, *Meth. Enzymol.*, *1*: 67.
91. Mellanby, J. (1905). Globulin, *J. Physiol.*, *33*: 338.
92. Dixon, M., and Webb, E. C. (1961). Enzyme fractionation by salting-out: A theoretical note, *Adv. Prot. Chem.*, *16*: 197.
93. Long, F. A., and McDevit, W. F. (1952). Activity coefficients of nonelectrolyte solutes in aqueous salt solutions, *Chem. Rev.*, *51*: 119.
94. Cohn, E. J. (1925). The physical chemistry of proteins, *Physiol. Rev.*, *5*: 349.
95. Salahuddin, A., Waseem, A., Yahiya Khan, M., Abul Qasim, M., and Sibghatullah. (1983). A possible relation between the salting-out behavior of proteins and their surface hydrophobicity, *Indian J. Biochem. Biophys.*, *20*: 127.
96. von Hippel, P. H., and Schleich, T. (1969). The effects of neutral salts on the structure and conformational stability of macromolecules in solution, *Biological Macromolecules*, vol. 2 (S. N. Timasheff and G. D. Fasman, eds.), Marcel Dekker, New York, p. 417.
97. von Hippel, P. H., and Hamabata, A. (1973). Model studies on the effects of neutral salts on the conformational stability of biological macromolecules, *J. Mechanochem. Cell Motility*, *2*: 127.
98. Foster, P. R., Dunnill, P., and Lilly, M. D. (1976). The kinetics of protein salting-out: Precipitation of yeast enzymes by ammonium sulfate, *Biotechnol. Bioeng.*, *18*: 545.
99. Czok, R., and Bucher, Th. (1960). Crystallized enzymes from the myogen of rabbit skeletal muscle, *Adv. Protein Chem.*, *15*: 315.
100. Hofmeister, F. (1888). Zur lehre von der wirkung der saltze, *Arch. Expt. Pathol. Pharmakol.*, *24*: 247.
101. Debye, P. (1927). The electric field of ions and salting out, *Z. physik. Chem.*, *130*: 56.

102. Melander, W., and Horvath, C. (1977). Salt effects on hydrophobic interactions in precipitation and chromatography of proteins: An interpretation of the lyotropic series, *Arch. Biochem. Biophys.*, *183*: 200.

103. Przybycien, T. M., and Bailey, J. E. (1989). solubility-activity relationships in the inorganic salt-induced precipitation of α-chymotrypsin, *Enzyme Microb. Technol.*, *11*: 264.

104. Przybycian, T. M., and Bailey, J. E. (1989). Structure-function relationships in the inorganic salt-induced precipitation of alpha-chymotrypsin, *Biochim. Biophys. Acta*, *995*: 231.

105. Timasheff, S. N., and Arakawa, T. (1988). Mechanism of protein precipitation and stabilization by co-solvents, *J. Crystal Growth*, *90*: 39.

106. Timasheff, S. N., and Arakawa, t. (1989). Stabilization of protein structure by solvents, *Protein Structure: A Practical Approach* (T. E. Creighton, ed.), IRL Press, Oxford, p. 331.

107. Arakawa, T., and Timasheff, S. N. (1984). Mechanism of protein salting in and salting out by divalent cation salts: Balance between hydration and salt binding, *Biochemistry*, *23*: 5912.

108. Arakawa, T., and Timasheff, S. N. (1982). Preferential interactions of proteins with salts in concentrated solutions, *Biochemistry*, *21*: 6545.

109. Arakawa, T., Bhat, R., and Timasheff, S. N. (1990). Preferential interactions determine protein solubility in three-component solutions: The $MgCl_2$ system, *Biochemistry*, *29*: 1914.

110. Arakawa, T., Bhat, R., and Timasheff, S. N., (1990). Why preferential hydration does not always stabilize the native structure of globular proteins, *Biochemistry*, *29*: 1924.

111. Breslow, R., and Guo, T. (1990). Surface tension measurements show that chaotropic salting-in denaturants are not just water-structure breakers, *Proc. Nat. Acad. Sci. USA*, *87*: 167.

112. Hardy, W. B. (1905). Colloidal solution; The globulins, *J. Physiol.*, *33*: 251.

113. Sorensen, S. P. L., and Sladek, I. (1929). On W. O. Ostwald's "Bodenkörper-Regel" and the solubility of casein in sodium hydroxide, *Compt. rend. Trav. Lab. Carlsberg*, *17*: 1.

114. Edsall, J. T. (1930). studies in the physical chemistry of muscle globulin. II. On some physicochemical properties of muscle globulin (myosin), *J. Biol. Chem.*, *89*: 289.

115. Green, A. A. (1931). Studies in the physical chemistry of the proteins. IX. The effect of electrolytes on the solubility of hemoglobin in solutions of varying hydrogen ion activity with a note on the comparable behavior of casein, *J. Biol. Chem.*, *93*: 517.

116. Collins, K. D., and Washabaugh, M. W. (1985). The Hofmeister effect and the behavior of water at interfaces, *Q. Rev. Biophys.*, *18*: 323.

117. Voet, A. (1937). Quantitative lyotropy, *Chem. Rev.*, *20*: 169.

118. Robinson, D. R., and Jencks, W. P. (1965). The effect of concentrated salt solutions on the activity coefficient of ATGEE, *J. Amer. Chem. Soc.*, *87*: 2470.

119. Nandi, P. K., and Robinson, D. R. (1972). The effects of salts on the free energies of nonpolar groups in model peptides, *J. Amer. Chem. Soc.*, *87*: 2470.

120. Schrier, E. E., and Schrier, E. B. (1967). The salting-out behavior of amides and its relation to the denaturation of proteins by salts, *J. Phys. Chem.*, *71*: 1851.
121. Fredericq, E., and Neurath, H. (1950). The interaction of insulin with thiocyanate and other anions. The minimum molecular weight of insulin, *J. Amer. Chem. Soc.*, *72*: 2684.
122. Reis-Kautt, M. M., and Ducruix, A. f. (1989). Relative effectiveness of various ions on the solubility and crystal growth of lysozyme, *J. Biol. Chem.*, *264*: 745.
123. Bruins, E. M. (1934). The lyotropic number and its elucidation, *Rec. trav. chim.*, *53*: 292.
124. Bull, H. B., and Breese, K. (1980). Protein solubility and the lyotropic series of ions, *Arch. Biochem. Biophys.*, *202*: 116.
125. Franks, F., and Eagland, D. (1975). The role of solvent interactions in protein conformation, *Critical Reviews in Biochem.*, *3*: 165.
126. Taylor, R. P., and Kuntz, I. D., Jr. (1972). Proton acceptor abilities of anions and possible relevance to the Hofmeister series, *J. Amer. Chem. soc.*, *94*: 7963.
127. Muller, N. (1988). Is there a region of highly structured water around a nonpolar solute molecule, *J. Solution Chem.*, *17*: 661.
128. Jain, S. M. (1982). Fractionation of protein mixtures, *U. S. Patent No. 4,351,710.*
129. Nemethy, G., and Scheraga, H. A. (1962). The structure of water and hydrophobic bonds in proteins, *J. Phys. Chem.*, *66*: 1773.
130. Alderton, G., Ward, W. H., and Fevold, H. L. (1945). Isolation of lysozyme from egg white, *J. Biol. Chem.*, *157*: 43.
131. Laki, K. (1951). The polymerization of proteins: The action of thrombin on fibrinogen, *Arch. Biochem. Biophys.*, *32*: 317.
132. Chen, C.-C., Zhu, Y., and Evans, L. B. (1989). Phase partitioning of biomolecules: Solubilities of amino acids, *Biotechnol. Prog.*, *5*: 111.
133. Keller S., and Block, R. J. (1960). Separation of proteins, *A Laboratory Manual of Analytical Methods of Protein Chemistry*, vol. 1 (P. Alexander and R. J. Block, eds.), Pergamon Press, New York, p. 2.
134. Pennell, R. B. (1960). Fractionation and isolation of purified components by precipitation methods, *The Plasma Proteins*, vol. 1, (F. W. Putnam, ed.), Academic Press, New York, p. 9.
135. Schultze, H. E., and Heremans, J. F. (1966). *Molecular Biology of Human Proteins, With Special Reference to Plasma Proteins*, vol. 1, Elsevier, New York.
136. Sandor, G. (1966). *Serum Proteins in Health and Disease*, William and Wilkins, Baltimore, Md.
137. Reid, A. F., and Jones, F. (1951). Fractionation of blood plasma proteins using ion exchange resins—Revised techniques, *Ind. Eng. Chem.*, *43*: 1074.
138. Nitschmann, H., Kistler, P., Renfer, H. R., Hassig, A., and Joss, A. (1956). A heat stable human plasma protein solution obtained by desalting (PPL), *Vox. Sang.*, *1*: 183.
139. Bing, D. H., DiDonno, A. C., Regan, M., and Strang, C. J. (1986). Blood plasma processing by electrodialysis, *Membrane Separations in Biotechnology* (W. C. McGregor, ed.), Marcel Dekker, New York, p. 135.
140. Edsall, J. T. (1947). The plasma proteins and their fractionation, *Adv. Protein Chem.*, *3*: 384.

141. Taylor, J. F. (1953). The isolation of proteins, *The Proteins*, vol. 1, part A (H. Neurath and K. Bailey, eds.), Academic Press, New York, p. 2.

142. Mosse, J. (1959). Sur la séparation des proteines du serum sanguin par précipitation au sulfate d'ammonium, *Compt. rend. Acad. Sci.* (Paris), *249*: 2638.

143. Heide, K., and Schwick, H. G. (1973). Salt fractionation of immunoglobulines, *Handbook of Experimental Immunology*, vol. 1 (D. M. Wier, ed.), 2d ed., Blackwell Scientific, Oxford, p. 6. 1.

144. Harms, A. J. (1946). Abnormal precipitation of proteins from antitoxic horse plasma in the presence of phenolic compounds, *Nature, 157*: 514.

145. Harms, A. J. (1953). Studies on the blood proteins of hyperimmune horses. I. The effect of high concentrations of phenolic substances on the proteins of plasma, *J. Sci. Food Agric., 4*: 65.

146. Schilling, K. (1953). Serum protein fractionation by means of ammonium sulfate in the presence of phenolic compounds, *Acta Chem. Scand., 7*: 1007.

147. Michon, J., and Arnaud, R. (1964). Fractionation of plasma proteins by phenol and ammonium sulfate, *Proteides of the Biological Fluids, Proc. 11th Colloq.* (H. Peeters, ed.), Elsevier, Amsterdam, p. 437.

148. Kazal, L. A., Amsel, S., Miller, O. P., and Tocantins, L. M. (1963). The preparation and some properties of fibrinogen precipitated from human plasma by glycine, *Proc. Soc. Exp. Biol. Med.* (N.Y.), *113*: 989.

149. Straughn, W., III, and Wagner, R. H. (1966). A simple method for preparing fibrinogen, *Thrombos. Diathes. Haemorrh.* (Stuttg.), *16*: 198.

150. Zahn, R. K., and Stahl, I. (1953). Die kontinuierliche extraction von stoffgemischen unter änderung eines parameters nach dem volum-erzatsprinzip, *Z. Physiol. Chem., 293*: 1.

151. Zahn, R. K., and Stahl, I. (1955). Die kontinuierliche extraction von stoffgemischen unter beliebiger änderung beliebiger parameter nach dem prinzip der diagramm-abtastung, *Z. physiol. Chem., 302*: 204.

152. Keil, B., Keilova, H., and Bartosek, I. (1962). Column gradient extraction of proteins, *Coll. Czech. Chem. Commun., 27*: 2940.

153. King, T. P. (1972). Separation of proteins by ammonium sulfate gradient solubilization, *Biochemistry, 11*: 367.

154. Sargent, R. N., and Graham, D. L. (1964). Salting-out chromatography of serum proteins, *Anal. Chim. Acta, 30*: 101.

155. von der Haar, F. (1976). Purification of proteins by fractional interfacial salting out on unsubstituted agarose gels, *Biochem. Biophys. Res. Commun., 70*: 1009.

156. Porath, J. (1962). Zone precipitation, *Nature, 196*: 47.

157. Rickets, C. R. (1952). Interaction of dextran with fibrinogen, *Nature, 169*: 970.

158. Laurent, T. C. (1963). The interaction between polysaccharides and other macromolecules 5. The solubility of proteins in the presence of dextran, *Biochem. J., 89*: 253.

159. Laurent, T. C. (1963). The interaction between polysaccharides and other macromolecules 6. Further studies on the solubility of proteins in dextran solutions, *Acta Chem. Scand., 17*: 2664.

160. Kroll, J., and Dybkaer, R. (1964). In vitro precipitations in plasma by low molecular weight dextran, *Scand. J. Clin. Lab. Invest., 16*: 31.

161. Dudman, W. F. (1966). Precipitation of tobacco mosaic virus by macromolecules: A method for estimating molecular volumes, *Nature, 211*: 1049.

162. Iverius, P. H. (1968). Solubility of low density (beta-lipoproteins in the presence of dextran, *Clin. Chim. Acta.*, *20*: 261.
163. Rampling, M. W. (1974). The solubility of fibrinogen in solutions containing dextrans of various molecular weights, *Biochem. J.*, *143*: 767.
164. Perkins, H. A., Rolfs, M. R., Thatcher, C. and Richards, V. (1966). Effect of polyvinyl pyrrolidone on plasma coagulation factors, *Proc. Soc. Exper. Biol. Med.* (N.Y.), *123*: 667.
165. Casillas, G., and Simonetti, C. (1982). Polyvinylpyrrolidone (PVP): A new precipitating agent for human and bovine factor VIII and fibrinogen, *British J. Haemat.*, *50*: 665.
166. Garcia, L. A., and Ordonez, G. A. (1976). The use of pluronic polyols in the precipitation of plasma proteins and its application in the preparation of plasma derivatives, *Transfusion*, *16*: 32.
167. Stocking, C. R. (1956). Precipitation of enzymes during isolation of chloroplasts in Carbowax, *Science*, *123*: 1032.
168. Polson, A., Potgieter, G. M., Largier, J. F., Mears, G. E. F., and Joubert, F. J. (1964). The fractionation of protein mixtures by linear polymers of high molecular weight, *Biochim. Biophys. Acta*, *82*: 463.
169. Fried, M., and Chun, P. W. (1971). Water-soluble nonionic polymers in protein purification, *Meth. Enzymol.*, *22*: 238.
170. Juckes, I. R. M. (1971). Fractionation of proteins and viruses with polyethylene glycol, *Biochim. Biophys. Acta*, *229*: 535.
171. Foster, P. R., Dunnill, P., and Lilly, M. D. (1973). The precipitation of enzymes from cell extracts of *Saccharomyces cerevisiae* by polyethyleneglycol, *Biochim. Biophys. Acta*, *317*: 505.
172. Hao, Y. L., Ingham, K. C., and Wickerhauser, M. (1980). Fractional precipitation of proteins with polyethylene glycol, *Methods in Plasma Protein Fractionation* (J. Curling, ed.), Academic Press, New York, p. 57.
173. Ingham, K. C. (1984). Protein precipitation with polyethylene glycol, *Meth. Enzymol.*, *104*: 351.
174. Laurent, T. C. (1966). Solubility of proteins in the presence of polysaccharides, *Federation Proc.*, *25*: 1127.
175. Ogston, A. G. (1958). The spaces in a uniform random suspension of fibres, *Trans. Faraday Soc.*, *54*: 1754.
176. Ogston, A. G., and Phelps, C. F. (1960). The partition of solutes between buffer solutions and solutions containing hyaluronic acid, *Biochem. J.*, *78*: 827.
177. Edmond, E., and Ogston, A. G. (1968). An approach to the study of phase separation in ternary aqueous systems, *Biochem. J.*, *109*: 569.
178. Ogston, A. G. (1970). On the interaction of solute molecules with porous networks, *J. Phys. Chem.*, *74*: 668.
179. Atha, D. H., and Ingham, K. C. (1981). Mechanism of precipitation of proteins by polyethylene glycols, *J. Biol. Chem.*, *256*: 12108.
180. Hermans, J. (1982). Excluded volume theory of polymer-protein interactions based on polymer chain statistics, *J. Chem. Phys.*, *77*: 2193.
181. Knoll, D, and Hermans, J. (1983). Polymer-protein interactions: Comparison of experiment and excluded volume theory, *J. Biol. Chem.*, *258*: 5710.
182. Hasko, F., Vaszileva, R., and Halasz, L. (1982). Solubility of plasma proteins in the presence of polyethylene glycol, *Biotechnol. Bioeng.*, *24*: 1931.

183. Polson, A. (1977). A theory for the displacement of proteins and viruses with polyethylene glycol, *Prep. Biochem.*, 7: 129.

184. Honig, W., and Kula, M.-R. (1976). Selectivity of protein precipitation with polyethylene glycol fractions of various molecular weights, *Anal. Biochem.*, 72: 502.

185. Lee, J. C., and Lee, L. L. Y., (1981). Preferential solvent interactions between proteins and polyethylene glycols, *J. Biol. Chem.*, 256: 625.

186. Arakawa, T., and Timasheff, S. N. (1985). Mechanism of poly(ethylene glycol) interaction with proteins, *Biochemistry*, 24: 6756.

187. Lee, L. L. Y., and Lee, J. C. (1987). Thermal stability of proteins in the presence of poly(ethylene glycols), *Biochemistry*, 26: 7813.

188. Comper, W. D., and Laurent, T. C. (1978). An estimate of the enthalpic contribution to the interaction between dextran and albumin, *Biochem. J.*, 175: 703.

189. Knoll, D. A., and Hermans, J. (1981). Effect of poly(ethylene glycol) on protein denaturation and model compound pK_a's, *Biopolymers*, 20: 1747.

190. Bigelow, C. C. (1967). On the average hydrophobicity of proteins and the relation between it and protein structure, *J. Theor. Biol.*, 16: 187.

191. Eichele, G., Karabelnik, D., Halonbrenner, R., Jansonius, J. N., and Christen, P. (1978). Catalytic activity in crystal of mitochondrial aspartate aminotransferase as detected by microspectrophotometry, *J. Biol. Chem.*, 253: 5239.

192. Ingham, K. C., and Busby, T. F. (1980). Methods of removing polyethylene glycol from plasma fractions, *Chem. Eng. Commun.*, 7: 315.

193. Busby, T. F., and Ingham, K. C. (1980). Removal of polyethylene glycol from proteins by salt-induced phase separation, *Vox. Sang.*, 39: 93.

194. Hardy, W. B., and Gardiner, Mrs. S. (1910). Proteins of blood plasma, *J. Physiol.*, 40: lxviii.

195. Dean, H. R. (1913). An attempt to preserve haemolytic complement in a permanent form, *J. Path Bact.*, 18: 118.

196. Hartley, P. (1925). Observations on the role of the ether-soluble constituents of serum in certain serological reactions, *Brit. J. Exper. Path.*, 6: 180.

197. Felton, L. D. (1931). The use of ethyl alcohol as precipitant in the concentration of antipneumococcus serum, *J. Immunol.*, 21: 357.

198. Merrill, M. H., and Fleisher, M. S. (1933). Factors involved in the use of organic solvents as precipitating and drying agents of immune sera, *J. Gen. Physiol.*, 16: 243.

199. Liu, S.-C., and Wu, H. (1934). Fractional precipitation of serum proteins with methyl alcohol, *Chinese J. Physiol.*, 8: 97.

200. Cohn, E. J., Leutscher, J. A., Jr., Oncley, J. L., Armstrong, S. H., Jr., and Davis, B. D. (1940). Preparation and properties of serum and plasma proteins. III. Size and charge of proteins separating upon equilibration across membranes with ethanol-water mixtures of controlled pH, ionic strength, and temperature, *J. Amer. Chem. Soc.*, 62: 3396.

201. Cohn, E. J., Strong, L. E., Hughes, W. L., Jr., Mulford, D. J., Ashworth, J. N., Melin, M., and Taylor, H. L. (1946). Preparation and properties of serum and plasma proteins. IV. A system for the separation into fractions of the protein and lipoprotein components of biological tissues and fluids, *J. Amer. Chem. Soc.*, 68: 459.

202. Strong, L. E. (1948). Blood fractionation, *Encyclopedia of Chemical Technology*, vol. 2 (R. E. Kirk and D. F. Othmer, eds.), Interscience Encyclopedia, New York, p. 556.
203. Oncley, J. L., Melin, M., Richert, D. A., Cameron, J. W., and Gross, P. M., Jr. (1949). The separation of the antibodies, isoagglutinins, prothrombin, plasminogen, and beta$_1$-lipoprotein into subfractions of human plasma, *J. Amer. Chem. Soc.*, *71*: 541.
204. Pillemer, L. (1943). The separation and concentration of the *iso*haemagglutinins from human serums, *Science*, *97*: 75.
205. Fasoli, A. (1949). Curve di solubilità delle proteine plasmatiche in miscele acqua-meanolo a freddo, *Experientia*, *5*: 406.
206. Dubert, J. M., Slizewicz, Rebeyrotte, P., and Macheboeuf, M. (1953). Nouvelle méthode de séparation des proteines sériques par le méthanol. Application aux sérums de lapin et de cheval, *Annales de L'Institut Pasteur*, *84*: 370.
207. Askonas, B. A. (1951). The use of organic solvents at low temperature for the separation of enzymes. Application to aqueous rabbit muscle extract, *Biochem. J.*, *48*: 42.
208. Mackay, M. E. (1955). The fractionation of mammalian serum proteins with ether, *Biochem. J.*, *60*: 475.
209. Sumner, J. B., and Dounce, A. L. (1937). Crystalline catalase, *J. Biol. Chem.*, *121*: 417.
210. Blomback, B., Blomback, M., and Holmberg, E. (1966). A new method for fractionation of proteins, *Acta Chem. Scand.*, *20*: 2317.
211. Schneider, M. (1978). Process for extracting a polypeptide from an aqueous solution, *U.S. Patent No. 4,066,505*.
212. Schneider, M., Guillot, C., and Lamy, B. (1981). The affinity precipitation technique. Application to the isolation and purification of trypsin from bovine pancreas, *Ann. N.Y. Acad. Sci.*, *369*: 257.
213. Taniguchi, M. Kobayashi, M. Natsui, K., and Fujii, M. (1989). Purification of Staphylococcal Protein A by affinity precipitation using a reversibly soluble-insoluble polymer with human IgG as a ligand, *J. Ferment. Bioeng.*, *68*: 32.
214. Nguyen, A. L., and Luong, J. H. T. (1989). Syntheses and applications of water-soluble reactive polymers for purification and immobilization of biomolecules, *Biotechnol. Bioeng.*, *34*: 1186.
215. Senstad, C., and Mattiasson, B. (1989). Affinity precipitation using chitosan as ligand carrier, *Biotechnol. Bioeng.*, *33*: 216.
216. Senstad, C., and Mattiasson, B. (1989). Precipitation of soluble affinity complexes by a second affinity interaction: A model study, *Biotechnol. Appl. Biochem.*, *11*: 41.
217. Bradshaw, A. P., and Sturgeon, R. J. (1990). The synthesis of soluble polymer-ligand complexes for affinity precipitation studies, *Biotechnol. Tech.*, *4*: 67.
218. Green, A. A. (1938). The amphoteric properties of certain globulin fractions of normal horse serum, *J. Amer. Chem. Soc.*, *60*: 1108.
219. Oncley, J. L., Ellenbogen, E., Gitlin, D., and Gurd, F. R. N. (1952). Protein-protein interactions, *J. Phys. Chem.*, *56*: 85.
220. Osborne, T. B., and Harris, I. F. (1905). The solubility of globulin in salt solution, *Amer. J. Physiol.*, *14*: 151.

221. Cohn, E. J., Surgenor, D. M., Schmid, K., Batchelor, W. H., Isliker, H. C., and Alameri, E. H. (1953). The interaction of plasma proteins with heavy metals and with alkaline earths, with specific anions and specific steroids, with specific polysaccharides, and with the formed elements of the blood, *Discussions Faraday Soc., 13*: 176.

222. Gurd, F. R. N. (1954). The specificity of metal-protein interactions, *Ion Transport Across Membranes* (H. T. Clarke and D. Nachmansohn, eds.), Academic Press, New York, p. 246.

223. Gurd, F. R. N., and Wilcox, P. E. (1956). Complex formation between metallic cations and proteins, peptides and amino acids, *Adv. Protein Chem., 11*: 311.

224. Astrup, T., Schilling, K., Birch-Anderson, A., and Olsen, E. (1954). Fractional precipitation of serum proteins by heavy metal ions, *Acta Chem. Scand., 8*: 1361.

225. Uriel, J. (1961). Interaction entre des proteines sériques et des cations métalliques, *Biol. Med., 50*: 27.

226. Aoki, K., and Hori, J. (1964). Effect of metallic cations on human serum: Study by starch-gel electrophoresis I. Effect of Pb^{++}, Cu^{++} and NH_4^+, *Arch. Biochem. Biophys., 106*: 317.

227. Aoki, K., Hori, J., and Kawashima, K. (1967). Effect of metallic cations on human serum: Study by starch-gel electrophoresis II. Effect of Hg^{++}, Cr^{++}, Ag^{++}, Ni^{++}, Cd^{++}, Zn^{++}, Ba^{++}, Mg^{++}, Al^{+++} and Fe^{+++}, *Arch. Biochem. Biophys., 120*: 255.

228. Steven, F. S., Griffin, M. M., Brown, B. S., and Hulley, T. P. (1982). Aggregation of fibrinogen molecules by metal ions, *Int. J. Biol. Macromol., 4*: 367.

229. Maeda, H., Kishi, T., Ikeda, S., Sasaki, S., and Kito, K. (1983). Interaction of human fibrinogen with divalent metal chlorides, *Int. J. Biol. Macromol., 5*: 159.

230. Escribano, J. (1964). Emploi de l'acétate de cuivre pour la séparaton des gamma-globulines sériques, *Vox Sang., 9*: 463.

231. Van Dam, M. E., Wuenschell, G. E., and Arnold, F. H. (1989). Metal affinity precipitation of proteins, *Biotechnol. Appl. Biochem., 11*:492.

232. Lewin, J. (1954). Techniques de préparation des gamma-globulines au Centre national de Transfusion sanguine. Nouvelles méthods, *Thérapie, 9*: 523.

233. Lewin J., and Steinbuch, M. (1955). Modifications apportées aux méthodes de fractionnement par l'alcool en vue de la préparation des gamma-globulines destinées a l'emploi clinique, *Les Gamma Globulines et la Médecine des Enfants*, Masson, Paris, p. 75.

234. Rejnek, J., and Skvaril, F. (1957). Untersuchung der einwirkung von metallen auf plasmaeiweisstoffe I. Einfluss von aluminum auf die eiweisstoffe aus plasma, serum und die Fraktionen II + III, *Coll. Czech. Chem. Commun., 22*: 1489.

235. Rejnek, J., and Skvaril, F. (1958). Untersuchung der einwirkung von metallen auf plasmaeiweisstoffe II. Anwendung der kombination von Zn^{2+}- und Al^{3+}-ionen für die isolierung von gamma-globulin aus Fraktion II + III und menschlichem plasma, *Coll. Czech. Chem. Commun., 23*: 733.

236. Rejnek, J., and Skvaril, F. (1959). Untersuchung der einwirkung von metallen auf plasmaeiweisstoffe III. Isolierung der alpha- und beta-globulinfraktionen aus der ethanol Fraktion II + III, *Coll. Czech. Chem. Commun., 24*: 1327.

237. Heremans, J. F., Heremans, M.-Th., and Schultze, H. E. (1959). Isolation and description of a few properties of the beta$_{2A}$-globulin of human serum, *Clin. Chim. Acta, 4*: 96.

238. Cambier, J. C., and Butler, J. E. (1974). A rapid method for the purification of immunoglobulin M (IgM) from the sera of certain mammalian species, *Prep. Biochem., 4*: 31.

239. Cohn, E. J., Gurd, F. Rn. N., Surgenor, D. M., Barnes, B. A., Brown, R. K., Derouaux, G., Gillespie, J. M., Kahnt, F. W., Lever, W. F., Liu, C. H., Mittelman, D., Mouton, R. F., and Schmid, K., and Uroma, E. (1950). A system for the separation of the components of human blood: Quantitative procedures for the separation of the protein components of human plasma, *J. Amer. Chem. Soc., 72*: 465.

240. Surgenor, D. M., Pennell, R. B., Alameri, E., Batchelor, W. H., Brown, R. K., Hunter, M. J., and Mannick, V. L. (1960). Preparation and properties of serum and plasma proteins, XXXV. A system of protein fractionation using zinc complexes, *Vox Sang., 5*: 272.

241. Zaworski, P. G., and Gill, G. S. (1988). Precipitation and recovery of proteins from culture supernatants using zinc, *Anal. Biochem., 173*: 440.

242. Collingwood, T. N., Daniel, R. M., and Langdon, A. G. (1988). An M(III)-facilitated flocculation technique for enzyme recovery and concentration, *J. Biochem. Biophys. Methods, 17*: 303.

243. Collingwood, T. N., Shanmugam, M., Daniel, R. M., and Langdon, A. G. (1989). M(III)-facilitated recovery and concentration of enzymes from mesophilic and thermophilic organisms, *J. Biochem. Biophys. Methods, 19*: 281.

244. Michael, S. E. (1939). The precipitation of proteins with complex salts, *Biochem. J., 33*: 924.

245. Brown, M. E., and Rothstein, F. (1967). Fibrinogen from human plasma: Preparation by precipitation with heavy-metal coordination complex, *Science, 155*: 1017.

246. Mannuzza, F. J., and Rothstein, F. (1971). The isolation of fibrinogen with mercury complexes and their interaction, *Vox Sang., 20*: 480.

247. Horejsi, J., and Smetana, R. (1954). The effect of "Rivanol" on plasma proteins, *Coll. Czech. Chem. Commun., 19*: 1316.

248. Horejsi, J., and Smetana, R. (1956). The isolation of gamma globulin from blood-serum by Rivanol, *Acta Med. Scand., 155*: 65.

249. Scheiffarth, F., Gotz, H., and Zicha, L. (1958). Vergleichende elektrophoretische und immunologische untersuchungen an isoliertem gamma-globulin, *Z. Immunforsch. Exp. Therap., 115*: 92.

250. Saifer, A., and Lipkin, L. E. (1959). Electrophoretic and immunologic studies of Rivanol-fractionated serum proteins, *Proc. Soc. Exp. Biol. Med., 102*: 220.

251. Neurath, A. R., Malik, Z., and Altaner, C. (1961). Immunochemisches studium eines modifizierten verfahrens zur gewinnung von immuno-globulinen mittels Rivanol, *Z. Immunoforsch. Exp. Therap., 121*: 239.

252. Korinek, J., and Paluska, E. (1961). Immunochemical studies of Rivanol-soluble serum proteins, *Folia Biologica, 7*: 185.

253. Schatz, H. (1965). Untersuchungen an mittels Rivanol gewonnenen serumfraktionen, *Acta Med. Scand., 177*: 427.

254. Boettcher, E. W., Kistler, P., and Nitschmann, Hs. (1958). Method of isolating the beta$_1$-metal-combining globulin from human blood plasma, Nature, 181: 490.

255. Patras, B., and Stone, W. H. (1961). Partial purification of cattle serum transferrin using Rivanol, Proc. Soc. Exp. Biol. Med., 107: 861.

256. Steinbuch, M., and Quentin, M. (1959). Preparation of ceruloplasmin, Nature, 183: 323.

257. Steinbuch, M., and Pejaudier, L. (1959). The behavior of haptoglobin during routine fractionation, Nature, 184: 362.

258. Miller, K. (1959). Rivanol, resin, and the isolation of thrombins, Nature, 184: 450.

259. Steinbuch, M., and Niewiarowski, S. (1960). Rivanol in the preparation of plasminogen (profibrinolysin), Nature, 186: 87.

260. Steinbuch, M., Quentin, M., and Pejaudier, L. (1965). Specific technique for the isolation of human alpha$_2$-macroglobulin, Nature, 205: 227.

261. Steinbuch, M., and Blatrix, Ch. (1970). Préparation de l'alpha$_2$-macroglobuline comme sous-produit du frationnement, Rev. Franc. Transf. Immuno. Hematol., 13: 141.

262. Rejnek, J., Bednarik, T., and Masek, J. (1961). Preparation of serum albumin by the Rivanol method (in Czech), Ceskoslov. farm., 10: 407.

263. Steinbuch, M., Granier, C., Tavernier, D., and Faure, A. (1979). Side products of routine plasma fractionation. I. Serum cholinesterase, Vox Sang., 36: 142.

264. Franek, F. (1986). Purification of IgG monoclonal antibodies from ascitic fluid based on Rivanol precipitation, Meth. Enzymol., 121: 631.

265. Dietzel, E., and Geiger, H. (1964). Gewinnung und eigenschaften therapeutisch wichtiger human-plasmaproteine, Behringwerke-Mitteil., 43: 129.

266. Heide, K., and Haupt, H. (1964). Darstellung noch nicht therapeutisch angewandter plasmaproteine, Behringwerke-Mitteil., 43: 161.

267. Schultze, H. E., and Heremans, J. F. (1966). Molecular Biology of Human Proteins, vol. 1, Elsevier, Amsterdam, p. 261.

268. Stastny, M., and Horejsi, J. (1961). The interaction of acridine dyes with blood plasma proteins, Clin. Chim. Acta, 6: 782.

269. Kaldor, G., Saifer, A., and Vecsler, F. (1961). The interaction of Rivanol with bovine serum albumin, Arch. Biochem. Biophys., 94: 207.

270. Matthaeus, W., and Matheka, H. D. (1963). Über die gewinnung von normal and MKS-immunoglobulinen aus entsprechenden seren vom rind und meerschweinchen mittels Rivanol. I. Mitteilung. Die fraktionierung und isolierung von rinderserumproteinen mit Rivanol und sein chemisches verhalten in proteinfreier und proteinhaltiger lösung, Zentr. Bakteriol. Parasitenk., Abt. I, Orig., 188: 6.

271. Neurath, A. R., and Brunner, R. (1969). Fractionation of proteins with different isoelectric points by Rivanol, Experientia, 25: 668.

272. Sutton, H. E., and Karp, G. W., Jr. (1965). Adsorption of Rivanol by potato starch in the isolation of transferrins, Biochem. Biophys. Acta., 107: 153.

273. Nelson, J. W. (1971). Process of removing acrinol from gamma globulin using siliceous material such as silica gel, U.S. Patent No. 3,607,857.

274. Kurioka, S., Inoue, F., and Nakada, F. (1975). Purification of fibrinogen using cationic detergent, J. Biochem., 77: 457.

275. Mylon, e., Winternitz, M. C., and de Suto-Nagy, G. J. (1942). The determination of fibrinogen with protamine, *J. Biol. Chem.*, *143*: 21.
276. Godal, H. C. (1960). The interaction of protamine with human fibrinogen and the significance of this interaction for the coagulation of fibrinogen, *Scandinav. J. Clin. Lab. Investigation*, *12*: 433.
277. Morawetz, H., and Hughes, W. L., Jr. (1952). The interaction of proteins with synthetic polyelectrolytes. I. Complexing of bovine serum albumin, *J. Phys. Chem.*, *56*: 64.
278. McKernan, W. M., and Ricketts, C. R. (1960). A basic derivative of dextran and its interaction with serum albumin, *Biochem. J.*, *76*: 117.
279. Boehringer Mannheim G. M. B. H. 1972). Process for the enrichment of proteins, *U. K. Patent No. 1,298,431.*
280. Snoke, R. E., and Klein, W. (1977). Purification of microbial enzyme extracts using synthetic polyelectrolytes, *U.S. Patent No. 4,055,469.*
281. Hodo, H. G., III, and Blatti, S. P. (1977). Purification using polyethylenimine precipitation and low molecular weight subunit analyses of calf thymus and wheat germ DNA-dependent RNA polymerase II, *Biochemistry*, *16*: 2334.
282. Hoch, H., and Chanutin, A. (1954). Albumin from heated human plasma. I. Preparation and electrophoretic properties, *Arch. Biochem. Biophys.*, *50*: 271.
283. Chanutin, A., and Curnish, R. R. (1960). The precipitation of plasma proteins by short-chain fatty acids, *Arch. Biochem. Biophys.*, *89*: 218.
284. Steinbuch, M., and Audran, R. (1965). Technique de purification des immunoglobulinés, *Transfusion* (Paris), *8*: 141.
285. Steinbuch, M., and Audran, R. (1969). The isolation of IgG from mammalian sera with the aid of caprylic acid, *Arch. Biochem. Biophys.*, *134*: 279.
286. Pejaudier, L., Audran, R., and Steinbuch, M. (1970). Caprylic acid as an aid for the rapid isolation of human ceruloplasmin, *Clin. Chim. Acta.*, *30*: 387.
287. Steinbuch, M., Audran, R., Balan, S., and Pejaudier, L. (1971). Méthode d'isolement de l'orosomucoide du plasma humain, *C. R. Acad. Sci.* (Paris), *272*: 655.
288. Fine, J. M., and Steinbuch, M. (1971). A simple technique for the isolation of monoclonal IgG and IgA, *Rev. Franc. Clin. Biol.*, *15*: 1115.
289. Steinbuch, M., and Audran, R. (1972). *C. R. Acad. Sci.* (Paris), *274*: 2805.
290. Steinbuch, M. (1980). Protein fractionation by ammonium sulfate, Rivanol, and caprylic acid precipitation, *Methods of Plasma Fractionation* (J. M. Curling, ed.), p. 53.
291. Faure, A., Tepenier, D., and Caron, M. (1983). Studies on plasma protein fractionation with fatty acids, *Affinity Chromatography and Biological Recognition* (I. M. Chaiken, M. Wilchek, and I. Parikh, eds.), Academic Press, New York, p. 467.
292. Habeeb, A. F. S. A., and Francis, R. D. (1984). Preparation of human immunoglobulin by caprylic acid precipitation, *Prep. Biochem.*, *14*: 1.
293. Russo, C., Callegaro, L., Lanza, E., and Ferrone, S. (1983). Purification of IgG monoclonal antibody by caprylic acid precipitation, *J. Immunol. Methods*, *65*: 269.
294. McKinney, M. M., and Parkinson, A. (1987). A simple, non-chromatographic procedure to purify immunoglobulins from serum and ascites fluid, *J. Immunol. Methods*, *98*: 271.

295. Reik, L. M., Maines, S. L., Ryan, D. E., Levin, W., Bandiera, S., and Thomas, P. E., A simple non-chromatographic purification procedure for monoclonal antibodies. Isolation of monoclonal antibodies against cytochrome P450 isozymes, *J. Immunol. Methods*, *100*: 123.

296. Ogden, J. R., and Leung, K. (1988). Purification of murine monoclonal antibodies by caprylic acid, *J. Immunol. Methods*, 111: 283.

297. Temponi, M., Kekish, U., and Ferrone, S. (1988). Immunoreactivity and affinity of murine IgG monoclonal antibodies purified by caprylic acid precipitation, *J. Immunol. Methods*, *115*: 151.

298. Allary, M., and Saint-Blancard, J. (1973). Utilisation du caprylate de sodium pour fractionner les proteines plasmatiques, *Ann. Pharm. Franc.*, *31*: 513.

299. Race, J. (1932). The determination of blood proteins by acid-acetone, *Biochem. J.*, *26*: 1571.

300. Levine, S. (1954). Solubilization of bovine albumin in nonaqueous media, *Arch. Biochem. Biophys.*, *50*: 515.

301. Delaville, M., Delaville, G., and Delaville, J. (1954). Caractère de solubilité de la fraction albuminique du sérum sanguin dans l'alcool trichloracétique. Son application au dosage des diverses fractions proteiques, *Ann. Pharm. Franc.*, *12*: 109.

302. Korner, A., and Debro, J. R. (1956). Solubility of albumin in alcohol after precipitation by trichloroacetic acid: A simplified procedure for separation of albumin, *Nature*, *178*: 1067.

303. Schwert, G. W. (1957). Recovery of native bovine serum albumin after precipitation with trichloroacetic acid and solution in organic solvents, *J. Amer. Chem. Soc.*, *79*: 139.

304. Kallee, E., Lohss, F., and Oppermann, W. (1957). Trichloressigsäure-aceton-extraktion von albumin aus seren und antigen-antikörper-präzipitaten, *Z. Naturforsch.*, *12b*: 777.

305. Michael, S. E. (1962). The isolation of albumin from blood serum or plasma by means of organic solvents, *Biochem. J.*, *82*: 212.

306. Dirr, K., and Faber, D. (1958). Über serumeiweissfraktionierung mit trichloressigsäure, *Z. Physiol. Chem.*, *313*: 296.

307. Sri Ram, J., and Maurer, P. H. (1958). Modified bovine serum albumin. V. Immunochemical and other studies of bovine serum albumin, after precipitation with trichloroacetic acid and solution in ethanol, *Arch. Biochem. Biophys.*, *76*: 28.

308. Rao, M. S. N., Sagar, A. J., Jahan, N. S., and Premsagar, K. D. A. (1965). A physico-chemical study of trichloracetic acid treated bovine serum albumin, *Indian J. Biochem.*, *2*: 47.

309. Liautaud, J., Pla, J., Debrus, A., Gattel, P., Plan, R., and Peyron, L. (1974). Préparation de l'albumine humaine a partir de sang hemolyse extrait de placentas congeles. I. Technique de préparation et qualité du produit, *Develop. biol. Standard.*, *27*: 107.

310. Winzler, R. J., Devor, A. W., Mehl, J. W., and Smith I. M. (1948). Studies on the mucoproteins of human plasma. I. Determination and isolation, *J. Clin. Invest.*, *27*: 609.

311. Schultze, H. E., Heide, K., and Haupt, H. (1962). Die mit perchlorsäure nicht fällbaren proteine des humanserums, *Clin. Chim. Acta*, 7: 854.

312. Astrup, T., Birch-Andersen, A., and Schilling, K. (1954). Fractional precipitation of serum proteins by means of specific anions, *Acta Chem. Scand.*, 8: 901.

313. Berry, E. R., Rosenfeld, L., and Chanutin, A. (1956). Influence of pH, tungstate, and picrate on precipitation of plasma proteins, *Arch. Biochem. Biophys.*, 62: 318.

314. Dolezalova, V., Brada, Z., and Kocent, A. (1964). Chromatography of sulphosalicylic acid-soluble substances from normal human serum, *Clin. Chim. Acta*, 9: 542.

315. Pavlu, J. (1964). Fractionation of the proteins from the sulphosalicylic acid filtrates of serum by chromatography on DEAE-cellulose, *Coll. Czech. Chem. Commun.*, 29: 2268.

316. Pavlu, J. (1965). Fractionation of proteins from the sulphosalicylic acid filtrates of human serum, *Coll. Czech. Chem. Commun.*, 30: 3211.

317. Burstein, M., and Morfin, R. (1969). Précipitation des alpha lipoproteines du sérum par le phosphotungstate de sodium en présence du chloure de magnésium, *Life Sci.*, 8: 345.

318. Burstein, M. Scholnick, H. R., and Morfin, R. (1970). Rapid method for the isolation of lipoproteins from human serum by precipitation with polyanions, *J. Lipid Res.*, 11: 583.

319. Burstein, M., and Legmann, P. (1982). *Lipoprotein Precipitation*, vol. 11, Monographs on Atherosclerosis (T. B. Clarkson, D. Kritchevsky, and O. J. Pollack, eds.), S. Karger, Basel.

320. Sternberg, M. Z. (1970). The separation of proteins with heteropolyacids, *Biotechnol. Bioeng.*, 12: 1.

321. Rane, L. and Newhouser, L. R. (1954). A method for the separation of protein fractions, *U.S. Armed Forces Med. J.*, 5: 368.

322. Etheridge, P. A., Hickson, D. W., Young, C. R., Landmann, W. A., and Dill, C. W. (1981). Functional and chemical characteristics of bovine plasma proteins isolated as a metaphosphate complex, *J. Food Sci.*, 46: 1782.

323. Nitschmann, Hs., Rickli, E., and Kistler, P. (1959). Über den einfluss der polyphosphate auf die löslichkeit einiger plasmaproteine und die möglichkeit der plasma-fractionierung mit polyphosphat, *Helv. Chim. Acta*, 42: 2198.

324. Nitschmann, Hs., Rickli, E., and Kistler, P. (1960). Fractionation of human plasma with polyphosphate, *Vox Sang.*, 5: 232.

325. Lee, Y.-Z., Sim, J. S., Al-Mashikhi, S., and Nakai, S. (1988). Separation of immunoglobulins from bovine blood by polyphosphate precipitation and chromatography, *J. Agric. Food Chem.*, 36: 922.

326. Coulthard, C. E., Michaelis, R., Short, W. F., Sykes, G., Skrimshire, G. E. H., Standfast, A. F. B., Birkinshaw, J. H., and Raistrick, H. (1945). Notatin: An antibacterial glucose-aerodehydrogenase from *Penicillium notatum* Westling and *Penicillium resticulosum* sp. nov., *Biochem. J.*, 39: 24.

327. Mejbaum-Katzenellenbogen, W. (1959). Studies on regeneration of protein from insoluble protein-tannin compounds. I. Removal of tannin from the protein-tannin compounds by caffeine, *Acta Biochim. Polon.*, 6: 350.

328. Kubicz, A., and Katzenellenbogen, W. (1964). On the use of tannin for the preparation of glycoprotein hormones from hog pituitary gland, *Acta Biochim. Polon.*, 11: 395.

329. Casillas, G., Simonetti, C., and Pavlovsky, A. (1960). Fibrinogène: Préparation à partir du complexe fibinogène-tannin, Rev. Franc. Etudes Clin. et Biol., 5: 925.
330. Simonetti, C., Cassillas, G., and Pavlovsky, A. (1961). Purification du facteur VIII antihémophilique (FAH), Hémostase, 1: 57.
331. Thomas, L., Smith, R. F., and von Korff, R. W. (1954). Cold-precipitation by heparin of a protein in rabbit and human plasma, Proc. Soc. Exper. Biol. Med., 86: 813.
332. Smith, R. F., and von Korff, R. W. (1957). A heparin-precipitable fraction of human plasma. I. Isolation and characterization of the fraction, J. Clin Investigation, 36: 596.
333. Godal, H. C. (1960). Precipitation of human fibrinogen with heparin, Scandinav. J. Clin Lab. Investigation, 12: 56.
334. Anderson, A. J. (1963). The formation of chondromucoprotein-fibrinogen and chondromucoprotein-beta-lipoprotein complexes, Biochem. J., 88: 460.
335. Weiland, Th., Goldmann, H., Kern, W., Schultze, H. E., and Matheka, H. D. (1953). Versuche zur fractionierung von proteingemischen mit polyacrylsäuren, Makromol. Chem., 10: 136.
336. Whitaker, D. R. (1953). Purification of Myrothecium verrucaria cellulase, Arch. Biochem. Biophys., 43: 253.
337. Berdick, M., and Morawetz, H. (1954). The interaction of catalase with synthetic polyelectrolytes, J. Biol. Chem., 206: 959.
338. Noguchi, H. (1956). Interactions of proteins with polymeric materials, Biochim. Biophys. Acta, 22: 459.
339. Isliker, H. C., and Strauss, P. H. (1959). The purification of antibody to PR8 influenza A virus, Vox Sang., 4: 196.
340. Sternberg, M., and Hershberger, D. (1974). Separation of proteins with polyacrylic acids, Biochim. Biophys. Acta, 342: 195.
341. Sternberg, M. (1976). Purification of industrial enzymes with polyacrylic acids, Process Biochem., 11(9): 11.
342. Caygill, J. C., Moore, D. J., and Kanagasabapathy, L. (1983). Concentration of plant proteases by precipitation with polyacrylic acids, Enzyme Microb. Technol., 5: 365.
343. Clark, K. M., and Glatz, C. E. (1987). Polymer dosage considerations in polyelectrolyte precipitation of protein, Biotechnol. Prog., 3: 241.
344. Isliker, H. C. (1957). Über die wechselwirkungen von polystyrolsulfonaten mit eiweissen, Helv. Chim. Acta, 40: 1628.
345. Astrup, T., and Piper, J. (1946). Interaction between fibrinogen and polysaccharide polysulfuric acids, Acta Physiol. Scand., 11: 211.
346. Walton, K. W. (1952). The biological behavior of a new synthetic anticoagulant (dextran sulfate) possessing heparin-like properties, Brit. J. Pharmacol., 7: 370.
347. Sasaki, S., and Naguchi, H. (1959). Interaction of fibrinogen with dextran sulfate, J. Gen. Physiol., 43: 1.
348. Bernfeld, P., Donahue, V. M., and Berkowitz, M. E. (1957). Interaction of human serum beta-lipoglobulin with polyanions, J. Biol. Chem., 226: 51.
349. Oncley, J. L., Walton, K. W., and Cornwell, D. G. (1957). A rapid method for the bulk isolation of beta-lipoproteins from human plasma, J. Amer. Chem. Soc., 79: 4666.

350. Cornwell, D. G., and Kruger, F. A. (1961). Molecular complexes in the isolation and characterization of plasma lipoproteins, *J. Lipid Res.*, 2: 110.
351. Kabat, E. A. (1976). *Structural Concepts in Immunology and Immunochemistry*, Holt, Rinehart, Winston, New York.
352. Harboe, M., Saltvedt, E., Closs, O., and Olsnes, S. (1975). Interactions between Ricinus agglutinin and human plasma proteins, *Scand. J. Immumol.*, 4: Suppl. 2, 125.
353. Latner, A. L., and Hodson, A. L. (1980). Differential precipitation with Concanavalin A as a method for the purification of glycoproteins: Human alkaline phosphatase, *Anal. Biochem.*, *101*: 483.
354. Bhattacharyya, L., Khan, M. I., and Brewer, C. F. (1988). Interactions of concanavalin A with asparagine-linked glycopeptides: Formation of homogeneous cross-linked lattices in mixed precipitation systems, *Biochemistry*, 27: 8762.
355. Pearson, J. C., Burton, S. J., and Lay, C. (1986). Affinity precipitation of lactate dehydrogenase with a triazine dye derivative: Selective precipitation of rabbit muscle lactate dehydrogenase with a Procion blue H-B analog, *Anal. Biochem.*, *158*: 382.
356. Buki, K. G., Kirsten, E., and Kun, E. (1987). Isolation of adenosine diphosphoribosyltransferase by precipitation with Reactive Red 120 combined with affinity chromatography, *Anal. Biochem.*, *167*: 160.
357. Pearson, J. C., Clonis, Y. D., and Lay, C. R. (1989). Preparative affinity precipitation of L-lactate dehydrogenase, *J. Biotechnol.*, *11*: 267.
358. Pearson, J. C. (1987). Fractional protein precipitation using triazine dyes, *Reactive Dyes in Protein and Enzyme Technology* (Y. D. Clonis, T. Atkinson, C. Bruton, and C. R. Lay, eds.), Macmillan Press, Basingstoke, U.K., p. 187.
359. Larsson, P. O., and Mosbach, K. (1979). Affinity precipitation of enzymes, *FEBS Letts.*, *98*: 333.
360. Flygare, S., Mannsson, M.-O., Larsson, P.-O., and Mosbach, K. (1982). Affinity precipitation of enzymes, *Appl. Biochem. Biotechnol.*, *7*: 59.
361. Flygare, S., Griffin, T., Larsson, P.-O., and Mosbach, K. (1983). Affinity precipitation of dehydrogenases, *Anal. Biochem.*, *133*: 409.
362. Hayet, M., and Vijayalakshmi, M. A. (1986). Affinity precipitation of proteins using bis-dyes, *J. Chromatogr.*, *376*: 157.
363. Nielson, A. E. (1964). *Kinetics of Precipitation*, Macmillan, New York.
364. Walton, A. G. (1967). *The Formation and Properties of Precipitates*, Wiley-Interscience, New York.
365. O'Rourke, J. D., and Johnson, R. A. (1955). Kinetics and mechanism in formation of slightly soluble ionic precipitates, *Anal. Chem.*, 27: 1699.
366. Ives, K. J. (1978). Rate theories, *The Scientific Basis of Flocculation* (K. J. Ives, ed.), Sijthoff & Noordhoff, Alphen aan den Rijn, The Netherlands, p. 37.
367. Spielman, L. A. (1978). Hydrodynamic aspects of flocculation, *The Scientific Basis of Flocculation* (K. J. Ives, ed.), Sijthoff & Noordhoff, Alphen aan den Rijn, The Netherlands, p. 63.
368. Gregory, J. (1978). Flocculation by inorganic slats, *The Scientific Basis of Flocculation* (K. J. Ives, ed.), Sijthoff & Noordhoff, Alphen aan den Rijn, The Netherlands, p. 89.

369. Bratby, J. (1980). *Coagulation and Flocculation*, Uplands Press Ltd., Croydon, England, ch. 7.
370. Willard, H. H. (1950). Separation by precipitation from homogeneous solution, *Anal. Chem.*, *22*: 1372.
371. Gordon, L. (1952). Precipitation from homogeneous solution, *Anal. Chem.*, *24*: 459.
372. Gordon, L. (1955). Slow precipitation processes; Application of precipitation from homogeneous solution to liquid-solid distribution studies, *Anal. Chem.*, *27*: 1704.
373. Gordon, L., Salutsky, M. L., and Willard, H. H. (1959). *Precipitation From Homogeneous Solution*, John Wiley, New York.
374. Stine, C. r., and Gordon, L. (1953). Precipitation of iodates from homogeneous solution, separation of thorium iodate, *Anal. Chem.*, *25*: 1519.
375. Chan, M. Y. Y., Hoare, M., and Dunnill, P. (1986). The kinetics of protein precipitation by different reagents, *Biotechnol. Bioeng.*, *28*: 387.
376. Grabenbauer, G. C., and Glatz, C. E. (1981). Protein precipitation—Analysis of particle size distribution and kinetics, *Chem. Eng. Commun.*, *12*: 203.
377. Petenate, A. M., and Glatz, C. E. (1983). Isoelectric precipitation of soy protein: II. Kinetics of protein aggregate growth and breakage, *Biotechnol. bioeng.*, *25*: 3059.
378. Nelson, C. D., and Glatz, C. E. (1985). Primary particle formation in protein precipitation, *Biotechnol. Bioeng.*, *27*: 1434.
379. Glatz, C. E., Hoare, M., and Landa-Vertiz, J. (1986). The formation and growth of protein precipitates in a continuous stirred-tank reactor, *AIChE J.*, *32*: 1196.
380. Fisher, R. R., and Glatz, C. E. (1988). Polyelectrolyte precipitation of proteins: II. Models of the particle size distributions, *Biotechnol. Bioeng.*, *32*: 786.
381. Lawson, E. Q., Brandau, D. T., Tra P. A., Aziz, S. E., and Middaugh, C. R. (1987). Kinetics of the precipitation of cryoimmunoglobulins, *Molec. Immunol.*, *24*: 897.
382. Przybycien, T. M., and Bailey, J. E. (1989). Aggregation kinetics in salt-induced protein precipitation, *AIChE J.*, *35*: 1779.
383. Parker T. G., and Dalgleish, D. G. (1977). The use of light-scattering and turbidity measurements to study the kinetics of extensively aggregating proteins: alpha$_s$-casein, *Biopolymers*, *16*: 2533.
384. Kam, Z., Shore, H. B., and Feher, G. (1978). On the crystallization of proteins, *J. Mol. Biol.*, *123*: 539.
385. Baldwin, E. T., Grumley, D. V., and Carter, C. W., Jr. (1986). Practical, rapid screening of protein crystallization by dynamic light scattering, *Biophys. J.*, *49*: 17.
386. Carter, C. W., Jr., Baldwin, E. T., and Frick, L. (1988). Statistical design of experiment for protein crystal growth and use of precrystallization assay, *J. Cryst. Growth*, *90*: 60.
387. Mikol, V., Hirsch, E., and Giege, R. (1990). Diagnostic of precipitant for biomacromoleculer crystallization by quasi-elastic light-scattering, *J. Mol. Biol.*, *212*: 187.

388. Kadima, W., McPherson, A., Dunn, M. F., and Jurnak, F. A. (1990). Characterization of precrystallization aggregation of canavalin by dynamic light scattering, *Biophys. J.*, *57*: 125.
389. Bell, D. J., Heywood-Waddington, D., and Hoare, M. (1982). The density of protein precipitates and its effect on centrifugal sedimentation, *Biotechnol. Bioeng.*, *24*: 127.
390. Grabenbauer, G. C., and Glatz, C. E. (1981). Protein precipitation—Analysis of particle size distribution and kinetics, *Chem. Eng. Commun.*, *12*: 203.
391. Hoare, M. (1978). Dependence of precipitate particle size distribution on mixing and aging technique, *Proceedings of the International Workshop on Technology for Protein Separation and Improvement of Blood Plasma Fractionation* (H. E. Sandberg, ed.), DHEW Publication No. (NIH) 78-1422, U.S. Govt. Printing Office, Washington, D.C., p. 44.
392. Virkar, P. D., Hoare, M., Can, M. Y. Y., and Dunnill, P. (1982). Kinetics of the acid precipitation of soya protein in a continuous-flow tubular reactor, *Biotechnol. Bioeng.*, *24*: 871.
393. Bell, D. J., and Dunnill, P. (1982). Shear disruption of soya protein precipitate particles and the effect of aging in a stirred tank, *Biotechnol. Bioeng.*, *24*: 1271.
394. Chan, M. Y. Y., Bell, D. J., and Dunnill, P. (1982). The relationship between the zeta potential and the size of soya protein acid precipitate particles, *Biotechnol. Bioeng.*, *24*: 1897.
395. Bell, D. J., and Dunnill, P. (1982). The influence of precipitation reactor configuration on the centrifugal recovery of isoelectric soya protein precipitate, *Biotechnol. Bioeng.*, *24*: 2319.
396. Hoare, M. (1982). Protein precipitation and precipitate aging. Part I: Salting-out and aging of casein precipitates, *Trans. IChemE*, *60*: 79.
397. Hoare, M. (1982). Protein precipitation and precipitate aging. Part II: Growth of protein precipitates during hindered settling or exposure to shear, *Trans. IChemE*, *60*: 157.
398. Hoare, M., Narendranathan, T. J., Flint, J. R., Heywood-Waddington, D., Bell, D. J., and Dunnill, P. (1982). Disruption of protein precipitates during shear in Couette flow and in pumps, *Ind. Eng. Chem. Fundam.*, *21*: 402.
399. Hoare, M., Dunnill, P. and Bell, D. J. (1983). Reactor design for protein precipitation and its effect on centrifugal separation, *Biochemical Engineering III* (K. Venkatasubramanian, A. Constantinides, and W. R. Vieth, eds.), Ann. N.Y. Acad. Sci., vol. 413, p. 254.
400. Twineham, M., Hoare, M., and Bell, D. J. (1984). The effects of protein concentration on the break-up of protein precipitate by exposure to shear, *Chem. Eng. Sci.*, *39*: 509.
401. Glatz, C. E., Hoare, M., and Landa-Vertiz, J. (1986). The formation and growth of protein precipitates in a continuous stirred-tank reactor, *AIChE J.*, *32*: 1196.
402. Petentate, A. M., and Glatz, C. E. (1983). Isoelectric precipitation of soy protein: I. Factors affecting particle size distribution, *Biotechnol. Bioeng.*, *25*: 3049.
403. Nelson, C. D., and Glatz, C. E. (1985). Primary particle formation in protein precipitation, *Biotechnol. Bioeng.*, *27*: 1434.

404. Glatz, C. E., and Fisher, R. R. (1986). Modeling of precipitation phenomena in protein recovery, *Separation, Recovery, and Purification in Biotechnology*, A. C. S. Symposium Series *314* (J. A. Asenjo, J. Hong, eds.), American Chemical Society, Washington, D.C., p. 109.

405. Brown, D. L., and Glatz, C. E. (1987). Aggregate breakdown in protein precipitation, *Chem. Eng. Sci.*, *42*: 1831.

406. Fisher, R. R., and Glatz, C. E. (1988). Polyelectrolyte precipitation of proteins: I. The effects of reactor conditions, *Biotechnol. Bioeng.*, *32*: 777.

407. Fisher, R. R., and Glatz, C. E. (1988). Polyelectrolyte precipitation of proteins: II. Models of the particle size distributions, *Biotechnol. Bioeng.*, *32*: 786.

408. Michaels, A. S., and Bolger, J. C. (1962). Settling rates and sediment volumes of flocculated kaolin suspensions, *Ind. Eng. Chem. Fundam.*, *1*: 24.

409. Foster, P. R. (1978). Protein precipitation. Formation of the solid phase and conditioning by acoustic vibration, *Proceedings of the International Workshop on Technology for Protein Separation and Improvement of Blood Plasma Fractionation* (H. E. Sandburg, ed.), DHEW Publication No. (NIH) 78-1422, U.S. Govt. Printing Office, Washington, D.C., p. 54.

410. Watt, J. G. (1970). Automatically controlled continuous recovery of plasma protein fractions for clinical use, a preliminary report, *Vox Sang.*, *18*: 42.

411. Watt. J. G. (1972). Automatic fractionation of plasma proteins, *Vox Sang.*, *23*: 126.

412. Foster, P. R., and Watt, J. G. (1980). The CSVM fractionation process, *Methods of Plasma Protein Fractionation* (J. M. Curling, ed.), Academic Press, New York, p. 17.

413. Foster, P. R., Dickson, A. J., Stenhouse, A., and Walker, E. P. (1986). A process control system for the fractional precipitation of human plasma proteins, *J. Chem. Tech. Biotechnol.*, *36*: 461.

414. Mitra, G., and Lundblad, J. (1978). Continuous fractionation of human plasma, *Biotechnol. Bioeng.*, *20*: 1037.

415. Chang, C. E. (1988). Continuous fractionation of human plasma proteins by precipitation from the suspension of the recycling stream, *Biotechnol. Bioeng.*, *31*: 841.

416. Salt, D. J., Leslie, R. B., Lillford, P. J., and Dunnill, P. (1982). Factors influencing protein structure during acid precipitation: A study of soya proteins, *Eur. J. Appl. Microbiol. Biotechnol.*, *14*: 144.

417. McMeekin, T. L. (1939). Serum albumin. I. The preparation and properties of crystalline horse serum albumin of constant solubility, *J. Amer. Chem. Soc.*, *61*: 2884.

418. Theorell, H. (1934). Kristallinisches myoglobin, *Biochem. z.*, *252*: 1.

419. Fisher, R. R., Glatz, C. E., and Murphy, P. A. (1986). Effects of mixing during acid addition on fractionally precipitated protein, *Biotechnol. Bioeng.*, *28*: 1056.

420. Jain, S. M. (1983). Electric membrane processes for protein recovery, *Biochemical Engineering III* (K. Ventkatasubramanian, A. constantinides and W. R. Vieth, eds.), Ann. N.Y. Acad. Sci., vol. 413, p. 290.

421. Brodkey, R. S. (1966). Fluid motion and mixing, *Mixing Theory and Practice*, vol. 1 (V. W. Uhl and J. B. Gray, eds.), Academic Press, New York, p. 7.

422. Brodkey, R. S. (1975). *Turbulence in Mixing Operations*, Academic Press, New York.

423. Brodkey, R. S. (1981). Fundamentals of turbulent motion, mixing and kinetics, *Chem. Eng. Commun.*, *8*: 1.
424. Holland, F. A., and Chapman, F. S. (1966). *Liquid Mixing and Processing in Stirred Tanks*, Reinhold, New York.
425. Nagata, S. (1975). *Mixing: Principles and Applications*, Halsted Press, New York.
426. Oldshue, J. Y. (1983). *Fluid Mixing Technology*, McGraw-Hill, New York.
427. Harnby, N., Edwards, M. F., and Nienow, A. W., eds. (1985). *Mixing in the Process Industries*, Butterworths, London.
428. Khang, S. J., and Levenspiel, O. (1976). The mixing-rate number for agitator-stirred tanks, *Chem. Eng.*, October 11, 1976: 141.
429. Khang, S. J., and Levenspiel, O. (1976). New scale-up and design method for stirrer agitated batch mixing vessels, *Chem. Eng. Sci.*, *31*: 569.
430. Steinbuch, M. (1980). Protein fractionation by ammonium sulphate, Rivanol, and caprylic acid precipitation, *Methods of Plasma Protein Fractionation* (J. M. Curling, ed.), Academic Press, New York, p. 41.
431. Jewett, W. R. (1974). Method and apparatus for treating multi-phase systems, *U.S. Patent No. 3,826,740.*
432. Bell, D. J., and Dunnill, P. (1984). Mechanisms for the acoustic conditioning of protein precipitates to improve their separation by centrifugation, *Biotechnol. Bioeng.*, *26*: 691.
433. Hoare, M., Titchener, N. J., and Foster, P. (1987). Improvement in separation characteristics of protein precipitates by acoustic conditioning, *Biotechnol. Bioeng.*, *29*: 24.
434. Titchener-Hooker, N. J., Hoare, M., and Dunnill, P. (1990). New approaches to the more efficient purification of proteins and enzymes, *Biochemical Engineering VI* (W. E. Goldstein, D. DiBiaso, and H. Pedersen, eds.), Ann. N.Y. Acad. Sci., vol. 589, p. 157.
435. Titchener-Hooker, N. J., Hoare, M., McIntosh, R. V., and Foster, P. R. (1992). The effect of fluid-jet mixing on protein precipitate growth during low-frequency conditioning, *Chem. Eng. Sci.*, *47*: 75.
436. Titchener-Hooker, N. J., and McIntosh, R. V., (1992). Enhancement of protein precipitate strength and density by low-frequency conditioning, *Bioprocess Eng.*, in press.
437. McIntosh, R. V., Stenhouse, a., Woolard, D., and Foster, P. R. (1989). Improvements in the formation and separation of protein precipitates, *I. Chem. E. Symposium Series No. 113: Solid-Liquid Separation Practice III*, Institution of Chemical Engineers, Warwickshire, U.K., p. 77.
438. Muralidhara, H. S., Ensminger, D., and Putnam, A. (1985). Acoustic dewatering and drying (low and high frequency): State of the art review, *Drying Technology*, *3*: 529.
439. Ensminger, D. (1986). Acoustic dewatering, *Advances in Solid-Liquid Separation* (H. S. Muralidhara, ed.), Battelle Press, Columbus, Ohio, p. 321.
440. Muralidhara, H. S., Senapati, N., and Beard, R. B. (1986). A novel electro-acoustic separation process for fine particle suspensions, *Advances in Solid-Liquid Separation* (H. S. Muralidhara, ed.), Battelle Press, Columbus, Ohio, p. 335.

441. Muralidhara, H. S., Beard, R. B., and Senapati, N. (1987). Mechanisms of ultrasonic agglomeration for dewatering colloid suspensions, *Filtration Separation, Nov./Dec.*, 409.
442. Bien, J. (1988). Ultrasonic preparation of sludges to improve dewatering, *Filtration Separation, Nov./Dec.*, 425.
443. Oeser, H. C., and Ahrens, S. (1978). Apparatus for the precipitation of human blood plasma components, *U.S. Patent No. 4,066,549.*
444. Falke, J., Geiger, H., Grunbein, W., and Kandel, H. G. (1981). Verfahren zur herstellung von blutplasma-fractionen, *European Pattent No. 0,040, 397.*
445. Chang, C. E. (1984). Fractionation of blood plasma, *U.S. Patent No. 4,486,341.*

ADDITIONAL REFERENCES

Since submission of the manuscript, a number of important articles have been published or called to the author's attention. They are presented below under the title of the pertinent sections of the paper.

A. Forces of Intermolecular Interaction
    1. van Oss, C. J. (1990). Aspecific and specific interactions in aqueous media, *J. Mol. Recognition, 3*: 128.

B. Derived Interactions
    1. Preissner, R., Egner, U., and Saenger, W. (1991). Occurrence of bifurcated three-centered hydrogen bonds in proteins, *FEBS Lett., 288*: 192.
    2. Dill, K. A. (1990). The meaning of hydrophobicity, *Science, 250*: 297.
    3. Muller, N. (1990). Search for a realistic view of hydrophobic effects, *Acc. Chem. Res., 23*: 23.
    4. Doig, A. J., and Williams, D. H. (1991). Is the hydrophobic effect stabilizing or destabilizing in proteins, *J. Mol. Biol., 217*: 389.
    5. Sharp, K. A., Nicholls, A., Fine, R. F., and Honig, B. (1991). Reconciling the magnitude of the microscopic and macroscopic hydrophobic effects, *Science, 252*: 106.

C. Overview of Protein Structure
    1. Branden, C., and Tooze, J. (1991). *Introduction to Protein Structure*, Garland, New York.
    2. Chan, H. S., and Dill, K. A. (1991). Polymer principles in protein structure and stability, *Ann. Rev. Biophys. Biophys. Chem., 20*: 447.
    3. Rupley, J. A., and Careri, G. (1991). Protein hydration and function, *Adv. Protein Chem., 41*: 37.
    4. Teeter, M. M. (1991). Water-protein interactions: Theory and experiment, *Ann. Rev. Biophys. Biophys. Chem., 20*: 577.
    5. Ponnuswamy, P. K. (1993). Hydrophobic characteristics of folded proteins, *Prog. Biophys. Molec. Biol., 59*: 57.

D. Parameters of Protein Solubility
  1. Timasheff, S. N., and Arakawa, T. (1988). Mechanism of protein precipitation and stabilization by co-solvents, *J. Crystal Growth*, *90*: 39.
  2. Schein, C. H. (1990). Solubility as a function of protein structure and solvent components, *Bio/Technology*, *8*: 308.
  3. Wilkinson, D. L., and Harrison, R. G. (1991). Predicting the solubility of recombinant proteins in *Escherichia coli*, *Bio/Technology*, *9*: 443.
  4. Guo, M., and Narsimhan, G. (1991). Solubility of globular proteins in polysaccharide solutions, *Biotechnol. Prog.*, *7*: 54.
E. Salting-Out
  1. Przybycien, T. M., and Bailey, J. E. (1991). Secondary structure perturbations in salt-induced protein precipitates, *Biochim. Biophys. Acta*, *1076*: 103.
  2. Shih, Y., Prausnitz, J. M., and Blanch, H. W. (1992). Some characteristics of protein precipitation by salts, *Biotechnol. Bioeng.*, *36*: 1155.
F. Nonionic Polymeric Precipitation
  1. Thrash, S. L., Otto, J. C., Jr., and Deits, T. L. (1991). Effect of divalent ions on protein precipitation with polyethylene glycol: Mechanism of action and applications, *Protein Expression and Purification*, *2*: 83.
  2. Mahadevan, H., and Hall, C. K. (1992). Theory of precipitation of protein mixtures by nonionic polymer, *AIChE J.*, *38*: 573.
  3. Sharma, A., Anderson, K., and Baker, J. W. (1990). Flocculation of serum lipoproteins with cyclodextrins: Application to assay of hyperlipidemic serum, *Clin. Chem.*, *36*: 529.
  4. Sharma, A., and Janis, L. S. (1991). Lipoprotein-cyclodextrin interaction, *Clin. Chim. Acta*, *199*: 129.
G. Miscible Organic Solvent Precipitation
  1. Khmelnitsky, Y. L., Mozhaev, V. V., Belova, A. B., Sergeeva, M. V., and Martinek, K. (1991). Denaturation capacity: A new quantitative criterion for selection of organic solvents as reaction media in biocatalysis, *Eur. J. Biochem.*, *198*: 31.
  2. Khmelnitsky, Y. L., Belova, A. B., Levashov, A. V., and Mozhaev, V. V. (1991). Relationship between surface hydrophobicity of a protein and its stability against denaturation by organic solvents, *FEBS Lett.*, *284*: 267.
H. Synthetic Anionic Polyelectrolytes
  1. Strege, M. A., Dbin, P. L., West, J. S., and Flinta, C. D. (1990). Protein separation via polyelectrolyte complexation, *Protein Purification From Molecular Mechanisms to Large-Scale Processes*,

ACS Symposium Series 427 (M. R. Ladisch, R. C. Willson, C. C., Painton, and S. E. Builder, eds.), American Chemical Society, Washington, D.C., p. 66.

2. Clark, K. M., and Glatz, C. E. (1990). Protein fractionation by precipitation with carboxymethyl cellulose, *Downstream Processing and Bioseparation*, ACS Symposium Series 419 (J. P. Hamel, J. B. Hunter, and S. K. Sikdar, eds.), American Chemical Society, Washington, D.C., p. 170.

3. Parker, D. E., Glatz, C. E., Ford, C. F., Gendel, S. M., Suominen, I., and Rougvie, M. A. (1990). Recovery of a charged-fusion protein from cell extracts by polyelectrolyte precipitation, *Biotechnol. Bioeng.*, *36*: 467.

4. Zhao, J., Ford, C. F., Glatz, C. E., Rougvie, M. A., and Gendel, S. M. (1990). Polyelectrolyte precipitation of β-galactosidase fusions containing poly-aspartic acid tails, *J. Biotechnol.*, *14*: 273.

5. Ford, C. f., Suominen, H., and Glatz, C. E. (1991). Fusion tails for the recovery and purification of recombinant proteins, *Prot. Expr. Purif.*, *2*: 95.

I. Precipitation of a Soluble Affinity Complex
1. Bradshaw, A. P., and Sturgeon, R. J. (1990). The synthesis of soluble polymer-ligand complexes for affinity precipitation studies, *Biotechnol. Tech.*, *4*: 67.

2. Chen, J. P. (1990). Novel affinity-based processes for protein purification, *J. Ferment. Bioeng.*, *70*: 199.

3. Fujii, M., and Taniguchi, M. (1991). Application of reversibly soluble polymers in bioprocessing, *Trends Biotechnol.*, *9*: 191.

J. Metal Ions
1. Glusker, J. P. (1991). Structural aspects of metal liganding to functional groups in proteins, *Adv. Protein Chem.*, *42*: 1.

K. Affinity Precipitation
1. Morris, J. E., and Fisher, R. R. (1990). Complications encountered using Cibacron Blue F3G-A as a ligand for affinity precipitation of lactic dehydrogenase, *Biotechnol. Bioeng.*, *36*: 737.

L. Precipitation
1. Glatz, C. E. (1990). Precipitation, *Separation Processes in Biotechnology* (J. A. Asenjo, ed.), Marcel Dekker, New York, p. 329.

2. Richardson, P., Hoare, M., and Dunnill, P. (1990). A new biochemical engineering approach to the fractional precipitation of proteins, *Biotechnol. Bioeng.*, *36*: 354.

3. Iyer, H. V., and Przybycien, T. M. (1993). Protein precipitation: Effects of mixing on protein solubility, *AIChE J.*, in press.

7

Conventional Chromatography

John M. Simpson

Lederle Laboratories, American Cyanamid Company, Pearl River, New York

I. INTRODUCTION

The vast majority of protein purification processes involve at least one chromatography step, and with good reason, for chromatography is very well suited to the gentle separation of proteins of very similar structure. Indeed, chromatography is often the key to the success of a separation process. Given the technical importance of chromatography and its relatively high expense (1) in terms of equipment and manpower, it is obvious that great care should be taken to be sure that separations developed in the lab can be scaled up to become commercial successes.

This chapter is intended to aid in the design and operation of large-scale conventional chromatography for the purification of proteins and peptides. Conventional chromatography is taken to mean those operations that contact a liquid mixture of proteins or peptides with a particulate adsorbent packed in a bed for the purpose of separating a desired product from the mixture. Further characteristics of conventional chromatography are moderate pressure drop across the packed bed (<50 psig), batchwise operation, and a cyclical sequence of processing steps. Specifically excluded from consideration in this chapter are batch adsorption from a slurry, continuous chromatography, radial chromatography, HPLC, metal affinity chromatography, dye ligand chromatography, and the use of adsorbents based on antibodies or other biological interactions (affinity chromatography).

Many types of chromatography are available to the process engineer. The particular type chosen will depend on the type of protein being processed, the nature of the impurities, the yearly production required, the position of the step in the process, and many other factors. As a guide to making the proper choice, a brief description is given for each major type available, not with the intent of being exhaustive but rather to draw attention to those that are most useful and frequently applied.

II. TYPES OF CHROMATOGRAPHY

A. Ion Exchange

Ion exchange is one of the most frequently applied chromatographic steps. The reasons for this are not hard to understand. Ion exchange resin has a high capacity to adsorb protein. Higher-molecular-weight proteins are adsorbed less on a weight basis than lower-molecular-weight proteins, but for the average protein of 20,000 daltons a capacity of about 100 g/L of gel should be expected (2). Since virtually all proteins are charged at one pH or another, this method has very wide applicability. Even proteins with identical isoelectric points may be separated, for the protein attachment site to the matrix is determined by the surface charge of the protein and the proximity of other charges, not just by the integrated charge of the protein (3,4). Ion exchange has good selectivity. Very often, conditions can be found such that the desired protein is adsorbed while most impurities are not. By a judicious choice of the elution conditions the remaining impurities may be separated from the protein of interest. The proper choice of gel, pH, ionic strength, and other factors may be guided by the text of Scopes (2) and the electrophoretic titration method developed by Richey (5). Passage through an anionic gel is an extremely effective method to remove pyrogens from proteins (6). Depyrogenation is a must for all proteins derived from recombinant *E. coli* (7).

B. Gel Permeation

Gel permeation chromatography separates proteins and peptides on the basis of their molecular size (8). Separations can be achieved over the range of 10^2 to 10^7 daltons (9). It does have a place in larger-scale operations, but only under restricted conditions. The major factors limiting its use are low capacity and slow flow rate. If the impurities differ in molecular weight by a factor of five or more, ultrafiltration should be examined as a low-cost, high-throughput alternative or at least pretreatment. If the product commands a high price and must be ultrapure, a gel permeation step may be advantageous close to the end of the process. Low annual requirements (<10 kg/year) also favor GPC. Kelley (10) has estimated the cost of a typical GPC step as $5/g in 1987.

C. Hydrophobic Chromatography

Hydrophobic chromatography is based on the interaction of hydrophobic regions of the desired protein with a gel matrix possessing similar properties.

Generally the gels are coated with octyl or phenyl groups. The protein should be loaded in high salt concentration to encourage binding (11). For this reason, the step usually follows ion exchange or ammonium sulfate precipitation. Resolution in general is not as good as ion exchange, but the method does hold the considerable advantage of being based on an entirely different type of interaction compared to ion exchange. Bound protein is eluted by lowering the salt concentration of the eluent or by raising the organic solvent content. Protein denaturation through too strong an interaction with the matrix is sometimes a problem (12). In a few cases the protein is eluted by water alone. The gel is more expensive than ion exchange resin but less expensive than affinity or HPLC matrices. Capacity is somewhat lower than ion exchange (13).

D. Chromatofocusing

Chromatofocusing is a chromatographic technique, developed by Sluyterman (14) and commercialized principally by Pharmacia, that relies on a special ion exchange resin (polyethyleneimine-agarose), similar to a weak base anion exchange gel, but with a continuous range of titratable groups from high to low pH. The column is equilibrated to a pH higher than the highest expected isoelectric point (pI) of any of the sample components. A measured sample is injected onto the column, and a buffer of specially formulated ampholytes of high buffering strength and low ionic strength is fed to the column. The pH of the buffer must be less than the lowest pI expected in the sample. The action of the ampholyte mixture on the gel creates a linear pH gradient in the gel bed. Proteins are eluted from the column at or slightly above their isoelectric point. Sample volume is limiting and the height of the bed is important (13). Separation of isoforms of the same protein is possible with this technique, indicative of excellent resolving power. Resolution is affected most by gradient volume (15) and the range of pI to be covered. The major drawbacks are the high expense of the gel and special eluent, and the nuisance of having to remove the ampholyte after the chromatography is over. Application is usually limited to the final stages of purification of a high-value-added product (16).

E. Affinity and Large-Scale HPLC

Affinity chromatography and process scale HPLC are specialized types of chromatography that tend to be very expensive but can be appropriate in some applications. A few comments will be made on the application of these technologies compared to conventional chromatography. For small-volume high-value products containing closely related impurities, large-scale HPLC should be considered if resolution by conventional chromatography is inadequate (17). Scale-up from analytical separation to preparative scale to large scale is well established and has the advantage of minimizing development work and rushing the product to market. There is, however, an upper limit of about 2 to 10 kg/day productivity for each production machine, each of which costs hundreds of thousands of dollars. To obtain the maximum resolution, loading must be carefully controlled, generally resulting in a large volume of dilute eluent, which requires concentrating before further processing. The cost of the concentrating equipment is substantial. Expensive explosion-proof equipment is required to safely handle the solvents present in the elution buffers. The high pressures involved and the special requirements of the absorbent (low-micron-size particles, special coating, and particle-size uniformity) mean high operation and maintenance costs. Adsorbent lifetime is a major concern.

Affinity techniques using antibodies are attractive on the basis of their exquisite resolution, which offers the possibility, on paper at least, of shortening the process considerably. The method selects for molecules with the proper folding to interact with antibodies attached to the gel. Counter-balancing these advantages are a number of serious disadvantages that tend to limit industrial applications (18,19). The capacity of antibody columns is low, typically around 2 g/L of gel (2), while the cost to prepare the antibodies and attach them to the matrix is high. Robustness and column hygiene are other concerns in a production setting. These columns represent a consider-able investment, which can be easily destroyed by mistakenly washing the column with a strong reagent; they can also be irreparably fouled by contacting with process streams that are too crude (20). If a series of related proteins are to be developed into products, a new affinity column will be needed for each one unless the antibody interacts with a region common to all the members of the family. Convential chromatography is much easier to adapt to a series of related new products. The final disadvantage of affinity techniques is the need to monitor leaching of the ligand from the column. Assays must be developed to follow the fate of the released ligand through the remainder of the process (16,20). The best position for affinity chromatography is in the middle of the process. This placement maximizes the resolving power of the method while protecting the adsorbent from premature fouling. Any ligand that leaches off the column can be handled by the remaining refining steps.

III. MODES OF OPERATION

In addition to the type of chromatography, the mode of operation must also be considered.

A. Elution Chromatography

The elution mode is the one traditionally associated with chromatography. A small portion of material is introduced onto the column and adsorbs lightly to it. As the eluting solvent flows through the column, the differing components in the feed desorb from the matrix, flow for a short time with the solvent, and adsorb again. Each of the components in the feed differs in the strength of adsorption. Consequently, migration through the column separates the feed into a number of bands that emerge from the column. The weakly bound components emerge first and the strongly bound ones last. This type of chromatography is typical of analytical, isocratic HPLC analysis. It calls for a very delicate balance of solvent-feed-matrix interactions that cannot be obtained easily in the case of proteins. Advantages are constant eluent composition, ease of operation, the possibility of repetitive injections without intervening reequilibrations, and good correspondence to design models. Its disadvantages are limited use of the adsorbent capacity (it works best at very light loading), dilution of the feed stream, the need for long columns with accompanying high pressure drops and packing problems, the tendency to drift in repeatability due to the effects of irreversible adsorption on the matrix, and the difficulty, if not impossibility in practical situations, of finding the right combination of operating conditions for isocratic elution. Elution with an eluent of increasing strength (gradient elution) is a way around the last disadvantage, but it introduces a new debit in the form of added time for equilibration.

B. On-Off Chromatography

On-off chromatography accounts for almost all of protein and large-scale peptide chromatography. The feed stream is loaded onto the column at conditions that cause the desired component to stick strongly to the matrix. After all of the feed has been adsorbed, the composition of the eluent is changed so that the desired protein moves off the adsorbent and into the fluid or mobile phase. The change in eluent composition depends on the type of chromatography. For ion exchange, increasing ionic strength or changing pH is appropriate. In practice, changing pH is not very successful in supplying the required resolution unless the protein is adsorbed very strongly in the first place (2). A much surer way to elute adsorbed proteins selectively is to raise the ionic strength either stepwise or in a gradient. As the ionic strength increases, an ion in the eluent can either displace the protein by directly occupying the site occupied by the protein or, if the ion is a substrate for adsorbed enzyme, it can bind directly to the protein and reduce the affinity of the protein for the adsorbent (2). This latter type of elution can be quite specific and is called "affinity elution." In hydrophobic chromatography (also called hydrophobic interaction chromatography), a method of elution that generally does not denature proteins is to lower the ionic strength. This shifts the equilibrium of the protein between the adsorbent and fluid phases so that at a certain ionic strength, the protein is entirely in the fluid phase.

Chromatography of proteins by ion exchange with an increasing salt gradient is a typical application of this mode. Advantages are high use of gel capacity, ability to load dilute feed streams with no fear of heavy losses, concentrated product streams, greater flexibility in design of operating conditions to optimize the separation, only short columns required because the separation is based on the changing eluent strength rather than many exchanges between eluent and matrix over the length of a long column, and good reproducibility. The disadvantages are that it requires reequilibration before the next cycle can begin, and it is rather complicated operationally.

C. Frontal Chromatography

Frontal chromatography, also known as flow-through or breakthrough chromatography, is a mode in which conditions are chosen such that the desired component very quickly saturates the column and emerges from the column shortly after the feed is started. Impurities, on the other hand, are strongly retained by the adsorbent. Feeding is continued until the front of the adsorbed impurities approaches the column outlet. At this point the feed to the column is discontinued and a wash is introduced to maximize product recovery. After the wash is collected, the column is regenerated for the next cycle. Advantages are exceedingly high apparent capacity (capacity is limited by impurities, which are usually a small fraction of the feed, rather than by the desired component), and simple operation—no gradients or step changes in eluent, and unusually high recovery of desired product because it is never absorbed. Disadvantages are that the product stream is diluted, that feed must be concentrated if the column is to be used efficiently, and that impurities must bind more strongly than the desired protein.

D. Displacement Chromatography

Displacement chromatography is a cyclical mode of operation characterized by equilibrating the column to a weak mobile phase, loading the column to a fraction of its capacity with a feed that is strongly retained, eluting the column by continuously introducing an even more strongly adsorbed substance, known as the displacer, and finally regenerating the column by reequilibrating it to the starting mobile phase (21). A unique feature of this mode is the formation of a train of rectangular-shaped product bands with practically no overlap that is formed under the proper conditions of column length, displacer concentration, and feed and displacer isotherm shapes (22). The displacer for ion exchange applications is often a charged polymer, which can be expensive, hard to remove from the column, and may give rise to worrisome residues in the product.

Although displacement chromatography has been known for a long time, it has received more attention lately because it offers numerous apparent advantages over elution chromatography. Chief among these are the higher concentration of the eluted fractions and the higher purity of the fractions resulting from the elimination of tailing of one component into the other (23). On the negative side is the need to identify an appropriate displacer from the standpoint of the strength of its interaction with the adsorbent and the proper concentration to feed to the column, the need to regenerate the column, and the cost of recovering the often expensive displacer.

Recently Felinger and Guiochon (24) compared the maximum production rates of overloaded elution chromatography with those of displacement chromatography for the separation of small molecules. They concluded that in almost all cases the elution mode was more productive. The greater productivity is due to the much shorter cycle time of the elution mode. Unlike displacement chromatography, with elution chromatography new feed can be introduced before the previous injection has exited the column. Their intention is to extend the analysis to cover the case for large molecules, such as proteins. For the moment, one must be content to weigh the merits of each mode qualitatively with regard to the particular application at hand.

IV. PRELIMINARY BENCH-SCALE EXPERIMENTATION

A. Choosing the Type and Mode of Chromatography

For most separations there are many types and modes of chromatography that will work. The real question is how to pick the method that will cost the least, can be developed fastest, and will be the easiest and most reliable to operate. The guiding principle for this selection should be to examine the high-capacity mainstays (ion exchange, hydrophobic, and dye ligand chromatography) first and only go with the more exotic or low-capacity methods (affinity, gel permeation, chromatofocusing, and high performance chromatography) if a real need exists. There is no advantage to employing technology at the cutting edge solely for its own sake. In the vast majority of cases, ion exchange and the other familiar forms of conventional chromatography will easily meet the requirements of the separation. The actual procedure for screening methods is outside the scope of this chapter. It is nicely presented by Scopes and others (2,4,15,25) and will not be repeated here.

Right from the beginning, special attention should be given to working within the constraints of industrial practice. This will ensure a smooth scale-up. The number of variables that are changed on scale-up should be kept to a minimum with exceptions agreed to by the development team before they are adopted. A checklist is a good way to address all of the variables. It is helpful at this point to work with an automated lab-scale chromatographic system such as the Pharmacia FPLC system. This allows a series of experiments to be carried out under well controlled conditions while requiring only a minimum of operator attention. Inlet and outlet column pressure gages and automatic solenoid valves for flow reversal are useful additions to the basic FPLC configuration. This is the time to be wide-ranging in the scope of experimentation. As the process progresses toward final production, the opportunity for change becomes less and less.

Once a crude separation has been attained, it should be possible to estimate the number of columns required (see Section V.C.4). Discussion of the results of the calculations among the development team will point out the areas in need of further development and immediately suggest some improvements. A number of cycles of experimentation, estimation, discussion, and testing of improved conditions should develop the separation to the point that it is ready for final scale-up.

The lab protocol should be developed to the point that the behavior of the chromatography can be predicted reliably. The effect of excursions in the major process variables should be known as well as the required number of plates (column height) for adequate resolution. Typical chromatograms and a complete protocol should be provided indicating the windows for the various fractions to be collected. The degree of separation between the desired protein and the closest impurity of concern should be maximized and at least a fair understanding of the factors affecting the critical separation should be in hand.

The choice of the mode of chromatography seldom receives the attention it deserves. The most frequent choices are on-off and elution. In view of its inherently low capacity, elution chromatography should be reserved for those cases where an exacting separation is necessary and other modes have proved inadequate. Many times the on-off mode is not exploited fully, in that only a small fraction of the capacity is actually loaded with protein. As part of the early bench work, it should be determined just how far the resin can be loaded while still retaining acceptable yield and quality. Though seldom considered initially, frontal chromatography offers a number of decided advantages that may win out in the final selection process. Frontal chromatography should be considered in every case to see if conditions can be found such that the impurities are retained while the product passes through the column.

B. The Importance of Yield and Purity

Although yield and purity are the hardest attributes to predict, they cannot be neglected in the scale-up program. Any change that affects yield or purity will, in the majority of cases involving biotechnology, be far more important than the capital and productivity saved by optimizing the physical variables of the separation. The reason for this is the high unit cost and emphasis on quality characteristic of therapeutic proteins.

While yields may theoretically approach 100%, in practice they seldom do. The reasons for the shortfall are not well understood. They are often ascribed to such catchalls as nonspecific adsorption or denaturation of the protein on the adsorbent. Whatever the cause, the best course is to include yield and quality as responses in every experiment. One can expect differences among various brands of the same type of adsorbent. Likewise, the various modes of chromatography will exhibit different patterns of behavior.

V. SIZING OF COLUMNS TO PRODUCTION NEEDS

A. External Influences Affecting the Design

The design of a chromatographic separation is heavily influenced by other aspects of the total project. Such factors as the production capacity, selling price of the product, required purity, and timing of market introduction are all important in providing the best design. If the product is an extremely potent human therapeutic with life-saving potential for a previously untreatable disease, it is going to be handled very differently from a commodity-type enzyme designed to increase chemical processing efficiency. Many recombinant proteins are so potent that annual production ranges from several grams to several hundred kilograms (26). When such small volumes are involved, scale-up of the chromatography step is relatively straightforward. The emphasis is on moving the product through the regulatory approval process as quickly as possible. If the bench-scale separation produces a safe and effective product, simple duplication or modest scale-up is the best course. Time saved at this stage is worth much more than the lower production cost of a fully optimized chromatography step. On the other hand, proteins that are needed in ton quantities, or that must compete against existing products, or whose price is constrained by the value of the effect they produce are the ones that need careful design to insure commercial success. By deciding which group the new protein falls into, the appropriate development path may be chosen. Often certain types of chromatography can be immediately eliminated based on these consider-ations.

Extreme purity requirements can alter the development plan. It may become apparent that a single conventional chromatography step will not have the power to produce a product of high enough purity. Affinity or multiple conventional chromatography will be necessary. The sooner these factors are recognized the better will be the final design. It makes good sense to involve biochemical engineers at a very early stage of development. As soon as possible a scalable process should be conceptualized. This focuses development work on separation techniques that can be scaled up to a commercial process.

B. General Approach

Two approaches are available in scaling up chromatography. The first relies heavily on mathematical analysis involving the solution of partial differential equations. It attempts to discover the controlling mechanism for each part of the cycle and to construct a valid mathematical model. The model is manipulated to arrive at a suitable design (27). The loading phase has been well analyzed in the literature. Regeneration, elution, and washing, however, have received little attention as has the operation considered as a whole. Extensive mathematical analysis and experimentation are necessary to model the process adequately. Although some factors can be definitely ruled out by this approach, in many cases the results are ambiguous. The second approach is a more empirical and practical one that focuses on the total cycle and progresses naturally out of early and continuing development work. Column bed height, protein and buffer concentration, and adsorbent particle size and brand are kept constant with the idea of simplifying the analysis and minimizing the chance of significant scale-up effects. As a result, the design process is relatively uncomplicated, involves only algebraic equations, and the effects of each portion of the cycle can be seen in a single unifying equation.

As a rule, the scale-up factors for protein separations are much smaller than those typical of the petrochemical and chemical industries. Even high-volume products, such as proteins from sweet whey or albumin from human plasma, do not require columns over 700 to 2000 liters in volume (1,28). Consequently, it is not normally necessary to change bed height or adsorbent particle size to meet the practical requirements of large scale operation. Simply put, protein columns will not be 100 ft. tall and 30 ft. in diameter.

Perhaps the best solution is a preliminary design based on the second approach followed by a review of the crucial parts of the design with the more fundamental analytical techniques. In this way attention is focused on the process as a whole and the most important parts of it. If the separation is very exacting it is worthwhile, as a final check, to make sure that the best chemistry for the separation has been chosen. Many times the answer to a separation problem is improved chemistry rather than refinements in physical conditions or timing of an inferior process scheme.

C. Formulation of the Design Problem

The design problem is to determine the number and size of columns needed to produce economically a desired protein at a specified rate and purity. It is assumed that the chromatographic separation has been established at the bench scale. The problem can be broken down into two parts. The first part concerns relating the number of columns to production demand, column productivity per cycle, and the number of column cycles per day (29). The analysis is developed for on-off chromatography with indications as to how the results can be applied to elution, gel permeation, and frontal chromatography. The second part, treated later in this chapter, is concerned with the mechanical design of the column and choosing the best operating conditions.

1. Basic Design Equation

We start by expressing the production rate in terms of three factors. The total production rate is the product of the number of columns, the number of cycles per day, and the output of a single column in a single cycle.

$$\frac{\text{kg protein}}{\text{day}} = \text{No. of col.} \times \frac{\text{kg protein}}{\text{cycle col.}} \times \frac{\text{No. of cycles}}{\text{day}} \qquad (1)$$

Rearranging to solve for the number of columns gives

$$\text{No. of col.} = \frac{\dfrac{\text{kg protein}}{\text{day}}}{\dfrac{\text{kg protein}}{\text{cycle column}} \times \dfrac{\text{cycles}}{\text{day}}} \qquad (2)$$

The numerator in Eq. (2) is the desired production rate of protein, specified by the constant Q:

$$\frac{\text{kg protein}}{\text{day}} = Q \qquad (3)$$

Its value will depend on market forecasts, the number of working days per year, and the fraction of time the columns are on-line. Note that this is the final production rate, not the rate at the chromatography step. (See the Appendix at the end of the chapter for the definition and units of symbols.)

2. Column Productivity per Cycle

The first term of the denominator of Eq. (2), the column productivity per cycle, is expressed in terms of other known variables as given in equation (4).

$$\frac{\text{kg protein}}{\text{cycle col.}} = C \left(\frac{\text{kg protein}}{\text{L resin cycle}} \right) \times \frac{\pi D^2 \, h}{4000} \left(\frac{\text{L of resin}}{\text{column}} \right) \times U \qquad (4)$$

$$\frac{\text{kg protein}}{\text{cycle col.}} = \frac{\pi CUD^2 \, h}{4000} \qquad (5)$$

where D = column diameter in cm, h = bed height in cm, and U = fraction of the column saturation capacity that will be loaded on each cycle.

Fifty percent utilization is a reasonable figure in the absence of known adverse or beneficial effects of loading on yield or quality (13). The column saturation capacity C must be determined under flow and mobile phase conditions that are identical to the proposed process. This quantity should be determined experimentally. Care should be taken to ensure that the measured capacity truly reflects the dynamic capacity of the resin. The feed should be identical to that of the full-scale process. Reconstituted pure protein will not contain the same proteinaceous and ionic impurities as the genuine feed. The flow velocity must match the anticipated value, otherwise problems are likely. As flow velocity increases, dynamic capacity decreases due to kinetic and mass transfer effects. For the same reason, batch adsorption tests are not as useful as those conducted in a flow system.

For this analysis, the capacity is expressed in terms of the final product adsorbed per liter of resin. This establishes the capacity on two well-defined quantities: the weight of final product and the volume of the resin. The only drawback to this convention is the need to include yield estimates for the chromatography and all subsequent processing steps. These yields, however, are often high and well-defined. Chromatography is usually one of the last process steps and produces essentially pure protein. The other option—basing the capacity on an analysis of the feed stream—often leads to confusing inconsistencies and high variability: impure protein solutions are notoriously hard to characterize with a single assay.

3. Column Cycles per Day

The second term of the denominator of Eq. (2) is simply the working hours per day divided by the time to complete a single cycle. Continuous 24 h/day operation is assumed.

$$\frac{\text{No. of cycles}}{\text{day}} = \frac{24 \text{ h/day}}{\text{Time for one cycle, h}} \tag{6}$$

Column chromatography is a serial operation. The total cycle time is the sum of the loading, washing, elution, and regeneration times, as in Eq. (7).

$$\text{Total time for one cycle, h} = T_L + T_W + T_E + T_R \tag{7}$$

$$= \frac{4000}{\pi D^2} \left(\frac{L_L}{V_L} + \frac{L_W}{V_W} + \frac{L_E}{V_E} + \frac{L_R}{V_R} \right) \tag{8}$$

where L = liters processed at that step and V = superficial velocity through the bed, cm/h. (Superficial velocity is the linear flow velocity through the column, assuming it is empty.) The concept of bed volumes leads to useful simplifications at this point. A bed volume is the total of the resin and interstitial volumes occupied by the column packing. The loading, washing, eluting, and regenerating volumes can be represented in terms of dimensionless bed volumes as

$$B \text{ (bed volumes)} = \frac{\text{Liters processed} \times 4000}{\pi D^2 h} \tag{9}$$

$$\text{Liters processed} = \frac{\pi D^2 h}{4000} \times B \tag{10}$$

While the volumes of the various column feeds depend on the size of the column, bed volumes are independent of the scale of operation. Expressing each of the volumes processed in terms of bed volumes leads to

$$\text{Total time for one cycle, h} = h \left(\frac{B_L}{V_L} + \frac{B_W}{V_W} + \frac{B_E}{V_E} + \frac{B_R}{V_R} \right) \quad (11)$$

For many cases $V_L = V_W = V_E = V_R = V$, i.e., the flow velocity through the column is constant over the various steps. If it is not, an equivalent bed volume may be defined as

$$B_i = \left(\frac{V_L}{V_i} \right) \quad (12)$$

where i = subscript L, W, E, or R. The velocity at the loading step is taken as the reference value. For simplicity's sake, the velocity will be taken as constant for the remainder of this analysis. Hence

$$\text{Total time for one cycle, h} = \frac{h}{V} \left(B_L + B_W + B_E + B_R \right) + T_H \quad (13)$$

B_W, B_E, and B_R are constants specific to each process. If the wash step is a simple displacement, 2 to 5 bed volumes will usually suffice. Elution often requires more volume, say 3 to 7 bed volumes in normal cases, to accommodate peak tailing and to maximize yield. For large-scale work step elution patterns are favored over gradients (30). The regeneration volume is the sum of each of the volumes of regeneration and equilibration buffers, e.g., strong salt solution, sanitizing agent, strong buffer, and start buffer. Normally, between 6 and 12 bed volumes are required. The final term T_H allows for a constant hold period in a sanitizing agent at zero flow. The loading bed volume is a variable and depends on the potency of the feed stream and the working capacity of the bed.

$$\text{Liters processed in loading step} = \frac{\text{Working capacity of the column}}{\text{Potency of the feed}} \quad (14)$$

$$\text{Liters processed in loading step} = \frac{\pi C U D^2 h}{4P} \quad (15)$$

where P is the protein concentration in the feed in grams of final protein per liter. Substituting Eq. (15) into equation (13) gives

$$= \frac{h}{V}\left(\frac{1000\ CU}{P} + B_W + B_E + B_R\right) + T_H \qquad (16)$$

$$\frac{\text{No. of cycles per column}}{\text{day}} = \frac{24}{\frac{h}{V}\left(\frac{1000\ CU}{P} + B_W + B_E + B_R\right) + T_H} \qquad (17)$$

4. Final Design Equation

All of the necessary factors in equation (2) can now be expressed in terms of knowns to calculate the required number of columns.

$$\text{No. of columns} = \frac{53.05\,Q\left(\frac{h}{V}\left(\frac{1000\ CU}{P} + B_W + B_E + B_R\right) + T_H\right)}{CUD^2 h} \qquad (18)$$

5. Limiting Cases

Two limiting cases are of interest. The first is the situation where T_H, the hold time, is zero or negligible.

$$\text{No. of columns} = 53.05\,Q\frac{\left(\frac{1000\ CU}{P} + B_W + B_E + B_R\right)}{CUD^2 V} \qquad (19)$$

In this case the number of columns is independent of the bed height. A shallow bed cycling frequently is equivalent to a deep bed cycling slowly. The real factors that determine bed height are the desired resolution, cycle time, and pressure drop. The trend in industry is toward relatively short bed heights, say 15 to 45 cm. Classical chromatography theory predicts that resolution should be directly proportional to the square root of the bed height (31); however, changes in buffer pH, ionic strength, gradient shape, or choice of resin are far more flexible and attractive ways to improve resolution. A fuller discussion on the proper choice of bed height is addressed later in this chapter.

The second limiting case is the situation where the loading step dominates all others. This is encountered when the potency of the feed stream is very low. Eq. (18) reduces to

$$\text{No. of columns} = \frac{53050\,Q}{D^2 VP} \qquad (20)$$

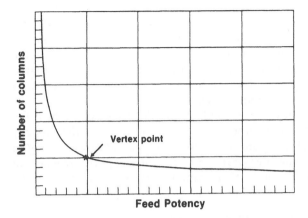

Figure 1 The effect of feed potency on the number of columns required to purify a set amount of protein. The vertex point is given by Eq. (21).

At low feed potency the number of columns is independent of bed height and capacity. The column's primary role has changed from separation to concentration. If the number of columns given by Eq. (18) is plotted as a function of feed concentration, the curve in Fig. 1 is obtained. Concentrating the feed to a potency to the right of the curve's "knee" will significantly reduce the number of columns required and the total expense. The location of the "knee" is the vertex of the hyperbolic curve given by

$$\text{Potency knee} = \left(\frac{53050\,Q}{D^2 V}\right)^{\frac{1}{2}} \tag{21}$$

6. Application to Other Modes of Chromatography

Elution chromatography is distinguished by a very low value of U, the fractional approach to the total capacity. This corresponds to very light loading of the column with a small volume of relatively concentrated protein. The exact amount to be loaded is determined by lab or preparative scale tests. There is no washing or regeneration step. Gradient elution requires an equilibration step to ready the column for the next cycle. Isocratic elution requires no equilibration. In isocratic cases it may be possible to overlap the time cycles of successive batches to some degree (32).

Gel permeation chromatography is amenable to this analysis if U is set equal to one and C is set equal to 5 to 15% of the feed potency (8). A highly concentrated feed and much greater capacity are possible if desalting is the objective (8). There is no washing or regeneration step. Elution of the lowest-molecular-weight components is usually finished by about one bed volume. The highest-molecular-weight components elute no sooner than the void volume of the column, about 0.35 bed volumes. The fact that GPC has no regeneration step allows the next feed cycle to start before the previous batch has completely eluted. A decrease to about 0.6 bed volume for the elution volume (apparent) is possible. The scale-up of GPC has been treated by a number of authors (8,10). These references should be consulted for a fuller discussion of the unique requirements of GPC.

Frontal chromatography can be handled with the same equations if the capacity of the resin is specified in the correct way. In this case the capacity C is defined as the weight in grams of desired protein that flows through a one-liter column before the breakthrough of retained impurity reaches an unacceptable level. In this mode of operation, U is usually close to unity. Naturally, the elution time and volume are zero.

D. Determining the Rate Controlling Step

The adsorption process can be broken down into a number of steps that take place in series. As shown in Fig. 2, the protein dissolved in the bulk liquid must diffuse across a thin, stagnant liquid layer surrounding the outside of the adsorbent particle. Once at the surface of the particle, the protein must diffuse into a pore leading to the interior. Diffusion continues until an unoccupied adsorption site is encountered. The protein then adsorbs to the site at some finite rate. In most cases one step of this sequence is much slower than the others. This step is known as the rate determining or rate controlling step. It sets the overall adsorption rate because of the serial nature of the process.

A closer examination of the rate controlling step in the chromatography is in order once the number of columns has been estimated. With this knowledge one can gain a deeper understanding of the factors that influence the column productivity. Changes that are inevitably suggested by plant personnel can be reviewed more intelligently. Those that might affect the controlling mechanism deserve a closer look, while those that are predicted to have no effect can be adopted with minimal testing. One should remember that any changes that improve the controlling rate might switch control to a different step. Furthermore, the rate controlling step will likely change with the switch from adsorption, to wash, to elution, and regeneration.

Over the years there have been many attempts to model chromatographic operations. They have ranged from simple lumped parameter approaches to numerical integration of complex, coupled partial differential equations. Rather than review each of these solutions, one set that covers many biotechnological applications has been chosen for emphasis.

The papers of Arnold, Blanche, and Wilke (33,34,35,36) give a convenient and systematic way to determine the rate controlling step for chromatography operated in the on-off mode. As with any analytical treat-

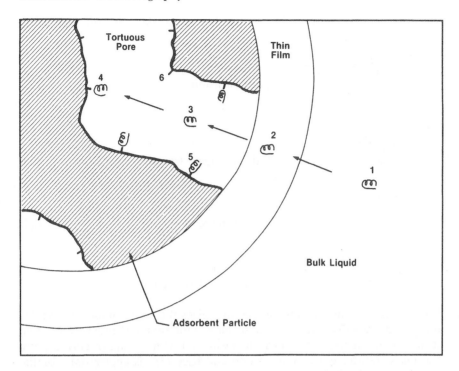

Figure 2 Pictorial representation of steps in the adsorption of protein. (1) Protein in well-mixed bulk liquid approaches adsorbent particle; (2) protein diffuses through thin film surrounding adsorbent particle; (3) protein diffuses through tortuous pore toward adsorbent site; (4) kinetic adsorption step; (5) adsorbed protein; (6) unoccupied adsorption site.

ment, numerous assumptions have to be made in order to make the problem tractable. It is assumed that the contribution of axial dispersion is small compared to the effects of pore diffusion, film resistance, or binding kinetics. Adsorption is taken to be essentially irreversible, and equilibrium is assumed between pore liquid and the internal surface of the adsorbent.

Finally, the concentration profiles are assumed to approach a constant shape as they make their way through the column. If all of these assumptions are satisfied, the breakthrough curve will depend solely on the rate determining step. If these assumptions are not satisfied, other appropriate solutions found in the literature should be applied. Another approach is to model the system with a set of computer programs such as those being currently developed by Sweetenham and coworkers (37) in Great Britain.

Pore diffusion, fluid film mass transfer, axial dispersion, and slow binding kinetics are considered as possible candidates for the rate controlling step.

The following expressions give the number of transfer units for each of the possibilities.

$$N_{\text{pore}} = \frac{15D_i \, (1 - \epsilon)L_B}{R^2 u_o} \qquad \text{pore diffusion} \qquad (22)$$

$$N_f = \frac{k_f \, a_p \, L_B}{u_o} \qquad \text{fluid film mass transfer} \qquad (23)$$

$$N_d = \frac{Pe L_B}{d_p} \qquad \text{axial dispersion} \qquad (24)$$

$$N_k = \frac{\mu_f \rho_B Q_{\text{max}} L_B}{u_o} \qquad \text{kinetic adsorption control} \qquad (25)$$

The rate determining step is the one that gives the least number of transfer units when evaluated with the data specific to the situation under study. Two of the equations (N_f and N_d) can be evaluated with the aid of correlations. The mass transfer correlation of Foo and Rice (38) is appropriate for the estimation of the fluid film mass transfer coefficient.

$$\frac{k_f d_p}{D_L} = 2 + 1.45 \left(\frac{d_p \rho \, u_o}{\mu} \right)^{0.50} \left(\frac{\mu}{\rho D_L} \right)^{0.33} \qquad (26)$$

For uniform spheres, the specific external area is given by $a_p = 3(1-\epsilon)/R$. The diffusion coefficient of the protein in a free liquid can be estimated from (39)

$$D_L = 8.34 \times 10^{-8} \, \frac{T_k}{\mu_c (MW)^{0.33}} \qquad (27)$$

or handbook data can be used. The Peclet number can be estimated from the work of Miller and King (40), who showed that the product ϵPe approaches a constant value of about 0.2 at low Reynolds number in packed beds. The number of transfer units for pore diffusion or binding kinetics can only be estimated with the help of data from experiments. Column runs with pulse inputs of different concentrations and at different flow rates will give the desired information (34). Measurement of the position of the pulse as it exits the column along with a measure of the peak spreading can be used to deduce the adsorption isotherm and effective diffusivity for transport within the pores. What is the likely rate determining step for adsorption in most conventional protein chromatography? In all but extremely short beds, axial dispersion will be negligible. Restriction due to slow mass transfer across the stagnant fluid film surrounding each particle is seldom a problem either, unless the feed is very dilute. The usual rate determining step is diffusion through the pores of the adsorbent (33). For such cases, the breakthrough curve for adsorption is given by

$$\frac{C}{C_o} = 1 - \left[\frac{2}{3} - 0.273 N_{\text{pore}} \, (T_D - 1)\right]^2 \qquad (28)$$

If the particles are extremely small or the protein-adsorbent interaction involves large molecules with exacting steric requirements, the possibility exists that binding kinetics may become dominant. Likewise, binding kinetics may control in the elution phase of the chromatography. Solutions are given by Arnold (33) for the various other rate controlling steps.

Once the rate determining step has been tentatively identified, it should be confirmed by further experimentation. Varying the size of the adsorbent particles is a good way to confirm the controlling step. If the response in N, the number of transfer units, is very strong, it is likely that pore diffusion controls (N is proportional to $1/R^2$). If the effect is moderate, stagnant film mass transfer or axial dispersion are confirmed (N is proportional to $1/R$). Lack of response would confirm slow binding kinetics.

Activation energies derived from temperature studies can aid in discriminating between physical mass transfer limitations (activation energies of 3 to 5 Kcal) and chemical reaction control (activation energies greater than 10 Kcal). None of these tests should be taken singly as proof of the identity of the rate controlling step. All available data must be considered as a whole to arrive at the best choice. In many real-life cases the data will not be clear-cut and will require careful interpretation.

E. Effect of Process Variables

1. Nature and Concentration of the Feed Stream

The composition and quantity of the feed stream can have a significant effect on the final design. Although the purpose of chromatography is purification, the job is made much easier the purer the feed stream is. Industrial chromatography must be robust, economical, and effective. To insure that these objectives are met, the following questions concerning the nature of the feed should be answered.

Is the feed in the right composition range? If it is too concentrated, density differences, inadequate buffering capacity, and high viscosity may cause problems. If it is too dilute, the column will be occupied all the time just adsorbing the product. For GPC the limits of protein concentration are 10 g/L to 70 g/L depending on the degree of resolution required (41). Simple desalting allows operation at the high end of the concentration range as well as increases in the volume of feed per cycle. For ion exchange the protein of interest should be at a concentration of 5 to 10 g/L with a total protein concentration no greater than 25 g/L (2). Solubility limits may lower these maxima. In no case should the viscosity of the feed be greater than twice the eluent viscosity. This corresponds to a protein concentration of about 70 g/L in a dilute aqueous buffer (13,42).

Does the feed need conditioning, e.g., filtration or a change in ionic strength or pH? Adsorbent beds are very efficient filters. Feeds to the column must be no more than very slightly hazy, otherwise the column may plug with solids. Aside from GPC, chromatography requires exacting control of ionic strength and pH. Even for GPC, the ionic strength should be above 0.15 if hydrohobic interaction is to be minimized (43). The higher feed concentrations typical of industrial chromatography often require increases in buffer strength compared to the original lab procedure. The buffer pK should be within 0.5 of the pH of the eluent. The feed must be brought to the conductivity and pH that were determined to be optimum in the lab. This requirement may prompt a change to a new sequence of process steps that minimizes transfers from one buffer to another.

Has the cleanest starting material been chosen? If not, fouling may be a problem and capacity will suffer. For crude feeds, a small guard column may be beneficial, or the chromatography might be better put off to a step later in the process.

The answers to all these questions depend to a great degree on the specific protein and process under review. A balance must be struck between the expense of chromatography and the expense of pretreatment or other alternatives. Generally, pretreatment will be less expensive.

2. Flow Velocity

The number of columns required to produce a set quantity of protein is directly related to the flow velocity through the columns. Velocity should be increased to the point that the upper pressure drop limit is approached or resolution deteriorates to an unacceptable degree. Flow velocity will influence the rate of mass transfer from the bulk liquid to the outer surface of the adsorbent. Higher velocity also increases the extent of eddy diffusion and backmixing. In extreme cases the flow can be increased to the point that the protein in the feed will be swept out of the column before it has a chance to adsorb.

Superficial velocities normally range from a low of 10–20 cm/h up to a high of about 400 cm/h for large-scale applications (19). Low-molecular-weight peptides and proteins and rigid adsorbents favor the high-velocity range. Very-high-molecular-weight proteins and compressible adsorbents are found at the low end. Smaller-scale operations based on freely permeable adsorbent particles (44), membrane chromatography, or small-diameter columns (particles given extra support by proximity to the wall) can be operated at velocities up to 5000 cm/h. The kinetics of adsorption can become a limiting factor under these conditions.

The effect of flow velocity on column efficiency is commonly illustrated with the Van Deemter (45) equation

$$\text{HETP} = a_1 + a_2 u_0 + a_3/u_0 \tag{29}$$

HETP or the height equivalent of a theoretical plate is directly related to the efficiency of the column. The smaller the HETP the greater the number of separation stages available to resolve mixtures. The plate height is influenced by three factors. The first term, a_1, accounts for undesired mixing due to imperfections in packing, liquid maldistribution, and dead volume in valves and lines. The second term, $a_2 u_0$, is directly proportional to the superficial velocity. It depends on the rate of mass transfer from the bulk liquid to the surface and interior of the adsorbent. It includes both the thin-film mass transfer resistance at the surface of the adsorbent and the intraparticle resistance due to diffusion within the particle. The final term, a_3/u_0, is proportional to the ratio of velocity of free diffusion in the direction of flow to the velocity due to convected flow. Macromolecular diffusion coefficients are so small that a_3/u_0 can be neglected in virtually all industrial applications.

The net result for the HETP analysis for practical cases is that plate height continually increases with increasing flow velocity. Mechanical design of the column system should be aimed at minimizing dead volume and maldistribution. The slope of the increase in HETP can be controlled by choosing adsorbents with properly tailored internal structures that do not impede the transport of the protein.

3. Temperature
Temperature can easily indirectly affect product purity or recovery. Often lab procedures will be carried out at 4°C just as a routine precaution against degradation of the protein. It is costly, however, to maintain 4°C throughout scale-up. Besides the obvious cost of cooling the column, there is the cost of air conditioning the surrounding room to prevent sweating of the cold equipment, the cost of insulation, and the cost to cool all the buffers, eluents, and regenerants. Additional factors are higher pressure drop due to increased liquid viscosity, and possible changes in the behavior of the adsorbent due to increased importance of hydrophobic forces at low temperature (46). Optimized, quick operation at room temperature will often give the same result as direct scale-up of a lengthy, preliminary lab process at 4°C.

The upper temperature limit of operation is set by the stability of the protein and the yield of the chromatography step. Diffusional processes are less of a problem at higher temperatures (47), but whether these effects are significant enough to warrant raising the temperature above ambient in production units can only be determined by experiments in the pilot plant.

The main point is to look at the effect of temperature closely and not follow the general rule of thumb that colder is better in all circumstances.

4. Properties of the Adsorbent

a.   Type of Adsorbent. There is a bewildering array of adsorbents on the market. The choice of a few candidates for further study can be guided by the discussion at the beginning of this chapter. In many cases, several types of chromatography can yield essentially equivalent results in terms of separation and cost. At this stage what is desired is to eliminate those types that are clearly not suited to the separation, rather than make a definitive choice of the "best." If two or more chromatography steps are involved in the process, it is a good idea to choose types that differ in their basis of separation. For example, one might choose hydrophobic chromatography (hydrophobic interaction) to follow anion exchange (electostatic interaction) in preference to two anion exchange steps.

Once several candidate types of chromatography have been identified, extensive lab experimentation should be done to develop a lab-scale separation process. Once the type of chromatography has been specified, choose three or four representative brands of adsorbent within that group for testing, because such factors as protein recovery and recyclability cannot be predicted. There is normally no need to test every available brand exhaustively.   Other factors to consider in picking adsorbents include cost, availability in bulk, thoroughness of documented manufacturing and quality control methods suitable for presentation to regulatory authorities, location of the source, customer service, and history of quality control.

b.   Capacity of the Adsorbent. Capacity has a direct and strong effect on the number of columns required to purify a protein. Consequently, it should be as high as possible consistent with good recovery. What matters is dynamic capacity rather than thermodynamic capacity. The capacity to adsorb the protein of interest must be determined under flow and buffer conditions identical to those specified for production (25). Capacities determined from acid-base titrations or other indirect methods should be taken as only suggestive of the dynamic capacity. In the preliminary design phase, the correlation of Scopes (2) is a useful tool to estimate the approximate ion exchange capacity for a protein of known molecular weight. For the final design, there is no substitute for experimental determination of the capacity employing the exact feed and flow conditions of the design.

The determination of the breakthrough curve is the best way to determine the dynamic capacity. A column is packed with the production adsorbent to the same height as will be used in the plant. A small-diameter column is suitable as long as the ratio of adsorbent particle diameter to column diameter is greater than 30. The bed is equilibrated to the eluent buffer. Next, feed of the same composition and history as that anticipated in production is pumped to the column at a specified superficial velocity in the range of 40 to 400 cm/h. The effluent from the column is continuously monitored for ultraviolet light absorption at a suitable wavelength, usually 280 nm. A curve similar to Fig. 3 should be obtained. If time zero is taken as the start of the feed, the curve may be broken up into five regions. The first is the portion covered by the time for the front of the feed to make its way through the bed. During this time the UV trace is unchanged from the buffer equilibration level. When the front of the feed reaches the end of the column there will usually be a small, rapid increase in UV response corresponding to the breakthrough of unadsorbed minor impurities in the feed. This is followed by region of shallowly increasing UV activity due to start of breakthrough of the desired component. At some point the UV trace starts to increase rapidly due to impending saturation of the adsorbent capacity. This sigmoid portion of the curve is followed by an asymptotic approach to the UV activity of the feed as the column is completely saturated. Lower superficial velocities give breakthrough curves approaching a step function.

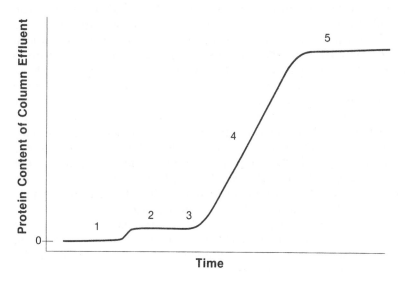

Figure 3 Breakthrough curve. (1) Dead time for feed to transit column assuming no adsorption; (2) breakthrough of unadsorbed impurities; (3) start of breakthrough of desired protein; (4) main portion of breakthrough; (5) final approach to total saturation.

Higher velocities give progressively shallower curves with lower dynamic capacities. The shallow curves reflect increasing mass transfer resistance.

Capacity can be defined in a number of ways. The first is taken to be the grams of protein fed to the column at the point that the UV trace reaches a certain percentage of the final UV level, usually 5%. A variant of this would be to choose the point that the integrated loss of desired product reaches a set value, again usually 5%. The number of grams of protein is divided by the bed volume in liters to obtain the specific capacity. Further adjustments for column and subsequent processing yields convert the capacity to the basis of grams of final protein per liter of adsorbent. The other popular definition is based on the final approach to saturation: either the 50% or the 95% level of the final UV activity. While perfectly legitimate, these latter definitions give capacities that are never approached in normal industrial practice. For this reason they are misleading, and their use should be avoided.

Dynamic capacity reflects the effects of mass transfer limitations as well as the ultimate capacity in the thermodynamic sense. Mass transfer limitations occur as the result of the interaction of flow velocity, particle size, pore size and pore size distribution, and the physical properties of the protein, buffer, and adsorbent.

Capacity is directly related to the accessible surface area of the gel and the density of adsorbent sites on the surface. If the ligand at the adsorbent site is small, it is possible to crowd too high a density of sites on the surface of the gel. If the protein interacts with too many sites, it will be very difficult to displace. With large ligands, such as monoclonal antibodies, it is hard to attach enough in the right configuration to give high capacity (20). Nonporous gel beads with adsorbent sites just on the surface (pellicular) have very low capacities (48). These gels, however, do have very fast mass transfer characteristics, which makes them popular for analytical applications. Porosity increases surface area and ultimate capacity dramatically, especially if the pores have a small diameter. There is a limit, however, to the degree of porosity that is practically attainable. Too high a porosity leads to poor mechanical strength of the particles. Arbitrarily decreasing the pore size ultimately leads to exclusion of the protein from the interior of the particle (see Section F below for a fuller discussion of pore size).

Capacity is often a strong function of pH, ionic strength, and polarity of the eluent. Concerns such as these affect the choice of strong vs. weak ion exchangers, the strength and pH of buffers, and the proper location in the process of the chromatography step.

c. *Particle Size, Particle Size Distribution, and Shape of the Adsorbent.* In general the particle should be as small as possible subject to pressure drop constraints and packing difficulties. Small particle diameter minimizes intraparticle diffusional resistances, which account in most practical cases for most of the mass transfer limitation of production scale chromatography.

Decreased diffusional path means less peak tailing and increased flow velocity before additional resistances come into play. Assuming an upper pressure drop of 50 to 100 psig and more typically 10 to 50 psig as a working value for aqueous solutions, the minimum particle size range is from 50 to 100 microns at bed depths of 15 to 60 cm. Pressure drop through an incompressible packed bed of solids can be predicted by the equation of Ergun (49) modified for laminar flow

$$\frac{\Delta P g_c}{L_B} = \frac{150 \mu u_o}{dp^2} \frac{(1 - \epsilon)^2}{\epsilon^3} \qquad (30)$$

Note that particle diameter appears in the denominator and is raised to the second power. Halving the particle size quadruples the pressure drop. Given that most gels on the market already are optimized to the 10 to 50 psig pressure drop at fast flow rates, this does not leave a lot of room to play with. Recently there has been a trend toward 30 to 50 micron particles for small-volume applications where the increased resolving power compensates for the higher pressure drop (50). The bed void volume is influenced by the tightness of the particle size distribution and the quality of the packing (13,31, 51). Very small changes in the void volume are rapidly reflected in changes in the bed pressure drop. Some manufacturers will supply, at extra cost, adsorbent with a narrow particle size distribution (52). The uniformity of particle size makes for sharper bands and greater resolving power. Viscosity of the feed and eluent also is directly reflected in increased pressure drop. Choice of solvent, concentration, and temperature of operation should be reviewed with this in mind. For dilute aqueous solutions, one can expect about twice the pressure drop at 4°C as would be obtained at 24°C (8).

d. *Particle Shape.* Spherical beads should be favored over irregularly shaped particles on the basis of greater permeability in packed beds and better bed stability on repeated use (51). Rough particles do have a price advantage over smooth spheres, which may warrant consideration in cases where the gel is used just once. Particles shaped like needles offer the advantage of faster adsorption kinetics by way of reduced diffusional distance compared to spheres of equivalent volume, but they raise concerns about packing and pressure drop.

e. *Compressibility and Swelling of the Adsorbent.* When protein chromatography first developed, many of the adsorbents available were easily compressed by very modest pressure gradients (53). In the most extreme cases, just the weight of the bed was enough to deform the particles on the bottom of the bed to the point that they completely blocked flow. The gels also dramatically expanded and contracted with changes in eluent composition, which led to the formation of voids and channels in the bed (16). Manufacturers of adsorbents have been very aware of these shortcomings and have introduced quite a number of improved adsorbents that hardly

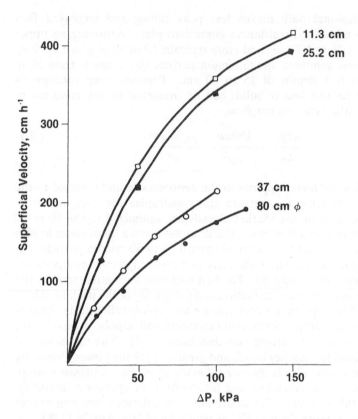

Figure 4   Pressure–flow rate relation for DEAE-Sepharose Fast Flow at a constant
bed height of 15 cm and different column diameters. (Adapted from Groundwater,
Ref. 131.)

compress under high flows or shrink or swell with changes in eluent
composition. Only in gel filtration of very-high-molecular-weight compounds
is the problem still evident. In this case the gel has to be very open with
large pores, which adversely affects its mechanical strength (54). Supports
that are derived from natural products tend to be more compressible than
those developed on inorganic bases. In small columns, wall effects definitely
reduce compressibility and the associated pressure drop. The effect can be
felt even up to a bed diameter of 37 cm (see Fig. 4). The pressure drop
relationship in the case of compressible beds is given by Janson and Hedman
(55).

$$\frac{\Delta P g_c}{L_B} = \frac{150 \mu u_o}{d_{p^2}} \exp\left[\frac{\alpha \Delta P}{L^B}\right] \tag{31}$$

The exponential term makes it clear that operation beyond a critical pressure drop per unit length of bed can lead to complete blockage of the column. Comparison of this equation to Eq. (30) shows that they are equal except for the last factor. The exponential term reflects a dependence of void volume on pressure as a result of deformation of the particles. Hysteresis and very slow recovery from high pressure drop excursion are typical of compressible adsorbents.

f. Porosity, Pore Size, and Pore Size Distribution. Since proteins are very large molecules, the issue of entry into the interior of the adsorbent cannot be overlooked. Pores should be large enough that free diffusion is not hindered significantly. This normally can be met with pores that are 10 to 20 times the diameter of the protein (56). Regnier (57) recommends 100 angstrom pores for small peptides and proteins, 300 angstrom pores for 50,000 to 100,000 dalton proteins, and 500 to 1000 angstrom pores for macromolecules larger than 200,000 daltons. The approximate diameter of globular proteins can be estimated from the equation shown below, which is adapted from Creighton (46).

$$\text{Diameter (angstroms)} = 1.344(\text{MW})^{0.33} \tag{32}$$

Alternatively, the manufacturer's tests of protein exclusion can be consulted to choose the appropriate gel. If pore size is increased indefinitely, mechanical strength will suffer and capacity will fall. The freedom to tailor the distribution of pore sizes has been exploited recently with the introduction of an ion exchange resin consisting of 10 to 20 micron particles with a bimodal pore size distribution (44). The larger pores at 6000–8000 angstroms are said to allow convective flow through the particle to some extent. The smaller pores at 500–1500 angstrom branch off the larger pores and contain most of the sites for adsorption. Concentration gradients within the particle are much reduced compared to conventional gels. High dynamic capacity is claimed at superficial velocities of up to 5000 cm/h.

g. Stability Toward Chemical and Microbial Attack. The gel under consideration should be stable to all the reagents that will contact it during the chromatographic cycle. All commercial gels are stable in aqueous media at slightly acidic to neutral pH. Most are stable to the common buffering salts and chaotropic agents such as guanidine hydrochloride, urea, and sodium dodecyl sulfate. Some, however, have difficulty with extremes of pH that may be required in the sanitizing and depyrogenation steps of the cycle. Sodium hydroxide has so many advantages as a cleansing, sanitizing, and depyrogenating agent (16) that short-term resistance of the resin to 0.5 N NaOH and long-term resistance to 0.1 N NaOH are very desirable properties. Cross-linked agarose will pass these tests. Silica based adsorbents (25,58) and cellulosic supports dissolve under these conditions. At times it may be necessary to treat the adsorbent with sodium phosphate, detergents, alcohol, or acetic acid in order to remove strongly adsorbed impurities (16,58). Stability toward these agents should be checked.

If the resin slowly degrades, it is important to determine at what rate and whether the degradation products are toxic. Mechanical strength of the gel may also suffer, leading to compression or the formation of fines. Breakdown of the attachment of the adsorbent ligand to the supporting gel or oxidation of the ligand may be a problem. All adsorbents should be freshly regenerated before use to be sure any breakdown products formed during long-term storage are washed from the gel.

Microbes will proliferate on most gels if nothing is done to suppress growth. The severity of the problem depends on the conditions of the chromatography and the incoming bioburden. Physiological pH and dilute phosphate buffers at room temperature favor growth (6). Low temperature, extreme pH (less than 3 and greater than 10), and mildly disinfecting buffers, such as borate, make it less likely. Feeds from earlier in the separation process tend to be more of a problem than those close to the end. The crude feeds usually have a higher bioburden and more nutrients for growth. In some cases the gel itself may serve as the food source (31). In others the adsorbent particles just serve as attachment sites.

h. Adsorbent Lifetime. The question of adsorbent lifetime is one for which there is no easy answer. Aside from the obvious extended use test, there is no way to predict the lifetime of a gel in a particular separation. What can be done easily is to perform a sensitivity analysis of the effect of gel lifetime on the economics of the process. If a small change in the estimated gel lifetime translates to a large cost increase, there is plenty of incentive to go ahead with the time trial or find a cheaper gel. If the effect is small, the pilot experience as it accumulates during development will suffice as an estimate of the gel lifetime. The data of Viljoen et al. (59) are illustrative of the approximate lifetime that has been reported in the literature. They report lifetimes of over 1000 regenerations for the purification of human albumin on a production scale. Total protein fed to the column may be a better gage of life expectancy than the number of regenerations or elapsed time (60). Fouling is usually a more important determinant of lifetime than chemical stability of the matrix (4). Estimates in the literature should be taken as nothing more than an indication of what is possible in some circumstances. There is no substitute for actual experience.

F. Optimization of Individual Steps

Chromatography is a cyclical operation. To prepare the best design, all steps of the cycle must be considered. The general cycle of operation consists of loading the column with feed solution, washing the residual feed off the column, eluting the column, and finally regenerating and sanitizing the column preparatory to the next cycle. Certain types of chromatography are simpler than the cycle given above.

The stepwise nature of chromatography offers opportunities for optimizing each of the steps separately. For instance, in the equilibration and regeneration steps much smaller molecules with faster transfer kinetics are being adsorbed and desorbed. This means that flow rates can be considerably higher than those specified for protein adsorption and elution. The faster equilibration and regeneration translates into faster turnaround time and fewer columns.

Flow direction may be changed if it is desired to remove very strongly bound impurities in a small volume and time (20). If impurities are bound strongly to the top of the column (assuming loading in downflow), regenerating upflow will sweep the impurities off the column without having to push them all the way through the bed.

It may also be possible entirely or intermittently to skip a sanitization cycle in cases of light fouling of the gel. Reequilibration can be started with high concentrations of buffer to take advantage of mass action to speed things up (19). The equilibration is finished with a relatively small volume of buffer whose strength matches that of the column feed.

The temperature of each step can be adjusted, but given the high thermal capacity of the column, usually only one step will be considered for change. A good candidate is the sanitization step. The effectiveness of the cleansing, sanitizing, or sterilizing agent is greatly increased by raising the temperature (1,30), thereby shortening the column turnaround time by hours.

VI. MECHANICAL DESIGN AND OPERATION

A. Column Geometry

Columns are available in diameters ranging from 0.5 cm up to 2 m and in lengths from 5 cm up to 1 m or more (61). Ion exchange columns of several thousand liters bed volume are in use today (13). For protein work, other than gel permeation, rather short columns of from 15 to 45 cm are favored, principally because the adsorption-desorption behavior of the protein negates almost all of the benefit of long columns, while the debits of high pressure drop and greater compression of the gel remain (20). The trend toward short squat columns means that excellent liquid distribution is a must. Vendors have gone to considerable effort to design liquid distributors that direct the flow evenly over the face of the column and minimize dead volume (31). They generally employ tortuous path, antijetting devices and stacked screens to insure proper operation. Two designs are shown in Figs. 5 and 6. In large diameter columns a fine screen over a coarse screen gives more reliable distribution than a porous plastic disk (31).

Fixed or movable head designs are available. The fixed head is less expensive, and easier to seal, but it is harder to pack and not as versatile as the movable head design. With the movable head, either one or both ends of the column are adjustable, so that the distributor can be brought down to the surface of the bed to eliminate dead volume.

O-ring seals prevent leakage past the movable distributor. In larger diameters, the problems of seal leakage, ease of adjustment, and parallel lowering of the distributor become more difficult. Newer designs address some of these problems.

Material of construction is usually glass or clear plastic for small columns (lab and pilot scale) and stainless steel or fluorocarbon-coated stainless steel for production columns. The plastic and glass designs are fragile and are limited to around 15 psig operating pressure in larger diameters (62,63). They do offer the advantage of seeing the bed at all times. Thicker wall designs are available on special order for higher pressure

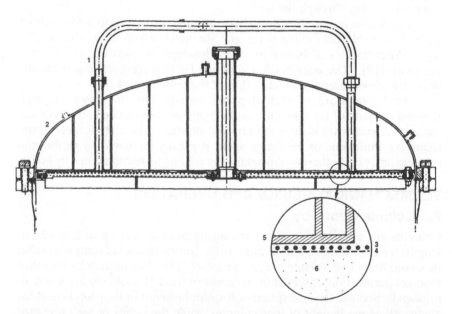

Figure 5 Cross-section of the upper part of a stainless steel Sephamatic Gel Filter belonging to the 08-series with a diameter of 80 cm. (1) Feed manifold of four pipes; (2) false head cover for structural strength; (3) coarse distributor screen; (4) fine screen to retain adsorbent; (5) true head plate; (6) adsorbent bed. (Adapted from Janson, Ref. 67.)

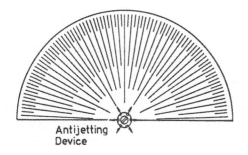

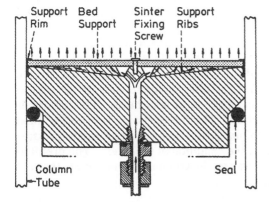

Figure 6 Amicon design of flow distributor for chromatography column. (Reprinted with permission from Amicon Division, W. R. Grace and Co.)

operation of large industrial columns (64). Adsorption of seemingly colorless protein solutions can cause a subtle change in the appearance of the gel that can be detected by the naked eye. Fissures or other gross abnormalities are easily spotted. Due to irregularities in concentricity, very large diameter glass columns are custom fitted to the distributor. If the glass wall of the column breaks, new end plates are needed in addition to a new glass tube. Plastic suffers from gradual darkening and crazing due to action of light and the aggressive chemicals used for sanitization and regeneration. If the crazing continues to the point of cracking the wall, sudden failure of the column is possible.

The stainless steel units are rugged and can operate at 45–60 psig or beyond with heavier construction. Stainless steel is susceptible to the corrosive action of buffer salts, especially chlorides. The more corrosion resistant type 316 should be specified in preference to type 304. Sanitary 3A construction with electropolishing minimizes crevices that promote corrosion and provides for easy cleaning. ASME or similar coded vessels are available if desired (65). The major disadvantage of the stainless units is that they are opaque. The transition from a clear pilot column to an opaque production column means giving up a process control that development personnel may have come to rely on heavily. On the other hand, large diameter columns of glass only show the condition of the bed in the vicinity of the wall. Visual appearance under these circumstances is not as reliable as periodic HETP determinations (26) (see Section J below). The final decision on the material of construction depends on the size of the production columns and the true usefulness of being able to observe the bed.

If the adsorbent is very compressible and yet a long bed is needed for resolution, shallow 15 cm beds may be stacked one above the other (66). Gel permeation chromatography of very high molecular proteins would fall in this category.

B. Column Prefilters

All chromatography columns should be protected from plugging by separately filtering all feeds to the column (67) The filter should retain particles smaller than 1/10 to 1/100 of the diameter of the adsorbent beads. Pleated depth-type cartridge filters are satisfactory. The filters should be sized to offer negligible pressure drop and minimal dead volume. Appropriate pressure gages should be installed to follow the condition of the filters. The prefilters need to be sanitized in the same way as the column. In-line filters that can be easily disassembled are best.

C. Tanks

If the chromatography step is close to the end of the process and represents the final purification step, type 316 stainless steel tanks that conform to the 3A sanitary code should be specified (30). An exception to this rule is tanks for buffers that are high in chlorides or other components corrosive to stainless steel. Plastic is usually a good alternative for such cases, provided it is impervious, nonleaching, smooth, and constructed to be free-draining. For production units, each feed stream to the column should come from a separate tank in order to minimize the chance of cross contamination. These tanks do not have to be any larger than the amount needed for a day's operation. Large inventories of dilute buffers at mild pH's should be avoided due to the possibility of the buildup of mold and bacteria. Stock buffer solutions may be prepared in highly concentrated form, which prevents spoilage. These concentrates are then fed from large holding tanks to the smaller feed tanks and diluted as needed. Ideally each tank should be equipped with agitation, a heating/cooling jacket, and load cells.

D. Pumps

The main requirements for pumps are that the flow be reproducible, pulse-free, and adjustable. For small lab or pilot columns, these conditions can be satisfied by peristaltic pumps (55). Their main advantages are the lack of moving seals, ease of cleaning, and gentle pumping action. Disadvantages are an upper pressure rating of 20 to 30 psig, slow drift in reproducibility of the flow as the pump tubing ages, slight pulsing in the flow, and a rather low upper limit to the flow capacity.

For large pilot or production columns, rotary lobe pumps, gear pumps, or double diaphragm pumps are good choices (30). In general these pumps are more rugged than the peristaltic type. They also have a better long term reproducibility of flow and can easily reach 100 psig. Flow capacity is not a problem. While pulsing is still present, it is usually less pronounced than that of a peristaltic pump. Disadvantages of these types of pump are that they have moving seals, they are harder to clean, they require pressure relief devices, and their corrosion resistance may be a problem.

Centrifugal pumps are not recommended because they require separate control systems to maintain constant flow under changing backpressure. Under certain flow conditions they may also subject the protein to elevated temperatures or slight cavitation that will probably cause aggregation or denaturation.

E. Detectors

The detection scheme that is almost universally specified for proteins is ultraviolet light absorption at 280 nm. The absorption is due primarily to tryptophan and tyrosine residues with a very small contribution from phenylalanine (46). Virtually any protein will contain at least some of these amino acids. The situation is not as sure for peptides. If absorption at 280 nm is inadequate, the wavelength can be dropped to 205 nm for a more universal response (68). Of course the lack of specificity at 205 nm means impurities may be falsely identified as peptides.

The detector light source is usually a long-life lamp and filter combination. Filters are available at wavelengths of 206, 226, 254, 280, 313, 365, and 405 nm. This setup has a much longer lamp lifetime (6000 vs. 200 h) than the deuterium lamp found in infinitely adjustable wavelength detectors.

Flow cells are available for all flows from the analytical scale to about 30 Lpm (30). Flow cells with a short and long path length are handy to get good sensitivity for impurities while still keeping the main component on scale. Appropriate flow cells for truly large-scale production are limited. The approach taken by vendors has been to split the flow and only send a small portion to the detector. While this can be made to work, it would be much better to have the total flow pass through the detector.

Another problem with commercial separations is that the concentration of protein coming off the column during elution will often saturate the response of the detector. Instead of Gaussian peaks the result is a peak with a flat top. Integration of the peak to determine the amount of protein is pointless. The total eluate has to be collected and sampled if an assay of the protein content is desired.

It is often useful to monitor conductivity and pH in addition to UV absorption. Various conductivity in-line flow cells are available for all scales of operation. Conductivity is a good way to verify the composition of buffers and monitor the progress of regeneration of ion exchangers. Units with temperature compensation and automatic range finding should be specified. Although pH changes are seldom used to displace proteins from absorbents (2), it is good practice to monitor the pH profile of the chromatography cycle. The profile can become part of the process validation. In-line pH probes are available for all scales of operation. Again temperature compensated units are preferred.

F. Air Traps

Air traps are necessary to prevent air from entering the column and interfering with proper flow distribution (30). The design is fairly simple. The trap is just an upright clear plastic or glass cylinder with inlet and outlet ports in the bottom head. Feed and entrained air enter the bottom of the cylinder where the air disengages and accumulates at the top. The liquid, free of bubbles, exits through the outlet port on the bottom of the cylinder. Periodically the air accumulated at the top of the trap is released by opening a vent valve. The trap must be big enough that the air can disengage from the liquid before the feed leaves the trap. An adequate design is to have the trap diameter 6 to 8 times the diameter of the inlet port. The height of the trap should be about 1.5 times the diameter. The trap is a fairly large dead volume. In situations where it is important to minimize backmixing, the trap can be drained just before switching over to the new feed. If the flow to the column can be reversed, design the plumbing so that the air trap is always on the feed side of the column.

G. Valves, Piping, and Plumbing Details

For lab and pilot scale equipment, plastic hose and tubing are adequate for piping. Ball valves or pinch clamps serve as the valves to control flow. For full production, stainless steel tubing and fittings that conform to the 3A sanitary code should be specified. Dead volume should be kept to a minimum. Velocities through the tubing should correspond to mildly turbulent flow if backmixing is to be kept to a minimum (55). Table 1, adapted from Johansson (30), shows the size required for different flows with aqueous solutions at room temperature. Sanitary diaphragm valves, butterfly valves, or special ball valves free of inaccessible pockets serve for production

Table 1 Pressure Drop and Flow Velocities for Water Flow at Room Temperature in Smooth Pipes at Reynolds Numbers of 2000 to 50,000

Pipe inner diameter (cm)	Flow rate (liters per minute)	Pressure drop (kPa per meter)
0.4	0.57–9.5	3–413
0.8	1.13–19	0.38–52
1.2	1.7–28.5	0.11–15
1.6	2.3–38	0.05–6.5
2.2	3.1–52	0.02–2.5
4.8	6.8–114	0.001–0.2

Source: Adapted from Johansson (30).

units. Three-way valves are also popular as a means of reducing the complexity of the piping involved in providing for flow in either direction through the column. Pressure gages should be installed as close to the column inlet and outlet as possible. This insures that the pressure drop reflects only the gradient across the bed. The column should be plumbed for flow in either direction by switching only a few valves.

Connections to the top head plate should be easily disconnected to allow the column to be packed. A vent valve is needed on each line leading to the head plates to allow for purging all the air from the lines on startup and column packing. If piping manifolds are installed, be sure any possible cross contamination can be tolerated, otherwise adequate checks for leaks have to be written into the operating procedure. The design should contain no dead legs or other plumbing that cannot be fully wetted by the sanitizing agent.

H. Flowmeters

On the lab or small pilot plant scale, flow rates are often just checked periodically with graduated cylinders and a stopwatch. For larger scale operation, rotameters, turbine flowmeters, or Coriolis effect flowmeters are preferred. Johansson (30) especially favors a bearingless flowmeter with a light reflective rotor sensed by a photodetector. Glass rotameters should not be exposed to sodium hydroxide sanitizing solution for long periods.

I. Fraction Collectors

Fraction collectors in the lab tend to be of the highly automated moving head type and thus easily adapted to the particular needs of the separation at hand. As the scale of operation increases, the number of models of fraction collectors to choose from decreases and the range of options narrows. For production columns the fraction collector is often not a separate unit. Rather it is a computer-controlled piping manifold. Once the program to control the valves in the manifold has been set, it is locked in.

It is possible to change it, but not as conveniently as with the pilot or lab units. Another feature of production fraction collectors is that the number of fractions is generally much fewer than those taken in a lab separation. By the time the separation has been scaled up, the number of fractions to take has been optimized. Each fraction from the large column goes to a separate tank.

J. Packing the Column

The column must be packed correctly if efficient chromatography is to be obtained. Although the specifics of packing vary depending on the type of gel and the manufacturer of the column, it is instructive to give two typical procedures for the lab and large scale as examples of the precautions necessary to achieve uniform packing. The lab procedure assumes a column with a movable head plate. The large-scale procedure assumes a fixed head plate.

The lab procedure starts with filling the column with buffer until liquid covers the lower bed support by about 2 inches. The bottom drain valve is opened, and buffer is run out until all air is purged from the bottom piping. Any air bubbles trapped under the bed support screen can be removed by vacuuming them out. This is done with a hose that sucks the bubbles through the screen into a trap bottle connected to a vacuum source. The gel is suspended in enough degassed buffer to make the slurry about 75% solids by volume (41). The buffer should match the composition of the process buffer that causes the greatest shrinkage of the gel. It has been found that packing a relatively heavy slurry gives a more uniform bed than packing a thin slurry. Care should be taken not to get air into the slurry either during stirring or upon addition to the column. The slurry is added quickly to the column containing about 2 inches of free buffer. The best results are obtained when the column is filled in a single pouring.

Always keep a head of buffer over the gel surface. The last portion of gel should settle to a height within the adjustment of the top bed support. Buffer is added to overflow the column. The vent on the top head plate is opened, and the top head is slightly tilted to the side before lowering it down onto the column. The tilt prevents air from getting caught under the top bed support, while the open vent allows air and water trapped in the head plate plumbing to escape. Once the head plate makes a complete seal on the column, it is straightened out and slowly lowered to the gel level. The head plate is secured to the column, and final adjustments in height are made before locking the support in place. The bed should have a uniform appearance, free of trapped air bubbles. In making the connections to the column make sure that all air has been purged from the lines. Further fine adjustments may be required after the bed has been equilibrated with buffer. The flow of buffer tends to consolidate the bed, producing a void at the entrance.

The packing procedure for a large-scale column is identical to the lab procedure except that the amount of gel added to the column has to be more carefully controlled. The fixed head means that the gel level has to be at precisely the top of the column for efficient packing. Normally several attempts will be required before the level is just right. To load gel to the top of the column, a short extension piece must be clamped onto the top of the column (31). The clamps should be of the type that can be snapped open and removed in a few seconds. Welder's vise grips are suitable. Gel slurry (75% v/v solids) is added to the extension piece in an amount estimated to bring the gel level to slightly above the joint between the extension piece and the top of the column. The extension piece is filled to the top with buffer. A rotary lobe pump is connected to the bottom drain of the column, and buffer is pumped out of the column at a rate greater than that of the flow at any step of the chromatography (16) until the buffer level is just above the gel. Exact recommendations for the flow rate are available from the adsorbent manufacturers. The pressure gradient caused by the pumping will compress the bed. If the gel estimate is correct, the gel level will be just below the top of the column. The pump is stopped, and the clamps holding the extension piece onto the column are quickly sprung and removed. As the extension is removed, excess gel and buffer cascade onto the floor and create quite a mess. The top head of the column is lowered very quickly onto the column. One must work quickly because the bed starts to expand as soon as the pumping stops. As soon as the lid is down, it is bolted in place. Buffer is pumped upward through the column to displace air from the top head and piping. The process required considerable skill and some luck.

The efficiency of the column can be checked by determining the HETP as described by Cooney and others (16,69).

VII. DEPYROGENATION AND COLUMN HYGIENE

A. Depyrogenation

Pyrogens are substances that cause a fever response when injected into man or other animals. The most common variety are endotoxins derived from the cell wall of Gram negative bacteria such as *E. coli*. Endotoxins are high-molecular-weight lipopolysaccharides of acidic character. Only tiny amounts, as little as 80 ng of *E. coli* pyrogen for the average man, are necessary to elicit the fever reaction (70).

Virtually all protein products will contain pyrogens unless positive steps are taken to control them. Proteins derived from recombinant *E. coli* will be heavily contaminated with pyrogens at the start of refining. Even in cases where *E. coli* is not involved, pyrogens can still be expected originating from other natural raw materials (70).

Although pyrogens are derived from bacteria, they are not living. Ordinary steam sterilization will not destroy them (71). Chemical destruction

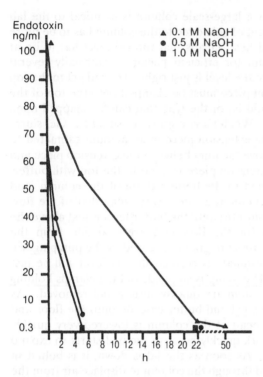

Figure 7 Destruction of *E. coli* endotoxin by sodium hydroxide at room temperature. The effect of sodium hydroxide concentration and time. (Reprinted with permission from Pharmacia LKB Biotechnology.)

requires extremes of temperature or pH that are far beyond the stability of proteins.

How then to control and remove pyrogens? One of the most effective ways of removing endotoxin is to pass the protein through an anion exchange column. Most pyrogens are strongly acidic in nature (6). They bind to the column even under conditions that would elute any adsorbed protein. The purification factor can easily be 10,000 or greater. While the purification factor may be impressive, it just suffices in the face of the extreme potency of pyrogens.

It is helpful to construct an endotoxin material balance across the total separation process. The balance will be crude because the assay for endotoxin is quite variable. Even with this problem, it will be instantly clear where to concentrate pyrogen removal and control. Usually pyrogen levels will reduced by many orders of magnitude as the protein is purified.

Once the pyrogens have been removed, great care must be taken to prevent recontamination. Pyrogens are ubiquitous. The most common sources are water and textiles made from natural fiber. The buffer for the elution step and all subsequent operations should be made up with water that is pyrogen-free. Water for Injection, USP (WFI) is suitable (72). All tanks and lines should be washed with WFI before introducing the eluted protein solution (73). Paper towels and cotton wipes should not be used to dry WFI-rinsed surfaces. Operators should wear surgical gloves for all operations. The column itself can be depyrogenated by exposure to sodium hydroxide for a length of time sufficient to hydrolyze the pyrogens. Figure 7 shows the time-concentration relationship for effective depyrogenation. A typical set of conditions would be 0.5 N NaOH for 6 h at room temperature. The hold period is important to allow time for complete chemical degradation.

B. Sanitization and Long-Term Storage

Columns must be sanitized between uses to prevent microorganisms from colonizing the equipment. The adverse effects of such colonization include breakdown of the column matrix, contamination of the product with unknown bacteria and their by-products, buildup of pyrogens, possible digestion of the product by proteases elaborated by the bacteria, and plugging of the column. In most cases, sanitization, i.e., the near total eradication of microbes, is sufficient to control the problem. Sterilization is not usually necessary. Sanitization is best implemented by a clean-in-place (CIP) procedure on a regular basis, preferable after every batch. With properly designed equipment (sanitary design to 3A standards) it should be unnecessary to unload the gel between uses. The most popular sanitizing agent is sodium hydroxide. It possesses the following set of advantages as first enumerated by Curling and Cooney (74) that put it far ahead of competing agents:

1. Its presence in the final product is of no consequence.
2. It is an effective disinfectant.
3. It has a solubilizing effect on proteins and lipids and will, therefore, remove such residues that can act as substrates for bacterial growth.
4. It is inexpensive.
5. It is easily disposed.
6. It is compatible with the separation media used.

Other chemicals such as ethanol, isopropanol, sodium azide, chlorbutanol, chlorhexidine, merthiolate, and bleach work perfectly well as disinfecting agents, but they fail on one or more of the questions regarding toxicity, reactivity, and carryover of residues to the final product. In special circumstances, such as resistance of the bacterial flora or instability of the gel toward base, it may be necessary to adopt one of these compounds in place of sodium hydroxide.

It is good practice to monitor the microbiological condition of the column on a regular basis. Later tests can be compared to the original work to demonstrate the continuing effectiveness of the sanitization procedure. Resistant strains can develop over time or be introduced with new lots of raw materials. If they are detected, switching to a different disinfectant or a much more concentrated solution of the same agent should clear up the problem. Time and temperature of contact are important variables in determining the effectiveness of the disinfection.

Long-term storage should be treated as a separate operation deserving careful consideration. Once the column has been sanitized it can be kept in that condition by holding the gel in a weak solution of disinfectant. As an example, sodium hydroxide at 0.05 N is commonly used for storage of ion exchange gels. Either the same or a different agent as that used for the main sanitization may be chosen (75). The choice depends primarily on effectiveness and lack of reactivity toward the gel over extended time. The dilute disinfectant maintains a bacteriostatic action while minimizing degradation of the gel over long periods of time. If convenient, the column may be held at 4°C to retard spoilage further. Certain gels can be completely dried for long-term storage (55).

When it is time to use the gel again, it should be put through a full regeneration cycle to remove any degradation products that might have been produced during storage.

C. Sterilization

In special circumstances it may be necessary to sterilize the adsorbent bed. In these cases very careful design of the entire system is essential to be sure that all surfaces are contacted effectively by the sterilizing agent. The preferred agent is live steam. Unfortunately, packed columns cannot stand this type of treatment. Chemical sterilants such as ethanol, sodium hydroxide, or formaldehyde are possible substitutes. Sodium hypochlorite and hydrogen peroxide should be avoided because they generate gas bubbles in the bed (30). The manufacturer of the adsorbent should be consulted for specific recommendations regarding the type and concentration of sterilant necessary to sterilize their media without adversely affecting their adsorptive properties. Naturally all piping, fittings, and solutions associated with the operation of the column must also be sterilized. All connections and takeoffs must be capable of aseptic operation.

The Food and Drug Administration (FDA) has deservedly very strict regulations covering aseptic operations (76). There are many technical papers that cover the *dos* and *don'ts* of aseptic operation (29,30,75). These sources should be consulted before attempting to design an aseptic chromatographic separation. Whatever method is finally decided on, it must be validated by extensive testing with appropriate challenges. Every aspect of the operation must be examined for possible sources of contamination.

Obviously the design, operation, and validation of an aseptic chromatography system is an expensive and time-consuming task. Every effort should be made to postpone the sterility requirement to as late in the process as is consistent with product quality. The best solution, if possible, is heat sterilization of the final product (76). Unfortunately, most proteins would be denatured by this treatment. More realistic alternatives are absolute filtration through a 0.22 micron filter or exposure to a sterilizing dose of radiation.

VIII. AUTOMATION

A. Pilot Plant Requirements and Systems

The distinguishing feature of the pilot plant is the need for flexibility (77). This translates to the need for an automation system that can be adapted on short notice with a minimum of programming skill. For serious development work, the control unit should be capable of duplicating the full chromatographic cycle anticipated in production. At the lab and pilot plant stage many automation systems are available that meet this requirement (78,79). They are available off-the-shelf and often include a dedicated microprocessor controller, pumps, and associated plumbing, all in one package. Most are quite flexible in adapting to the many different chromatographic separations that are encountered in pilot plant work. Peak detection, fraction collection, and step and gradient changes in eluent are easily handled. More troublesome, but still doable, are reverse flow, switching from one step in the chromatography to the next, and multiple buffers of very different composition. The control unit can be separated from the rest of the system if it is necessary to run the column in a refrigerated room. None of the systems on the market are temperature programmable as would be useful for quicker and more effective simulations of the sanitization cycle.

All of these units strive to be user-friendly. The best do succeed. The number of programs that can be stored is continually increasing with each new model. There is also a trend toward having the ability to request a complete operation with a single keystroke rather than having to key each of the individual valves that must be energized to accomplish the operation (79). Documentation of planned and ad hoc steps during the course of the separation is much better with recent machines. Paper tape indicating the position of the various valves has given way to a full video display of the ongoing chromatography in flowsheet form along with a complete history of the programmed and manual interventions. This reflects recognition by the vendors of the importance of good documentation as proof of compliance with FDA regulatory requirements. Some of the units can handle small production jobs, such as the purification of monoclonal antibodies. The upper limit of scale is set by the flow capacity of the valves, lines, and controlled pumps.

The alternative of a dedicated solid-state controller is cheaper for the hardware but decidedly user-unfriendly. At the other end of the spectrum, a multipurpose process computer does hold the advantage of being directly translatable to production. The control algorithm can be developed at the pilot stage, and operating personnel will be familiar with it prior to plant start-up. The disadvantages are the greater expense of the computer and the time lost to the learning curve before operation is smooth.

The final alternative is no automation at all. Depending on the turnaround time of the column, the frequency of production, and the complexity of operation, it is reasonable in many cases to operate columns manually. Most of these situations will arise at the pilot plant scale where supervision will be continuous with or without automation.

B. Production Requirements and Systems

Production automation must emphasize reliability, robustness, and a clearly documented history of each operation (77). The control of large-scale chromatography steps is usually handled as part of a computer system that oversees the operation of the entire process. The types of computers and software that are available for batch processing can quite easily handle the sequential steps of chromatography. Unlike the pilot plant models, the piping, valves, and pumps for the production system are usually custom designed and interfaced with the controlling computer. Input and output devices are designed for the higher loads and noisy electrical fields typically found in industrial operation.

The control language for plant systems is not as customized as that for pilot plant systems. The burden of dealing with a slightly less friendly system is compensated for by universal applicability once it is mastered. Production control programs are protected from tampering by passwords and key locks. While it does protect the integrity of the program, it also makes it more cumbersome to make a legitimate change. This is a feature common to all production systems. It is assumed that the control strategy has been well worked out before the protein is put into production. Changes occur much less frequently than in a pilot plant.

Accurate record keeping is one of the major advantages of automation. All production control systems must provide a good paper trail of all actions taken by the computer and operators. Chromatography in production should have already undergone an extensive validation study (80,81) to show that the purification is effective when certain operating parameters are maintained within prescribed limits. A major aim of automatic control is to prevent deviations outside of these limits. In cases where the system does go out of control, the deviation is documented and highlighted for corrective action.

Automation also nicely handles the logistical problems of running multiple columns that are not synchronized in operation.

The computer system itself should be validated following guidelines being developed by the FDA and the pharmaceutical industry (82). Proper validation assures that the program will perform as predicted, that proper backup and documentation is provided, that operators are properly qualified and trained, and that the system is secure and reliable.

C. Current Good Manufacturing Practices

The FDA has issued a set of regulations that are intended to insure the production of safe and effective drugs. These regulations, entitled *Current Good Manufacturing Practices* (CGMP) (83), cover the formulation and packing of the bulk drug into a finished dosage form. Over the years the agency has extended the published regulations back in the form of guidelines (84) to cover the preparation of the bulk drug. In the case of drugs derived from recombinant biotechnology, special points to consider (7) have been issued.

The approach in all cases is to foster a philosophy of building quality into every aspect of the process rather than just relying on the final quality control assay to detect problems. This is done through proper equipment design, training, validated procedures, and documentation proving continuing compliance. The significance of this with regard to scale-up of chromatography is that certain features must be designed into the system right from the start if compliance is to be assured. As the product gets closer and closer to its final purity, it becomes more important to protect that purity from contamination. Many times, chromatography steps are near the end of the process and represent the final purification. Subsequent steps just serve to concentrate or dialyze the product. In these circumstances, the design should protect against the introduction of foreign matter and cross-contamination with other products handled in the plant. The equipment must be designed so that it can be easily cleaned, and the gel must be reserved for one product only (19). The chromatography hardware must be dedicated to a single product or be cleaned by a method shown to be effective by actual test.

Water for the chromatography must be of the appropriate quality, in most cases WFI. A testing program must be in place to monitor the water quality (85), the pyrogen content of the eluate, and the bioburden of the buffers, column, and eluate. Closed systems are preferred over open tanks. In most situations, rated cleanrooms (86) are appropriate for the final steps of the process.

Every aspect of the operation and control of the chromatography must be properly documented with procedures and batch records. All raw materials must be covered by an inventory control system designed to insure their identity and potency.

APPENDIX: LIST OF SYMBOLS

a_1 HETP factor accounting for deviations from ideal plug flow
a_2 HETP factor accounting for thin-film and pore diffusion resistances
a_3 HETP factor accounting for axial diffusion
a_p external surface area of particles per unit packed volume (cm^{-1})
B bed volume defined by Eq. (9)
B' equivalent bed volume defined by Eq. (12)
c bulk liquid solute concentration (g cm^{-3})
c_o feed concentration (g cm^{-3})
C adsorbent saturation capacity [g final protein (liter adsorbent)$^{-1}$]
d_p particle diameter (cm)
D column diameter (cm)
D_i effective particle diffusion coefficient (cm^2 s^{-1})
D_L protein diffusivity in bulk liquid (cm^2 s^{-1})
E_z axial dispersion coefficient (cm^2 s^{-1})
F volumetric flow rate (cm^3 s^{-1})
g_c conversion factor [980 g cm ((g-wt)s^2)$^{-1}$]
h bed height (cm)
k_f fluid film mass transfer coefficient (cm s^{-1})
L liters processed (L)
L_B bed length (cm)
MW   molecular weight (daltons)
N_d number of transfer units assuming axial dispersion controls
N_f number of transfer units assuming fluid film mass transfer controls
N_k number of transfer units assuming kinetic control
N_{pore} number of transfer units assuming pore diffusion controls
P feed protein concentration [(g final protein) L^{-1}]
Pe $u_o d_p/E_z$, Peclet number
q_o sorbate concentration in equilibrium with c_o [g (g particle)$^{-1}$]
Q protein production rate [(kg final protein)day^{-1}]
Q_{max} maximum sorbate concentration [g (g particle)$^{-1}$]
R particle radius (cm)
S column cross-section (cm^2)
T time (h)
T_D $(V_T-\epsilon v)$ $(\Gamma v)^{-1}$, dimensionless throughput parameter
T_K temperature (°K)
u_o F/S, liquid superficial velocity (cm s^{-1})
U fraction of column capacity that will be loaded during each cycle
v bed volume (cm^3)
V superficial velocity through the bed (cm h^{-1})
V_T throughput volume (cm^3)

Subscripts

E elution phase
H holding phase
L loading phase
R regeneration phase
W washing phase

Greek

α adjustable parameter to account for bed compressibility in Eq. (31)
Γ $\rho_B q_o/c_o$, distribution parameter
ΔP pressure drop $[(\text{g-wt})\text{cm}^{-2}]$
ϵ void fraction, dimensionless
μ fluid viscosity (g cm^{-1} s^{-1})
μ_c fluid viscosity (centipoise)
μ_f adsorption rate constant (s^{-1} g^{-1} cm^3)
ρ density of the fluid (g cm^{-3})
ρ_B $(1-\epsilon)\rho_p$, particle bulk density [g cm^{-3}(bed volume)]
ρ_p particle density [g cm^{-3}(particle)]

REFERENCES

1. Sofer, G. K., and Nystrom, L. E. (1989). *Process Chromatography, A Practical Guide*, Academic Press, London, pp. 107–115, 65, 93–105.
2. Scopes, R. K. (1987). *Protein Purification Principles and Practice*, 2nd ed., Springer-Verlag, New York, pp. 100–126, 133, 161, 186–198.
3. Gooding, K. M., and Schmuck, M. N. (1983). Purification of trypsin and other basic proteins by high-performance cation-exchange chromatography, *J. Chromatogr.*, *266*: 633.
4. Regnier, F. E. (1984). High-performance ion-exchange chromatography, *Methods in Enzymology*, *104*: 170.
5. Richey, J. S. (1984). Optimal pH conditions for ion exchangers on macroporous supports, *Methods in Enzymology*, *104*: 223.
6. Sofer, G. (1984). Chromatographic removal of pyrogens, *Bio/Technology*, *2*: 1037.
7. *Points to Consider in the Production and Testing of New Drugs and Biologicals Produced by Recombinant DNA Technology* (1983). Draft, U.S. Department of Health and Human Services, Public Health Service, Food and Drug Administration, Bethesda, Maryland, November 7.
8. Delaney, R. A. M. (1980). Industrial gel filtration of proteins, *Applied Protein Chemistry* (R. A. Grant, ed.), Applied Science, Barking, England, pp. 233–280.
9. Gerstenberg, H., Sittig, W., and Zepf, K. (1980). Processing of fermentation products, *Ger. Chem. Eng.*, *3*: 313.
10. Kelley, J. J., Wang, G. Y., and Wang, H. Y. (1986). Large-scale gel chromatography: Assessment of utility for purification of protein products from microbial

sources, *Separation, Recovery, and Purification in Biotechnology*, A. C. S. Symposium Series, No. 314 (J. A. Asenjo and J. Hong, eds.), American Chemical Society, Washington, D.C., pp. 193–207.

11. Hammond, P. M.., Sherwood, R. F., Atkinson, T., and Scawen, M. D. (1987). Hydrophobic interaction chromatography for large scale purification of proteins, *Chim. Oggi*, *10*: 57.

12. Ingraham, R. H., Lau, S. Y. M., Taneja, A. K., and Hodges, R. S. (1985). Denaturation and the effects of temperature on hydrophobic-interaction and reversed-phase high performance liquid chromatography of proteins. Bio-Gel TSK-Phenyl-5-PW column, *J. Chromatogr.*, *327*: 77.

13. Groundwater, E. (1985). Guidelines for chromatography scale-up, *Lab. Pract.*, *34*: 17.

14. Sluyterman, L. A. A., and Wijdenes, J. (1981). Chromatofocusing IV. Properties of an agarose polyethyleneimine ion exchanger and its suitability for protein separations, *J. Chromatogr.*, *206*: 441.

15. Bergstrom. J., Sodenberg, L., Wahlstrom, L., Muller, R. M., Momicelj, A., Hagstrom, G., Stahlberg, R., Kallman, I., and Hansson, K. A. (1985). Recommendation for obtaining optimal separations on MONOBEAD™ ion exchangers, *Protides of the Biological Fluids* (H. Peeters, ed.), Pergamon Press, Oxford, vol. 30, pp. 641–646.

16. Cooney, J. M. (1984). Chromatographic gel media for large-scale protein purification, *Bio/Technology*, *2*: 41.

17. Kroeff, E. P., Owens, R. A., Campbell, E. L., Johnson, R. D., and Marks, H. I. (1989). Production scale purification of biosynthetic human insulin by reversed-phase high-performance liquid chromatography, *J. Chromatogr.*, *461*: 45.

18. Sadana, A. (1989). Protein inactivation during downstream processing, Part I: The processes, *BioPharm.*, *2*: 14.

19. Duffy, S. A., Moellering , B. J., Prior, G. M., Doyle, K. R., and Prior, C. P. (1989). Recovery of therapeutic-grade antibodies: Protein A and ion-exchange chromatography, *BioPharm*, *2*: 34.

20. Chase, H. A. (1984). Scale-up of immunoaffinity separation process, *J. of Biotechnol.*, *1*: 67.

21. Frenz, J., and Horvath, C. (1988). High-performance displacement chromatography, *High-Performance Liquid Chromatography*, vol. 5 (C. Horvath, ed.), Academic Press, San Diego, California, pp. 212–314.

22. Katti, A., and Guiochon, G. (1988). Prediction of band profiles in displacement chromatography by numerical integration of a semi-ideal model, *J. Chromatogr.*, *449*: 25.

23. Subramanian, G., Phillips, M. W., Jayaraman, G., Cramer, S. M. (1989). Displacement chromatography of biomolecules with large particle diameter systems, *J. Chromatogr.*, *484*: 225.

24. Felinger, A., and Guiochon, G. (1993). Comparison of maximum production rates and optimum operating/design parameters in overloaded elution and displacement chromatography, *Biotechnol. Bioeng.*, *41*: 134.

25. Curling, J. (1979). "Large-Scale Ion Exchange Chromatography of Proteins," Proceedings of FEBS Meet., *52*, pp. 45–57.

26. Van Brunt, J. (1988). Scale-up: How big is big enough, *Bio/Technology*, *6*: 479.

27. Chen, J. W., Buege, J. A., Cunningham, F. L., and Northam, J. I. (1968). Scale-up of a column adsorption process by computer simulation, *Ind. Eng. Chem. Process Design and Development, 7*: 26.

28. Cueille, G., and Tayot, J. L. (1985). "Ion Exchange as a Production Technique for Proteins," Proceedings of Biotech '85 Europe, Geneva, pp. 141–160.

29. Simpson, J. M. (1988). Preliminary design of ion exchange columns for protein purification, *Bio/Technology, 6*: 1158.

30. Johansson, H., Oesting, M., Sofer, G., Wahlstroem, H., and Low, D. (1988). Chromatographic equipment for large-scale protein and peptide purification, *Adv. Biotechnol. Processes, 8*: 127.

31. Janson, J. C., and Dunhill, P. (1974). "Factors Affecting Scale-Up of Chromatography," Proceedings of FEBS Meet., *30*, pp. 81–105.

32. Colin, A., Lowy, G., and Cazes, J. (1986). Design and performance of preparative-scale HPLC, *International Biotechnol. Laboratory, 4*:30.

33. Arnold, F. H., Blanch, H. W., and Wilke, C. R. (1985). Analysis of affinity separations I: Predicting the performance of affinity adsorbers, *Chemical Engineering J., 30*: B9.

34. Arnold, F. H., Blanch, H. W., and Wilke, C. R. (1985). Analysis of affinity separations II: The characterization of affinity columns by pulse techniques, *Chemical Engineering J., 30*: B25.

35. Arnold, F. H., Schofield, S. A., and Blanch, H. W. (1986). Analytical affinity chromatography I: Local equilibrium theory and measurement of association and inhibition constants, *J. of Chromatogr., 355*: 1.

36. Arnold, F. H., and Blanch, H. W. (1986). Analytical affinity chromatography II: Rate, theory, and measurement of biological binding kinetics, *J. of Chromatogr., 355*: 13.

37. Cowan, G. H., Gosling, I. S., Laws, J. F., and Sweetenham, W. P. (1986). Physical and mathematical modelling to aid scale-up of liquid chromatography, *J. Chromatogr., 363*: 37.

38. Foo, S. C., and Rice, R. G., (1975). Prediction of the ultimate separation in parametric pumps, *AIChE J., 21*: 1149.

39. Young, M. E., Carroad, P. A., and Bell, R. L. (1980). Estimation of diffusion coefficients of proteins, *Biotechnol. Bioeng., 22*: 947.

40. Miller, S. F., and King, C. J. (1966). Axial dispersion in liquid flow through packed beds, *AIChE J., 12*: 767.

41. Pharmacacia LKB Biotechnology, Piscataway, N. J. (1989). "Preparative Gel Filtration Goes High Performance," *Downstream: News and Views for Process Biotechnologists, 7*.

42. Pharmacia Fine Chemicals AB, Sweden (1979). *Gel Filtration- Theory and Practice*, p. 42.

43. Kopaciewicz, W., and Regnier, F. E., (1983). Nonideal size-exclusion chromatography of proteins: Effects of pH at low ionic strength, *High-Performance Liquid Chromatography of Proteins and Peptides*, (M.T.W. Hearn, F. E. Regnier, and C. T. Wehr, eds.), Academic Press, New York, pp. 151–159.

44. Afeyan, N. B., Fulton, S. P., Gordon, N. F., Mazsaroff, I., Varady, L., and Regnier, F. E. (1990). Perfusion chromatography, an approach to purifying biomolecules, *Bio/Technology, 8*: 203.

45. Van Deemter, J. J., Zuiderweg, F. J., and Klinkenberg, A. (1956). Longitudinal diffusion and resistance to mass transfer as causes of nonideality in chromatography, *Chem. Eng. Sci.*, *5*: 271.

46. Creighton, T. E. (1984). *Proteins*, W. H. Freeman, New York, p. 242.

47. Pfannkoch, E., Lu, K. C., Regnier, F. E., and Barth, H. G. (1980). Characterization of some commercial high performance size exclusion chromatography columns for water soluble polymers, *J. Chromatogr. Sci.*, *18*: 430.

48. Eveleigh, J. W., and Levy, D. E. (1977). Immunochemical characteristics and preparative application of agarose-based immunosorbent,*J. Solid-Phase Biochem*, *2*: 45.

49. Kunii, D., and Levenspiel, O. (1969). *Fluidization Engineering*, John Wiley, New York, p. 67.

50. Fulton, S. P. (1989). *The Art of Antibody Purification*, Pub. 868, Amicon Division, W. R. Grace, Danvers, Mass., p. 57.

51. Holdoway, M. J. (1989). The design of silica for HPLC, *Industrial Chromatography News*, *1*: 8.

52. *Industrial-Scale Chromatographic Separation with High Performance Dowex Monosphere Resins*, Form No. 177-1371-84, Dow Chemical USA, Specialty Chemicals Dept.

53. Yamamoto, S., Nakanishi, K., and Matsuno, R. (1988). *Ion Exchange Chromatography of Proteins*, Chromatographic Science Series No. 43, Marcel Dekker, New York, p. 306.

54. Scawen, M. D., and Hammond, P. M. (1989). Fractionation techniques in process biotechnology, *J. Chem. Tech. Biotechnol.*, *46*: 85.

55. Janson, J. C., and Hedman, P. (1982). Large-scale chromatography of proteins, *Advances in Biochemical Engineering, vol. 25*, Chromatography (A. Fiechter, ed.), Springer-Verlag, Berlin, pp. 43–99.

56. Satterfield, C. N., Colton, C. K., and Pitcher, W. H. (1973). Restriction diffusion in liquids within fine pores, *AIChE J.*, *19*: 628.

57. Regnier, F. E. (1982). Review: High performance ion-exchange chromatography of proteins: The current status, *High Performance Liquid Chromatography of Proteins and Peptides* (M. T. W. Hearn, F. E. Regnier, and C. T. Wehr, eds.), Academic Press, New York, pp. 1–7.

58. Pharmacia LKB Biotechnology, Piscataway, N.J. (1986). "Process Hygiene in Industrial Chromatographic Processes," *Downstream: News and Views for Process Biotechnologists*, Form 60-01-019 PD02.

59. Viljoen, M., Shapiro, M., Crookes, R., Chalmers, A., and Marrs, S. (1982). "Large-Scale Recovery of Human Serum Albumin by a Chromatographic Method," Abstract Th-131 of the Joint Meeting of the 19th Congress of the International Society of Haematology and the 17th Congress of the International Society of Blood Transfusion, Budapest, Aug. 1–7.

60. Knight, P. (1989). Chromatography: 1989 report, *Bio/Technology*, *1*: 243.

61. Amicon Division, W. R. Grace, Danvers, Mass. (1988). "Moduline Chromatography Columns for Pilot and Process Scale Chromatography," Pub. 852.

62. Amicon Division, W. R. Grace, Danvers, Mass. (1988). "Acrylic Columns for Pilot and Process Scale Chromatography," Pub. 853.

63. Amicon Division, W. R. Grace, Danvers, Mass. (1988). "Glass Columns for Pilot and Process Scale Chromatography," Pub. 854.

64. Keuer, T. A., and Ryland, J. R. (1990). "Industrial-Scale Ion Exchange Chromatography for Purification of Proteins," Abstract from Engineering Foundation Conference: Recovery of Biological Products V, St. Petersburg, Florida, May 13–18.
65. Amicon Division, W. R. Grace and, Danvers, Mass. (1988). "Stainless Steel Columns for Pilot and Process Scale Chromatography," Pub. 855.
66. Janson, J. C. (1971). Columns for large-scale gel filtration on porous gels, *J. Agr. Food Chem.*, *19*: 581.
67. Janson, J. C. (1978). "Large Scale Chromatography of Proteins," Proceedings Int. Workshop Technol. Protein Sep. Improv. Blood Plasma Fractionation, 1977, DHEW Publ. (NIH) (U.S.), NIH-78-1422, pp. 205–220.
68. Scopes, R. K. (1974). Measurement of protein by spectrophotometry at 205 nm, *Analytical Biochemistry*, *59*: 277.
69. Pharmacia LKB Biotechnology, Piscataway, N.J. (1989). "Get the Best from your Sephacryl HR," *Separation News*, *16.1*: 5–8.
70. Pearson, F. C. (1985). *Pyrogens: Endotoxins, LAL Testing and Depyrogenation*, Marcel Dekker, New York, pp. 11, 23, 37, 24.
71. Novitsky, T. J., and Gould, M. J. (1985). Depyrogenation by moist heat, *Depyrogenation*, Technical Report No. 7, Parenteral Drug Association Inc., Philadelphia, Penn., p. 109.
72. United States Pharmacopeial Convention, Rockville, Md. (1990). *United States Pharmacopeia*, p. 1456.
73. Weary, M. (1985). Depyrogenation, *Pyrogens: Endotoxins, LAL Testing and Depyrogenation* (F. C. Pearson, ed.), Marcel Dekker, New York, p. 209.
74. Curling, J. M., and Cooney, J. M. (1982). Operation of large-scale gel filtration and ion-exchange systems, *J. Parenteral Science and Technology*, *36*: 59.
75. Hasko, F., Kristof, K., Salamon, M., and Dobo, P. (1985). Large scale chromatographic experiments for plasma, *Dev. Hematol. Immul.*, *13*: 105.
76. U. S. Department of Health and Human Services, Public Health Services, Food and Drug Administration (1987). *Guideline on Sterile Drug Products Produced by Aseptic Processing*, June.
77. Johansson, J. (1985). "Automation of Chromatographic Processes," Proceedings of Biotech '85 Europe, Geneva, May, 1985, pp. 193–202.
78. Pharmacia LKB Biotechnology, Piscataway, N.J. (1988). *FPLC for Protein Chromatography*, Pub. No. FFPC 50-01-425.
79. OROS Instruments, Cambridge, Mass. (1989). *OROS Instruments Controlled Protein Liquid Chromatography*.
80. U.S. Department of Health and Human Services, Public Health Services, Food and Drug Administration, (1987). *Guidelines on General Principles of Process Validation*, May.
81. Jones, A. J. S., and O'Connor, J. V. (1985). Control of recombinant DNA produced pharmaceuticals by a combination of process validation and final product specifications, *Develop. Biol. Standard.*, *59*: 175.
82. Agalloco, J. (1989). Validation of existing computer systems, *Pharmaceutical Technology*, *Jan*: 38.
83. *Human and Veterinary Drugs Good Manufacturing Practices and Proposed Exemptions for Certain OTC Products* (1978). *Federal Register*, Part II, Sept. 29, 1978, *43 (190)*: 45013-45089.

84. U.S. Department of Health and Human Services, Public Health Service, Food and Drug Administration (1991). *Guide to Inspection of Bulk Pharmaceutical Chemicals*, Washington, D. C., September.

85. Pharmaceutical Manufacturers Association Deionized Water Committee (1985). Validation and control concepts for water treatment systems, *Pharmaceutical Technology, Nov*: 50.

86. Munson, T. E. (1988). "Regulatory View of Environmental Monitoring," Reprint from Pharm. Tech. Conference of September 1988.

8

Biospecific Affinity Chromatography

Nikos K. Harakas
Monsanto Company, St. Louis, Missouri

I. INTRODUCTION

The purpose of this chapter is to describe succinctly for the practicing chemical, biochemical, and process engineers and research and development scientists and investigators the powerfulness of biospecific affinity chromatography (BAC) to obtain highly purified proteins and enzymes that can be used for either in vivo or in vitro applications. BAC was championed in the late 1960s by Cuatrecasas, Wilchek, and Anfinsen (1). They demonstrated that enzymes could be purified using a specific competitor inhibitor immobilized on solid matrices covalently attached. This development followed the pioneering work in the early 1950s by Campbell, Leuscher and Lerman (2), who isolated nonprecipitating antibodies from immune serum by means of a cellulose-protein antigen. Later, in 1953, Lerman (3) extended the crude affinity technique for the isolation of the enzyme tyrosinase using azo dyes prepared by coupling an aromatic amine with phenol on cellulose, which inhibits the enzyme.

Since the paper of Cuatrecasas and collaborators, over 1000 proteins and enzymes have been purified by affinity chromatography, and probably over 10,000 papers have elaborated on the technique with major improvements. There have been three striking developments in affinity chromatography in the last two decades. First of these is the use of heavy metal ions such as Zn^{2+} and Cu^{2+} as affinity ligands immobolized appropriately as chelates on solid gels that bind selectively on histidine and cysteine residues on the surface of proteins, successfully demonstrated in 1975 by Porath and collaborators (4). Second is the use of monoclonal antibodies as ligands, first demonstrated in 1980 by Secher and Burke for the large-scale purification of human leukocyte interferon (5). Third is the very recent development of receptor affinity chromatography, which utilizes biological recognition by cell surface receptors, demonstrated in 1987 by Bailon and Weber and collaborators for the purification to homogeneity of only biologically active interleukin-2 (IL-2) in one step, using the IL-2 receptor as the affinity ligand (6,7).

The purification of proteins to homogeneity is a rather new science. It was only in the 1930s that Arne Tiselius first demonstrated that serum is comprised of many proteins using electrophoresis, a method which he invented and developed for his dissertation (8). In 1948, Tiselius was awarded the Nobel Prize in Chemistry for his pioneering work on the purification of proteins (9). Tiselius succinctly describes the discovery and development of the methods for purifying proteins under his aegis, at the Institute of Biochemistry at Uppsala University, Sweden, in two classical papers (10,11). The chromatography of proteins was initiated in the 1950s primarily by Sober and Peterson (12) for ion exchange and by Porath and Flodin (13–16) for size exclusion, or gel filtration. High performance liquid chromatography (HPLC) for size exclusion, which increased resolution greatly and decreased processing time, was significantly developed in 1975–1976 by Tsuji and Robertson (17) and by Regnier and collaborators (18,19), who also developed an appropiate system for ion exchange (20). The development of HPLC followed the earlier basic observations, in 1941, by Martin and Synge (21), that the stagnant mobile phase mass transfer contribution to band-spreading is inversely related to solute diffusivity, and that the time required for mass transport could be decreased by small microparticulate sorbents (22–24). HPLC utilizing affinity ligands and polyclonal antibodies was developed in 1978 by Mosbach and collaborators (25). HPLC using metal-ion affinity and other ligands is not very well developed. Reviewed recently by Porath and others (26,27), it is discussed later in this chapter. Some process developments in protein purification have recently been summarized (28–31). The general status of the purification of proteins and enzymes, by various chromatographic methods, has been reviewed recently by Regnier (32). Table 1 gives the various purification methods for proteins and enzymes, classified into five major categories (33). The investigator should consult the other chapters in this treatise for the current status of the practice of conventional chromatography and HPLC for the purification of proteins and peptides.

The selectivity of biospecific affinity chromatography has proven to be important in the isolation and purification to homogeneity of newly discovered proteins and enzymes. Examples of proteins and enzymes, first purified using biospecific affinity ligands during the last 15 years and which have proven to be of clinical importance, are the various thrombolytics and wound healers. Astrup and collaborators identified plasminogen activator biological activity in animal tissue in the late 1940s (34,35). The thrombolytic

Table 1 Protein Purification Processes

1. Solubility—Precipitation
   a. Salt
   b. Solvent
   c. Isoelectric
2. Ionization
   a. Ion-exchange chromatography
   b. Electrophoresis
3. Molecular Size-Shape
   a. Gel filtration
   b. Dialysis
   c   SDS electrophoresis
   d. Ultracentrifugation: Density-gradient
   e. Ultrafiltration
4. Partition Coefficient
   a. Countercurrent distribution
   b. Thin layer chromatography
   c. Paper chromatography
5. Special Methods
   a. Affinity chromatography
   b. Adsorption chromatography
   c. Immunologic methods

Source: Ref. 33.

human tissue type plasminogen activator (t-PA) was first partially purified using Zn^{2+} chelating affinity chromatography, in 1979 by Rijken (36). Human t-PA was purified to homogeneity by a second purification step, concanavalin A affinity chromatography, in 1980 by Rijken and Collen (37,38). The human endothelial plasminogen activator inhibitor (PAI-1) of t-PA was purified to homogeneity and partially sequenced directly from endothhelial cells by Sanzo (39), using the immunoaffinity of a monoclonal antibody against human t-PA. Others (40,41) determined the amino acid sequence of PAI-1 indirectly by first using the terminal sequences of bovine PAI-1 purified by Loskutoff (42) by concanavalin A affinity ligand that bound the t-PA/PAI-1 inhibitor complex; they constructed oligonucleotide probes that were used to isolate and sequence the cDNA clone of human origin. A decade of massive search for tumor angiogenesis, angiogenesis and wound healing proteins culminated in 1984 by Klagsbrun (43), who first used heparin affinity ligand to purify a tumor derived capillary endothelial cell growth factor. Later, in the 1984–1986 period, the heparin affinity technique was used by Gospodarowicz, Klagsbrun, and others (44–51), who purified, sequenced, and cloned the cDNA of the family of angiogenic proteins, termed basic and acidic fibroblast growth factors (bFGF and aFGF) from human and other sources. In 1987, Folkman and Klagsbrun (52) reviewed the major progress of the purification, amino acid sequencing, and cDNA cloning of angiogenic factors. The search began in 1845 by the clinician Thiersch to isolate the factor that allows tumors to grow and metastasize, and he published his twenty-year studies in 1865 (53). In 1988, Guillemin and collaborators (54) determined that the amino acid sequence of bFGF has cell surface receptor- and heparin-binding domains. The biological properties of heparin have been described (55). Shing (56) recently disclosed a heparin-copper bioaffinity system, which recognizes the various forms of FGF. Connolly and associates (57,58) have just isolated, purified to homogeneity, sequenced, and cloned the cDNA of a new human vascular permeability factor (hVPF), which is also mitogenic (angiogenic) for endothelial cells, using Cu^{2+} chelating affinity chromatography, a key purification step.

Proteins and enzymes purified using BAC methods to be used for either pharmaceutical or industrial applications, in manufacturing quantities, are very limited. It is highly possible that the manufacturers are reluctant to disclose their proprietary BAC technology (59).

Especially since the advent of recombinant DNA cloning and expression, numerous BAC studies to purify proteins, enzymes, and antibodies have been described (60–111); a significant number of studies have also been done in the emerging exploratory area for the purification of the various glycoforms of proteins and enzymes that have different oligosaccharide structure, composition and function (112–121). This work has been directed not only toward obtaining a purer protein or enzyme that is biologically active but also toward improving the economics of BAC, which has to date limited its use at large scale.

II. BIOSPECIFIC AFFINITY CHROMATOGRAPHY

A. Basic Concept

Two critical developments were achieved in 1967 and earlier by Porath and collaborators that impacted protein purification: (1) chemical coupling of proteins to solid matrices by means of cyanogen halides (122,123), and (2) availability of Sephadex (*se*paration *pha*rmacia *dex*tran) and Sepharose (ag*arose*) solid matrices with appropriate chemical functionality, porosity, and surface and fluid dynamic characteristics (124). Both were used in 1968 by Cuatrecasas and collaborators to develop BAC (1). In 1970, Cuatrecasas (125–128) improved the technique significantly with the incorporation of the spacer-arm principle, minimizing protein-matrix interactions. Figure 1 demonstrates the basic concept of affinity chromatography. Figure 2 shows the spacer-arm concept.

The general process of BAC is comprised of four or five sequential steps. First, the ligand is chosen for the protein or enzyme (ligate) to be purified on the basis of its biospecificity and selectivity. The complex formed

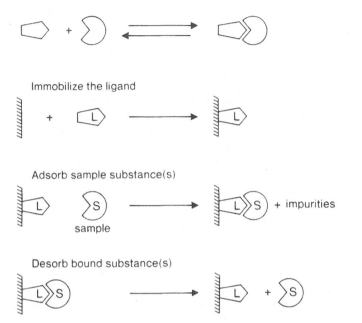

Figure 1 Basic concept of biospecific affinity chromatography. (Courtesy Pharmacia LKB Biotechnology, Ref. 62, modified.)

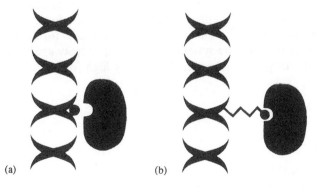

Figure 2 Spacer-arm concept for biospecific affinity chromatography. (a) Ligand attached to matrix; (b) spacer-arm attached to matrix. (Courtesy Pharmacia LKB Biotechnology, Ref. 62, modified.)

between ligand and protein must be reversible. In certain cases, a covalent bond may be formed, but it should be of such type that after the protein or enzyme has been purified from the biological stream, a selective cleaving agent must be available to cleave the ligand-protein complex. Second, the ligand is immobilized on a solid inert matrix, preferably in most cases a type of Sepharose, using in most cases cyanogen bromide. In certain cases, a spacer-arm is used between the matrix and the ligand, which can be attached covalently either to the matrix or to the ligand before its covalent immobilization. Third, the biological fluid stream, containing the protein or enzyme specific for the ligand, is contacted with the matrix-ligand system in either batch or column mode for the appropriate time, usually less than 1 h. The protein or enzyme is adsorbed, whereas the impurities stay in solution. Fourth, the protein is desorbed by appropriate elution methods. Fifth, the matrix-ligand system is regenerated and reequilibrated for the next batch to be purified. The schematic of the first four steps is shown in Fig. 1 (60,62,73,74,76,78,81,83).

B. Types

1. Bioselectivity

Bioselectivity can be classified into three major areas, as shown in Table 2, which are (1) affinity ligands, (2) immunoaffinity, and (3) receptors. The affinity ligands area includes enzyme inhibitors, enzyme substrates, lectins, carbohydrates, dyes, heavy metal-ion chelates and nucleic acids (80,83). They are charaterized for their biospecificity, but their selectivity may be for classes of proteins or enzymes. The purification of a protein using ligands can be achieved by controlling the composition of the biological stream, if possible, and by desorbing the bound proteins with a gradient of the eluting agent, selecting the desired protein or enzyme by collecting column fractions. In general, different proteins have different affinity constants for the same ligand, allowing different proteins to elute as separate activity entities or peaks. Immunoaffinity ligands are either polyclonal or monoclonal antibodies against a specific protein. The diversity of antibody formation indicates the diversity of the immune system and its biospecificity against a protein. The selectivity of polyclonal antibodies is very high for its corres-

Table 2 Biospecific Methods

Affinity ligands
Immunoaffinity
  + Polyclonal Abs
  + Monoclonal Abs (mcAb)
     Milstein and Kohler Nobel Prize in 1984
Receptors

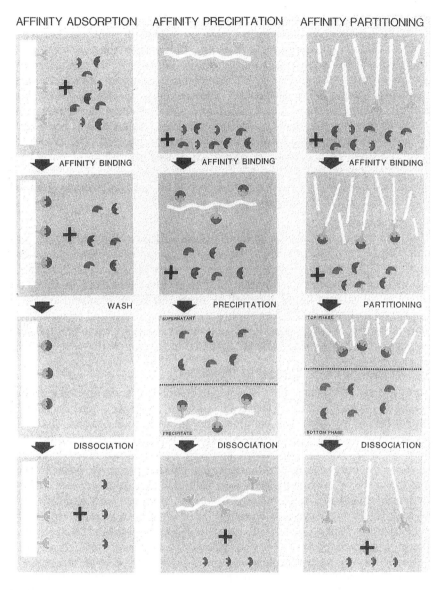

Figure 3 Biospecific affinity chromatography process modes. (From J.-C. Janson, Ref. 80, with permission.)

ponding protein, although nonspecific protein binding occurs. The production of monoclonal antibodies (MABs) in 1975 by Kohler and Milstein (129,130) provided a unique ligand for a given protein. The bioselectivity is unique. However, inhibitor complexes, biologically inactive protein, or fragments of the protein are recognized by the specific antigenic determinant(s) of the particular MAB. All the complexes and the fragments whose molecular weight Mr is sufficiently different from the Mr of the purified protein can be separated by subsequent size exclusion chromatography, resulting in a homogeneously purified protein. In 1984, Milstein and Kohler received the Nobel Prize for their work on MABs (131,132). Use of cell surface receptors of a protein as ligand has solved the inhibitor complexes, protein fragment and biologically inactive protein problems of MABs, as developed in 1987 by Bailon and Weber (6,7). Each bioselectivity area will be discussed separately in other sections.

2. Processing

BAC can be accomplished in either batch or column mode adsorption. The batch mode is preferred when the feed is viscous or contains particulate matter. Other ways that biospecific affinity separations can be carried out are by precipitation or partitioning. Although these latter two methods are not chromatography *per se*, they will be discussed in this chapter because of their similarities to BAC. The three processes are illustrated beautifully by Janson in Fig. 3 (80). The significant implications of each method with respect to up-scaling BAC will be discussed in Section VIII.

C. Activation and Coupling Methods

Several procedures have been developed to activate solid porous matrices, primarily polysaccharide (cellulose, dextran, agarose) and polyamide (polyacrylamide) type, for coupling spacer arms and ligands, since the pioneering technique by cyanogen bromide of Porath (122,123,133,134). The methods explored functionalized matrices with various reactive groups. *Hydroxyl* can be activated with cyanogen halides (bromine is preferred), halotriazines, or epoxide; *amino* with isonitrile or isothiocyanate; *carboxyl* with acid anhydride, acid chloride, or azide; *carbonyl* with isonitrile; and *sulfhydryl* with homocysteine lactone. Another activation technique is the derivatization of agarose by *N*-hydroxysuccinimide esters that also provide a spacer arm, introduced in 1972 by Cuatrecasas and Parikh (135). It was later developed as the Affi-Gel affinity supports (136). Affi-Gel 10 and Affi-Gel 15 have been proven to be very useful products for purification of proteins, including monoclonal antibodies and immobilization of ligands deduced from peptide libraries (137–139). All these and many other functionalities and activation methods are elaborated in detail by Porath and Kristiansen (76), Dean et al. (69), Scouten (63), Mohr and Pommerening (70), and others (140–145).

1. Cyanogen Bromide

Although more than 50 different methods have been attempted for activation and coupling of the matrices, cyanogen bromide remains the preferred agent (78,81,83). The CNBr technique has been studied and improved significantly over the 25-year period that it has been used. Wilchek and collaborators (81,146–148) have studied in detail the chemistry of CNBr activation and coupling, and they have improved it using organic solvents (81,149). However, the use of mild conditions in predominantly aqueous media with CNBr is still the most common and reliable method (83). The leaching problem of the ligand is still a major concern, not only for limiting the life of the affinity column but also for product contamination, e.g., with MABs, which may induce an immune response clinically.

2. New Promising Methods

Kohn et al. (150) have developed a method that substitutes p-nitrophenylcyanate for CNBr to activate OH- groups and does not require special hoods, eliminating the CNBr hazardous conditions. The generation of thiol functional groups using sequential chemical treatments on agarose is a technique used in early studies (125,151) with some success, and the method has been modified and improved by Kincaid and Vaughan (152) recently with much promise. The most recent method is the generation of carbonate functional groups in matrices with hydroxyl groups using a carbonochloridate that shows improved stability (153). Hydrazide-preactivated hydrophilic hollow fiber membranes have been shown to be useful and stable for monoclonal antibody immobilization (154,155), or on other solid supports for glycoproteins in general (156,157). The method has also been demonstrated for use in coupling membrane based receptors for affinity chromatography purification of the target protein (158). Membrane and receptor chromatography are discussed in subsequent sections of this chapter. The activaton of insoluble polysaccharide matrices with 1,1'-carbonyldiimidazole(CDI) show good stability and ease of processing compared to CNBr (159–161). A new activating method was just developed for application with high performance liquid affinity chromatography. The method is based on the use of 4,6-diphenylthieno[3,4-*d*]-1,3-dioxol-2-one-5,5-dioxide(TDO) esters on acrylic polymers (162). The TDO activation could be extended to any hydroxylated matrix. The ligand leakage problem from supports activated by several methods has been reported (163,164). Currently, chemical engineers are investigating processing conditions to minimize the ligand leakage problem (165).

D. Spacer-Arm and Protein-Matrix Interactions

Since the developments to use dextran (166) and agarose (167) for the chromatographic purification of proteins, matrix-protein interactions have been studied extensively (63,70,168–173). The concept of the spacer-arm in affinity purification is to allow unimpeded access of the protein to the ligand, minimizing steric hindrance interactions (125,126,174–176).

To purify a protein successfully using BAC, the ligand must be far enough from the matrix backbone to minimize steric restrictions for interactions between the ligand and the protein to be purified. It was demonstrated by Cuatrecasas that hydrocarbon extension arms between the solid matrix and the ligand are very effective in minimizing or eliminating completely such interactions. Hexamethylenediamine (HMD), $H_2N(CH_2)_6$ NH_2, is a reasonable choice for a spacer-arm. One amine is attached to the matrix and the other to the ligand. However, HMD generates some nonspecific protein binding. Agarose derivatives commonly used with various spacer arms are shown in Fig. 4 (83,125,126). The theoretical quantitation of affinity chromatography has been reported recently that can be used in the future to predict spacer-arm length, and ligand length and type for the protein to be used with certain physicochemical properties (177).

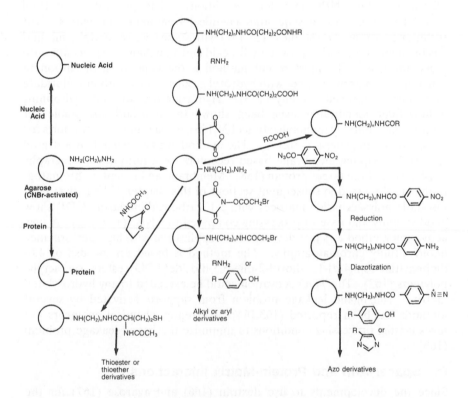

Figure 4 Reactions for coupling ligands to derivatized agarose. (From I. Parikh and P. Cuatrecasas, Ref. 83, with permission.)

E. Matrices and Biospecific Ligands

1. Matrices

Many types of matrices have been evaluated for use in affinity chromatography ranging from silica glass to polyacrylamide to agarose (60,64,76,78,83, 178). Agarose based matrices are preferred because they are hydrophilic, exhibit low protein binding, and are relatively easy to derivatize (76,78,83, 126,179–182). Exploratory and developmental research is a continuous venture by investigators to find better matrices for affinity chromatography to solve specific problems, related to ligand immobilization, flow characteristics, nonspecific protein binding, elution of the purified protein without denaturation, etc. Two recently developed matrices are a polyethyleneimine-substituted polymer (183) and porous chitosan granules (184). The use of various hollow fibers made from different polymers is a major area of research of several biotech based processing ventures, which will be discussed in the last section of this chapter.

2. Biospecific Ligands

The selection of a biospecific ligand to purify a newly discovered protein is a major exploratory venture and decision by the investigator. The biological activity and function of the protein to be purified can be used as guides in the selection of biospecific ligand(s), but there are no general rules for this difficult decision. In the next decade, the demand to sequence proteins for the human genome project will require a great deal of ingenuity by the investigators to purify the other 100,000 proteins coded and expressed under certain conditions of either development or physiologic requirements by the various differentiated human cells (185). Besides enzyme inhibitors and other known substrates for certain proteins, many types of dyes have been demonstrated to be useful ligands for classes of proteins. The use of dyes as ligands in BAC resulted from the early observations that Cibacron Blue Dextran bound phosphofructokinase (PFK), with no change of its enzymatic activity (186). Blue Dextran is used to determine the void volume and to calibrate with protein standards packed chromatographic size exclusion columns, and to check visually their packing quality. It was used in the experiments with PFK, and it was observed that the elution position of PFK had shifted, indicating PFK binding to it. Hence Cibacron Blue-Sepharose was developed as a very useful affinity medium in the mid-1970s (187). Many dyes are used as ligands including triazines, procion type (red, blue, green, brown), proflavine, thionine, bromothymol blue, and biomimetic type (188–195).

3. Commonly Used Matrix-Ligands

CNBr-activated agarose is available commercially (196,197). Most of the agarose derivatives shown in Fig. 4 are available including with six carbon spacer-arm, epoxy-activated, thiol-activated, and tresyl-activated (196,198, 199). Other matrix-ligands useful for affinity purification are available,

Table 3 A Separation Guide for Biospecific Affinity Chromatography

Target molecules	Type of gel	Examples of applications/specificity for
Immunoglobulins	Protein A Sepharose CL-4B	IgG, IgG subclasses, some IgM and IgA
	Protein G Sepharose 4 Fast Flow	IgG, IgG subclasses
	Con A Sepharose	IgM
Growth factors	Heparin Sepharose CL-6B	Fibroblast growth factor (FGF), endothelial cell growth factor (ECGF)
Protein synthesis factors	Heparin Sepharose CL-6B	Initiation factors, elongation factors (EF-1)
Hormones and hormone receptors	Con A Sepharose	Follicle-stimulating hormone, chorionic gonadotropin
	Heparin Sepharose CL-6B	Estrogen and androgen receptors
Coagulation proteins	Heparin Sepharose CL-6B	Antithrombin III[a], factors IX, X, XI, XII, XIIa, prothrombin, thrombin
	Blue Sepharose CL-6B	Prothrombin, factor IX
	Arginine Sepharose 4B	Prothrombin
Nucleic acids	Lysine Sepharose 4B	Ribosomal RNA, double-stranded DNA
Polysaccharides and glycoproteins	Con A Sepharose	α-D-glucosyl, α-D-mannosyl
	Lentil Lectin Sepharose 4B	α-D-glucosyl, α-D-mannosyl
	Agarose-Wheat Germ Lectin	N-acetyl-glucosaminyl residues
	Agarose-Peanut Lectin	Galactose β(1-3)N-acetyl-D-galactosaminyl
Membrane proteins	Lentil Lectin Sepharose 4 B	See above
	Con A Sepharose	See above
Lipoproteins	Heparin Sepharose CL-6B	β-lipoprotein
	Con A Sepharose	Low density lipoproteins
Enzymes		
Nucleic acid binding	Heparin Sepharose CL-6B	Restriction endonucleases, DNA ligase, DNA and RNA polymerases
	Blue Sepharose CL-6B	DNA polymerase, restriction endonucleases
NAD+-independent	5'AMP Sepharose 4B	Aldehyde dehydrogenase, formate dehydrogenase
	Blue Sepharose CL-6B	Alcohol dehydrogenase, lactate dehydrogenase

Category	Adsorbent	Enzyme/Protein
NADP⁺-dependent	AGNAD Type 3	Glyceraldehyde-3-phosphate dehydrogenase
	AGATP Type 3	Alcohol dehydrogenase, malate dehydrogenase
	2'5'ADP Sepharose 4B	Glucose-6-phosphate dehydrogenase
	Blue Sepharose CL-6B	6-Phosphogluconate dehydrogenase
	Red Sepharose CL-6B	Aldehyde reductase, dihydrofolate reductase
	AGNADP Type 3	Glucose-6-phosphate dehydrogenase
	AGCoA Type 5	HMG-CoA reductase
ATP-dependent	5' AMP Sepharose 4B	cAMP-dependent protein kinase
	Blue Sepharose CL-6B	Adenylate kinase, pyruvate kinase, hexokinase
	Calmodulin Sepharose 4B	Adenylate cyclase, cyclic nucleotide phosphodiesterase
	AGATP Type 2	Glutathione synthetase, adenylate cyclase
	AGATP Type 3	Creatine kinase, pyruvate kinase
	AGATP Type 4	Adenosine kinase
	AGGTP Type 4	Phosphoenolpyruvate carboxykinase
CoA-dependent	AGATP Type 4	Citrate synthase
	AG3',5', ADP Type 2	Succinate thiokinase
Protease binding	Benzamidine Sepharose 6B	Trypsin, urokinase, prekallikrein, kallikrein
	Arginine Sepharose 4B	Prekallikrein, clostripain
	Red Sepharose CL-6B	Carboxypeptidase G

Other proteins

Protein	Adsorbent
α_1-antitrypsin	Con A Sepharose
α_2-macroglobulin	Blue Sepharose CL-6B, Chelating Sepharose Fast Flow
Fibronectin	Gelatin Sepharose 4B, Heparin Sepharose CL-6B
Plasminogen and plasminogen activator	Lysine Sepharose 4B, Red Sepharose CL-6B, Arginine Sepharose 4B
Albumin	Blue Sepharose CL-6B
Interferon	Con A Sepharose, Heparin Sepharose CL-6B, Blue Sepharose CL-6B, Red Sepharose CL-6B, Calmodulin Sepharose 4B, Chelating Sepharose Fast Flow

[a] A patent for large-scale purification of AIII by use of immobilized heparin is held by AB Kabi, S-11287 Stockholm, Sweden, to whom application should be made for permission to use this process.

Source: Pharmacia LKB Biotechnology.

including concanavalin A–agarose, arginine-agarose, lysine-agarose, and heparin-agarose (200–204). Recently, a borate-agarose became available that can be used in the purification of glycosylated proteins (205,206). A BAC purification guide for matrix-ligands and classes of proteins for which they can be used effectively is given in Table 3.

F. Ligand BAC: Early and Recent Applications

Arsenis and McCormick (207,208) used flavin-cellulose to purify flavokinase and mononucleotide-dependent enzymes in the early 1960s, before the development of affinity chromatography by Cuatrecasas (1). Some of the first applications of BAC by Cuatrecasas and collaborators was to purify in one step avidin from egg white with biocytin-Sepharose (209) and beta-galactosidase from *E. coli* using the spacer-arm concept (128). Deutsch and Mertz (210) purified plasminogen from human plasma using lysine-Sepharose, a method still in use. Porath and collaborators (211) purified trypsin inhibitor from *Vicia cracca* with trypsin-Sepharose 2B using the bag method (80). In 1972, Allen and Majerus (212–214) isolated vitamin B_{12}-binding proteins by use of a vitamin B_{12}-Sepharose affinity column. They purified transcobalamin II from the Cohn III fraction of 1400 L of human plasma using the vitamin B_{12} affinity column. The 34 kg of protein of the Cohn III fraction was dissolved in 300 L of buffer, and following an ion-exchange step the isolated fraction was applied to the affinity column, isolating 24.7 mg of homogeneous transcobalamin II. Only affinity chromatography can accomplish such feats. The isoenzymes of carbonic anhydrase and lactate dehydrogenase were purified and separated in 1972–1973 by affinity ligands (215,216). In 1975, Thy-1, a cell surface glycoprotein, was purified both by lectin (ligand) or antibody affinity chromatography, a major development for cell surface antigens by Williams and associates (217). In 1981, human fibroblast interferon was purified with Cibacron Blue-Sepharose by Knight and Fahey (218,219). Recently, bovine fibroblast interferon was purified using Blue Sepharose CL-6B affinity chromatography (220). In some special experiments, about 1.5 mg human fibroblast t-PA was purified with sequential column affinity chromatography of Zn^{2+} chelated-Sepharose 6B, *p*-amino-benzamidine-agarose, MAB (against t-PA)-Sepharose 4B and size exclusion HPLC from 750 L of serum free cell culture conditioned media, recovering about 80% of the starting antigen (221). The procedure is modified from other experiments with the same cell strain (222). The result is an indication of the powerfulness of BAC. The years 1988–1989 witnessed an explosion in applications of BAC for protein purification (see, for example, Refs. 223–250).

III. METAL ION AFFINITY CHROMATOGRAPHY

A. Basic Concept

Histidine and cysteine form stable complexes with either Zn^{2+} or Cu^{2+} ions. Solid matrices chelated with either of these metal ions with excess binding capacity interact with surface-exposed imidazole and thiol groups of proteins as demonstrated in 1975 by Porath and collaborators (4) for human serum proteins. The affinity is not specific, but it allows the differential isolation of the metal-ion-binding proteins from a given biological stream, providing a significant increase in specific activity of the protein to be purified (222). The bound protein(s) can be eluted under mild conditions, using imidazole gradients or decreasing the pH from about 7.8 to 5.5, and the recovery is quantitative. Chelated agaroses are relatively inexpensive, compared to other affinity matrix-ligand media, and they can be regenerated easily. Other metal ions can be used, including Cd, Hg, Co, Ni, Fe (4,82,93). Several proteins have been partially purified using immobilized metal ion affinity chromatography (IMAC) including alpha(2)-SH glycoprotein, human fibroblast interferon, t-PA, and superoxide dismutase, (36,82,251–255). IMAC has been researched extensively concerning protein purification and surface properties during the last 18 years (256–269).

B. Applications and New Directions

IMAC has been demonstrated to provide a reliable and relatively inexpensive procedure to remove protein trace impurities from commercial human albumin after its initial purification by the Cohn method (270). The method has the potential to provide human albumin with a significant decrease in side effects, when it is used clinically. There is considerable interest to use IMAC in the high-performance (HP) mode, which not only will provide higher resolution and decreased processing time but also will make it a more popular method to purify newly discovered proteins (26,27,271). HP-IMAC will be discussed in Section VIII. A discovery direction of protein-metal-ion affinity is genetically to incorporate a polyhistidine-peptide to the gene of the protein of interest, produced by a vector-host. The fused protein is purified by IMAC, and the peptide is removed with carboxypeptidase A (272). The surface topography of histidine residues is being examined carefully (273). Haymore (274) has applied such topography cleverly in the production of both bovine and porcine somatotropin variants with histidine(s) strategically placed in the protein, providing efficient and cost-effective purification. Metal chelating agarose is available commercially that can be charged by the investigator with the desired metal ion (275–277).

IV. IMMUNOAFFINITY CHROMATOGRAPHY

A. Basic Concept

Polyclonal antibodies (Ab) and antigens (Ag) were purified using affinity matrices with either immobilized Ag or Ab, respectively (2,278,279). After the development of IMAC, the next major step forward for BAC resulted from the discovery of a way to produce MABs in 1975 by Kohler and Milstein (129). The first major application of an MAB immobilized on a solid matrix for affinity purification was for human leukocyte interferon (5). Subsequently, recombinant human leukocyte interferon was purified with MAB made against it (280,281), recA-based fusion proteins (282), superoxide dismutase (283), t-PA (222), and many more (284).   MABs recognize inhibitor complexes of the Ag, biologically inactive Ag, and certain fragments of the Ag. Most of these components can be purified by subsequent size exclusion chromatography, providing a homogeneous protein (222).

B. Development, Applications, and New Directions

The problem of obtaining MABs of sufficient purity has been addressed extensively by various methods including ion exchange, and size exclusion HPLC (285,286). Protein A-Sepharose CL-4B affinity purification (287,288), and HPLC adsorption purification (289) are the most widely used, providing homogeneous MABs, a requirement for either in vitro use for purification of the Ag and other applications or in vivo clinical use. The purification to homogeneity of IgM-type MABs has been difficult. A very promising affinity ligand has been developed recently, providing homogeneous murine IgM MABs. It is made from snowdrop (*Galanthus navalis*) bulb lectin (GNA), which is highly specific for D-mannose and immobilized on Sepharose 4B. The GNA-Sepharose 4B is prepared under special conditions to protect the lectin binding site during immobilization (290).

The production of MABs provided a major advance in immunology for isolating antibodies against each antigenic determinant of a protein (291). Hence mcAbs can be isolated that have low and high binding constants, and against specific domains of the protein that may have different physiologic functions. Desired MABs with specific properties have been produced and used effectively for purification and planned clinical applications from various proteins, including lysozyme (292–295) and t-PA (287,297,298). MABs have the potential to decipher the immune response and to provide many newer methods to purify and characterize proteins (295,299–302). MAB affinity purification ligands on agarose are available commercially (303–309).

V. RECEPTOR AFFINITY CHROMATOGRAPHY

A. Basic Concept

MAB purification came closer than any other chromatographic method in providing a uniquely recognized and homogeneous protein (28), until the development in November 1987 by Bailon and collaborators (6,7) of receptor affinity chromatography (RAC). Cell surface receptors recognize and bind only biologically active native protein. They do not recognize inactive molecules of the protein or inhibitor complexes. It is not known if they may recognize biologically active fragments of the protein, and variants that may be constructed only with certain of the domains of a protein. IL-2 receptor (310) immobilized on a solid matrix purified only biologically active recombinant IL-2 (6,7,311). The IL-2 receptor had been prepared using recombinant DNA methods (312), providing sufficient quantities for use as a ligand in affinity purification (6). The IL-2 receptor was used also to purify an IL-2-*Pseudomonas* exotoxin fusion protein (313,314). Others have also prepared the IL-2 receptor by recombinant DNA methods (315). In 1988, Phares (316) used RAC to purify a growth factor. The development of RAC will depend on the availability of receptors in reasonable quantities.

B. Expectations

Currently, there is intense activity in exploratory research of cell surface receptors for their isolation, purification, characterization, cDNA sequencing, and determination of their physiological structure-function (317,318). Several receptors (R) have been purified and sequenced and some were expressed in a vector-host during the last 2 to 7 years, including beta-2-adrenergic-R (319), beta-interferon-R (320), IL-1-R (321,322), IgE-R (323), IL-5-R (324), and various T cell receptors (325,326). The result of this type of activity may be wider application of RAC. RAC has the potential to provide proteins that are homogeneous, biologically active, and free of trace impurities. The clinical in vivo use of RAC purified proteins has the potential to minimize patient side effects. Recently, it was announced that epidermal growth factor (EGF) was shown to be clinically effective in the acceleration of wound healing (327). The low and high receptors of EGF have just been expressed in human hepatoma cells (328). Hence the RAC purification of EGF could be made possible, if necessary either clinically or economically.

VI. GLYCOPROTEINS: AFFINITY PURIFICATION OF GLYCOFORMS

A. Importance

Glycobiology is just now becoming a very exciting area of exploratory research to determine the biological function of oligosaccharides on proteins

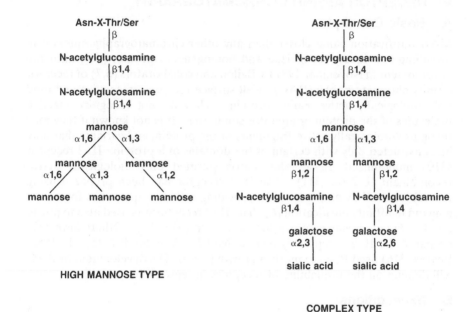

Figure 5   Typical forms of N-linked oligosaccharides. (Courtesy Dr. Joseph K. Welply.)

(113,114). A large number of human proteins are glycosylated; 62 of the 63 blood proteins are glycosylated (329). Most likely, the possible delineation of the physiological function of oligosaccharides on proteins and enzymes may be the third act in molecular biology, following the first and second acts of gene cloning and monoclonal antibodies of the 1970s, respectively. To achieve this expectation, significant effort is in progress in many laboratories to characterize the oligosaccharides of glycoproteins (114,118,119,330,331). Oligosaccharides are attached to proteins either on asparagine residues, N-linked to the nitrogen of the Asn side chain, with typical structures shown in Fig. 5, or to serine or threonine; or O-linked to the hydroxyl of Ser or Thr side chain, with typical structures shown in Fig. 6 (332–334).

B. Glycoform Ligand Purification

A number of glycoproteins are comprised of more than one glycoform, including plasminogen (335), t-PA (117–119), and others (113–116). Lectins and other affinity ligands have been used to purify glycoproteins, with concanavalin A lectin on agarose being specific for N-linked type (330,336–345). Recently, the two glycoforms of t-PA have been studied extensively because of the major clinical interest in the therapeutic potential of this

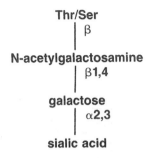

Figure 6 Typical form of *O*-linked oligosaccharide. (Courtesy Dr. Joseph K. Welply.)

physiological plasminogen activator. Type I t-PA is glycosylated at residues Asn-117, Asn-184, and Asn-448; Type II at Asn-117 and Asn-448, as shown schematically in Fig. 7 (117,119,331). Asn-218, a potential glycosylation site, is not glycosylated in either glycoform. The two glycoforms of t-PA were purified to homogeneity using lysine-Sepharose 4B affinity chromatography with differential gradient elution by Howard and associates; the results are shown for human melanoma derived in Fig. 8 (331). Lysine is an excellent ligand for t-PA, binding to certain structural domains of the enzyme. Type II t-PA has greater affinity for lysine than Type I (331). Purification of glycoforms and their subtypes will be a challenge to investigators with interest in the application and extension of BAC in the years ahead. Lectins have the potential to be used as key ligands to purify glycoforms and their subtypes (113,114,346).

VII. SALT-PROMOTED ADSORPTION OF PROTEINS

A. Basic Concept

Recently, Porath and associates (347–354) have been developing another protein chromatographic technique known by several names, including salting-out, hydrophobic interaction, zone precipitation, and interfacial salting-out. In 1948, Tiselius (355) first demonstrated that amino acids and proteins adsorb to neutral supports, e.g., on cellulose, in the presence of high concentrations of alkaline phosphates, and he coined the term salting-out chromatography. In 1973, Porath et al. (347) observed that under certain salting-out conditions, benzylated cross-linked agarose adsorbed certain proteins. These gels are amphiphilic. They are produced by introducing a limited number of hydrophobic groups into hydrophilic gels, yielding cross-linked polymers (170,347). The observation has been extended, with considerable success, by incorporating a number of selected adsorbents on

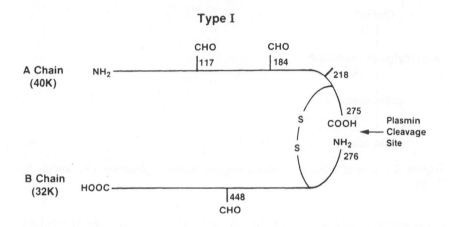

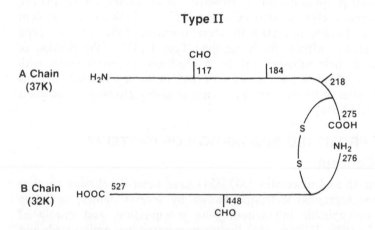

Figure 7 Structure of melanoma t-PA. Tissue-type plasminogen activator glycoforms. (Courtesy Dr. Daniel T. Connolly.)

neutral gels, primarily on Sepharose (350). The chemical composition and structure of the adsorbent are key elements for selective protein adsorption, shown for two immunoglobulin-binding agarose gels that include the propene-trinitrilo (PTN) group as part of the ligand in Fig. 9 (353). Other important ligand structures for certain protein adsorbents are shown in Fig.

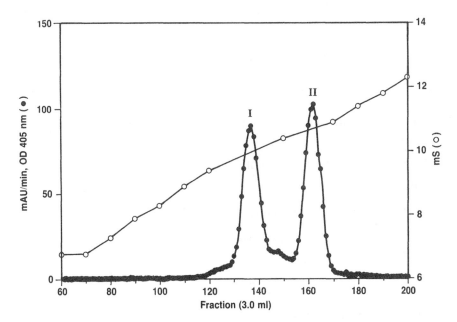

Figure 8 Lysine-Sepharose chromatography of Bowes melanoma tissue-type plasminogen activator. (Courtesy Dr. Susan C. Howard, Ref. 331.)

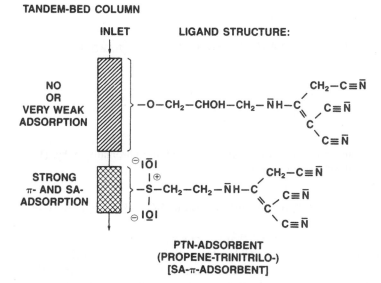

Figure 9 An S-site is required for strong enhancement of π-adsorption. Group specific adsorbents for affinity chromatography. (From J. Porath, Ref. 353, with permission.)

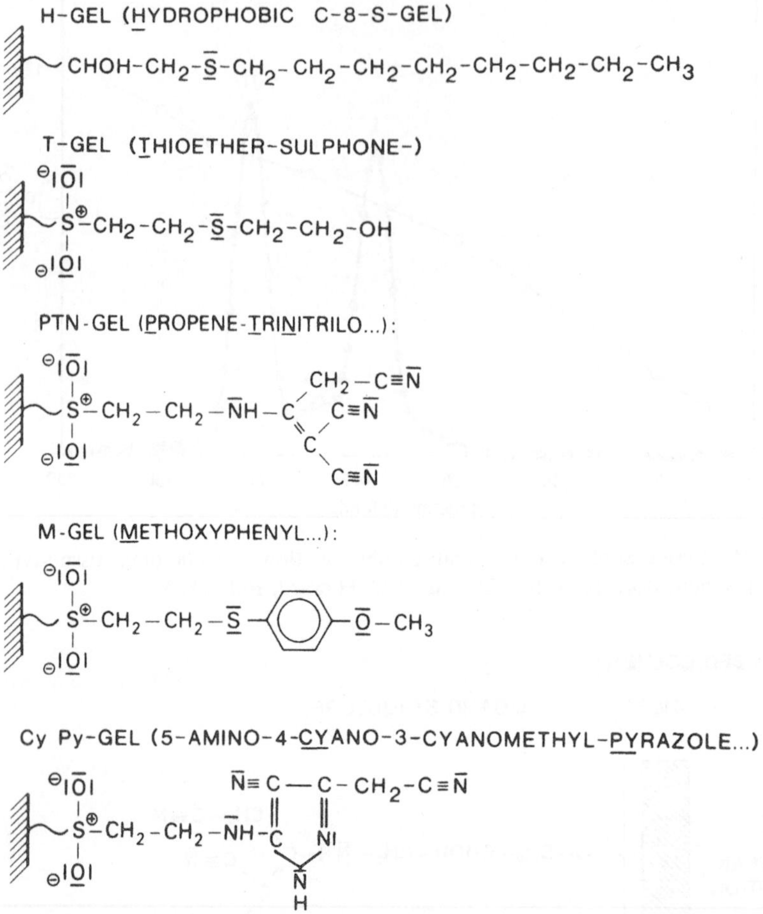

H-GEL (HYDROPHOBIC C-8-S-GEL)

⌇~CHOH-CH₂-S̄-CH₂-CH₂-CH₂-CH₂-CH₂-CH₂-CH₂-CH₃

T-GEL (THIOETHER-SULPHONE-)

⊖|Ō|
⌇~S⊕-CH₂-CH₂-S̄-CH₂-CH₂-OH
⊖|O̲|

PTN-GEL (PROPENE-TRINITRILO...):

⊖|Ō| CH₂-C≡N̄
⌇~S⊕-CH₂-CH₂-N̄H-C   C≡N̄
⊖|O̲| ⟍C⟍
                                   C≡N̄

M-GEL (METHOXYPHENYL...):

⊖|Ō|
⌇~S⊕-CH₂-CH₂-S̄-⟨◯⟩-Ō-CH₃
⊖|O̲|

Cy Py-GEL (5-AMINO-4-CYANO-3-CYANOMETHYL-PYRAZOLE...)

⊖|Ō| N̄≡C — C - CH₂-C≡N̄
⌇~S⊕-CH₂-CH₂-N̄H-C   N̄I
⊖|O̲| N
                              H

Figure 10 Group specific adsorbent structures for affinity chromatography. (From J. Porath, Ref. 350, with permission.)

10, including for T-Gel (Thioether-Sulfone-) and H-Gel (Hydrophobic C-8-S-Gel) (350).

It is important to understand that various salts can be used to elute or to adsorb proteins on neutral solids, depending on their position in the Hofmeister (lyotropic) series (356). The relative ability of salts to precipitate proteins in the Hofmeister series from aqueous solutions is phosphates > sulfates > acetates >chrolides > nitrates > thiocyanates. Proteins adsorb on solids with a strength that depends on the salt position in the Hofmeister series for precipitation. Salts at the start of the series, e.g., sulfates, are water-structuring or antichaotropic, and those at the end, e.g., thiocyanates, randomize the structure of liquid water or are chaotropic. Antichaotropic salts promote protein adsorption. Chaotropic salts facilitate protein elution in entropically driven adsorption-desorption processes. Within the Hofmeister series there is a shift from salt-promoted adsorption to salt-promoted desorption of proteins. The type of adsorbent used determines the location of the shift (350). The selectivity position of salt-promoted affinity adsorption of proteins is somewhere between bioaffinity, based on biological recognition, the highest selectivity position, and hydrophobic interaction and charged-charged attraction, the lowest position on the selectivity scale (350).

B. Applications and Expectations

The application of salt-promoted adsorption chromatography has been limited (354). Hutchens and Porath (348) and Belew et al. (352) have used T-Gels, thiophilic adsorbents, to purify MABs, IgG and IgM, either from serum-containing cell culture media or from ascites fluids in one step. The recovery for the IgG type was > 90%, but for the IgM it was considerably less. Porath (350) and Porath and Belew (354) have shown that tandem use of T-Gels and H-Gels, strategically placed, can selectively purify some of the component proteins of serum with good results. Further purification of the H-Gel fractions could be achieved by application of displacement chromatography, a method currently being developed by Horvath (357) and Cramer (358,359). Adsorption chromatography has potential for economical large-scale applications (350).

Exploratory research studies on the adsorption of proteins by salts will provide better understadning of the role that surface properties play in their purification by various chromatographic methods, including BAC. Protein adsorption exploits the surface molecular properties of proteins. In 1976, Chothia (171) determined for a number of proteins the surface location of amino-acid side chains by x-ray crystallography. Porath (350) used the work of Chothia and arrived at the following series for amino acids with respect to the order of descending solvent or solute accessibility: Arg > Lys > Gln > Asn = Tyr > His > Glu = Pro > Ser > Thr > Trp > Gly > Ala > 1/2 Cys = Met > Leu > Cys = Phe > Val > Ile. The recent studies of Haymore (274), Regnier (168), and Porath (273) to modify and use surface protein properties for their efficient and economical purification are examples of the direction of chromatography. These and other studies should lead to protein purification methods, in general, with better predictability.

VIII. LARGE-SCALE AFFINITY CHROMATOGRAPHY

Three topics will be discussed concerning large-scale processes for BAC. First, high-performance affinity chromatography, HPAC, is very likely to become a significant application for BAC not only for large-scale but also for a very sophisticated analytical technique. Second, affinity precipitation, partitioning, and adsorption in fluidized beds and other operational modes will be elaborated in terms of their potential for manufacturing processes to purify not only clinical products derived from biotechnology but also, equally important, biotech-based products of specialty chemicals, polymers, and fibers, in the late 1990s and beyond, a dream that is expected to become a reality. Third, BAC manufacturing processes for a number of proteins and enzymes, including interferons, dehydrogenases, Antithrombin III, and t-PA, will be summarized as much as the published literature permits, although it is very limited.

A. High-Performance Affinity Chromatography

HPAC is still underdeveloped (26), but rapid progress is underway, as indicated in a thorough 1988 review by Bergold, Muller, Hanggi, and Carr (27). The development of HPAC started in 1978, only two years after major improvements were made in size exclusion HPLC (17–19,22–24). Mosbach and associates (25) were the first to apply affinity chromatography in the HP mode, using both ligands and polyclonal antibodies. The operation of HPAC requires supports that can withstand high pressures. The inorganics silica (360) and glass can take high pressures, but they adsorb proteins nonspecifically. Mosbach minimized such adverse effects by using a method developed by Regnier (18) for HPLC: covalently bonding silica with a layer of glycerylpropylsilyl, upon which the ligands were also covalently attached. They demonstrated that enzymes, isoenzymes, and albumins could be purified to base-line resolution and in less than a few minutes using HPAC in columns with this derivatized silica (10 μm particles with 60 Å pore size), operating at pressures up to 27 atm. The columns were used repeatedly more than 20 times with no loss in resolution, rapidity of operation, or eluate biological activity recovery.

Borchert, Larsson and Mosbach (361,362) used epoxy-silane coupling agents as the interlayer between silica and ligands. Concanvalin A was used as the model ligand, immobilized directly on the epoxy-silica, via a diol-silica activated with tresyl chloride, or the diol-silica was converted to aldehyde-silica. These packings with immobilized con A were used in columns to purify various glycoproteins in 5–20 minutes with high resolution and were reused up to 60 times with no loss in performance. Other ligands have been immobilized using the epoxy-silane route (27,362). The mechanism of surface silanols in chromatography has been examined in detail by Nahum and Horvath (363). The use of other supports for HPAC including polysaccharides, polyacrylamides, and inorganics has been reviewed by Ernst-Cabrera and Wilchek (364) and others (27). Other coupling methods have also been used (27).

Porath (26), Rassi and Horvath (365), and very recently Chicz and Regnier (366) have demonstrated that HPAC with metal ion chelates has significant chromatographic advantages for purification. Under certain conditions, such columns can be used up to 1000 runs with no loss in performance. The specific activity is increased significantly, and occasionally up to 1000- to 10,000-fold. Site-specific variants of genetically engineered subtilisin were purified and separated using HPAC metal ion chelates (366).

During the last 2 to 7 years, HPAC has been applied in the purification and characterization of a number of proteins with success, demonstrating its potential to be used in large-scale purification for manufacturing purposes efficiently and economically (89,105,366–380). The fundamental aspects of HPAC have been reviewed and summarized recently (27).

B. Affinity Precipitation, Partitioning, and Adsorption

1. Precipitation and Partitioning

The three modes of operation for biospecific affinity separation are shown schematically in Fig. 3 (80); they are precipitation, partitioning, and adsorption in the probable order that they can be scaled up economically. Janson and others have reviewed large-scale affinity chromatography (80,179,381) and other scale-up chromatographic procedures (179). Reported work in precipitation and partitioning modes has been very limited (80,382,383,384). Precipitation is based on the use of a soluble ligand for the target protein in free solution inducing it to precipitate. The precipitation occurs either spontaneously by forming aggregates via oligomeric target proteins and oligomeric inhibitors, or via secondary functions of the inhibitor complex, which is not participating in the binding. In 1979, Larsson and Mosbach (382) first demonstrated the precipitation mode using lactate dehydrogenase and Bis-NAD(+pyruvate) as the ligand. The precipitating ligand can also be attached to gels such as agarose (382) and more recently on chitosan (384). Another mode is to attach the ligand to polymers that can form multifunctional soluble reagents. These reagents, after the product of interest has been complexed with them, are induced to precipitate by addition of a salt or by changing the pH (385). The last method has reportedly been used at the manufacturing scale (80). Partitioning is based on the preferential distribution of a solute ligand-protein system to one of the phases in an aqueous polymer two-phase solution. The ligand is attached covalently to a carrier polymer, usually polyethylene glycol (PEG) with M_r = 6000, which has low polarity. Proteins prefer the polar phase, usually high-M_r dextran. The protein for the ligand is selectively extracted and concentrated in the PEG phase (80,383). The theoretical aspects of partitioning have been addressed recently (386). More developments are likely in the use of affinity precipitation and partitioning of proteins, which have a good potential to be used in manufacturing purification processes.

2. Fluidized Bed Adsorption

Many attempts have been made to improve the operational dynamics of packed BAC columns, limited primarily by the flow characteristics of the gel (179,387). There have been attempts to (1) make monodisperse particles to improve flow (388); (2) use radial-flow cartridges (95); (3) use polyaldehyde microsphere beads to minimize leakage (389); and (4) divide a single column into two beds and operate in a periodic countercurrent mode, which improves the ligand utilization nearly four times compared to the single fixed bed mode (96). In early 1989, Somers, Van't Reit and associates (108) demonstrated convincingly that BAC can be effected in a fluidized bed mode. They successfully purified endopolygalacturonase from an industrial pectolytic enzyme using alginate as the ligand. Alginate is a substrate analog for the natural substrate pectate, and it was transformed by Ca^{2+}-complexation into beads that could be fluidized (390,391). A systematic study was made of the adsorption and desorption kinetics of the system, and the processing conditions were optimized with respect to pH, $CaCl_2$ concentration, and buffer ionic strength. The diffusion velocity of the enzyme in the alginate beads was determined. It was found that the desorption was controlled by the diffusion velocity of the enzyme and could be described by a diffusion model by standard chemical engineering methods in terms of equations. It was shown that the fluidized bed could be used for at least 100 cycles with no loss of adsorption capacity or fluid bed operability. The actual data for the 100 cycles are included in the paper, a milestone. The investigators have plans to use the technique in the fermentor to isolate the enzyme in a single process step. The study was made in cooperative work between the departments of engineering, genetics, and chemistry. The use of magnetic fields to stabilize fluidized beds for BAC adsorption to reduce back-mixing has been investigated previously (109,110).

3. Membrane Adsorption

Ultrafiltration and microporous membranes have been used in the affinity adsorption mode to purify proteins more efficiently and more economically than gel packed beds (392–398). Hollow fiber membranes with microporous cast structure, as reported in 1988 by Brandt and associates (393,394), have the highest potential to reduce the cost and improve purification efficiency significantly for affinity adsorption. According to Brandt et al. (393), the efficiency of ligand, a costly component in BAC, can be significantly increased by maximization of the rate of mass transfer of the purified protein to complex with the ligand. In packed gel affinity columns, the rate of mass transfer is limited by the time it takes for the protein to diffuse to the ligand, which lies in the interior of the gel beads. The binding kinetics in BAC are rapid. Hence the ligand can be used more efficiently if the time T_d for diffusion of the protein to be purified to the ligand could be reduced substantially as compared to its residence time in the column T_c, i.e., $T_d <<< T_c$. The dimensionless Peclet number Pe is a measure of transport

Table 4 Two Affinity Device Designs with Equal Mass Transfer Efficiency

	Hollow fiber membrane device	System packed with 100 μm agarose particles
Fluid residence time	0.014 min	34.7 min
Device volume	0.773 L	1,070 L
Average flow rate	1.4 L/min	1.4 L/min
Ligand loading	1.9 g	1,950 g

Source: Sepracor, Inc., from S. Brandt et al. (Ref. 393), with permission.

rate efficiency of either energy (390) or mass (399). It is the ratio of a characteristic length L_d, diffusion path length in this case, multiplied by the velocity of the fluid through the column, U, divided by the molecular diffusivity coefficient of the protein, D, i.e., $Pe = L_dU/D$. $Pe <<<< 1$ indicates high mass transport rate efficiency. For a packed column, the L_d is the mean particle diameter of the gel. Reducing L_d to improve mass transfer rate results in higher operating pressures, which gel particles cannot withstand without reduction in throughput. The hollow fiber microporous membrane provides a low L_d, by orders of magnitude, by allowing the protein to be purified to flow through the membrane support past the ligand, rather than diffusing through the gel particle to reach the ligand. Brandt et al. (393) showed that BAC adsorption is *diffusion*-limited, utilizing data and analysis by Olson and Yarmush (400). The result indicates that membrane-based affinity systems can be scaled up. Table 4 and Fig. 11 show clearly the advantages of hollow fiber membranes over either porous silica (360) or agarose (393). A very small membrane device (15 cm in length by 3.8 cm in diameter) is equivalent in processing capability to 24 agarose columns (60 cm in length by 25.2 cm in diameter), requiring only 0.1% of the ligand, which is very expensive. The purification efficiency of hollow fibers was demonstrated with fibronectin and compared to standard methods (393).

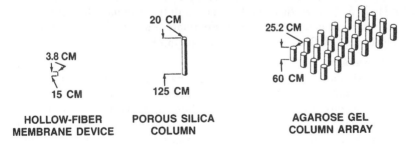

Figure 11 Three affinity purification devices of equivalent processing capability. (Courtesy Sepracor, Inc., from S. Brandt et al., Ref. 393, with permission.)

4. Other Adsorption Methods

Reversed micellar (401) and unilamellar vesicles (402) have been used very recently as a means to improve the economics of adsorption BAC, pursuing the current research theme to purify proteins directly from the biological stream by solution processes. Magnetic polymers were evaluated as supports for ligands several years ago, but currently there appears to be little interest in the approach (403–406).

5. Biospecific Affinity Separation Modes Summary

Significant theoretical and experimental work is in progress both in industry and in academia to make all biospecific affinity separation modes—precipitation, partitioning, and adsorption—economically attractive for manufacturing, utilizing the potential of the technique (80,92,381,387,407–415).

C. Affinity Purification of Various Proteins and Enzymes

1. Interferons

In the early 1980s, interferons (IFNs) attracted the attention of more than 80 biotechnology and pharmaceutical companies because of their potential therapeutic value for the patient. Many methods were used to purify IFNs, and major strides were made in obtaining highly purified IFNs that could be used clinically by use of either ligands or MABs (5,83,416–429). Reportedly (83), interferon (type not specified) was purified at the industrial scale by affinity chromatography (ligand not specified) since the early 1970s. In 1980, IFN-alpha was purified by a MAB against it on the large scale, as mentioned previously (5), with improvements for human recombinant IFN-alphaA and IFN-alpha2 reported in 1986 (420). Reportedly (416,417), the recombinantly produced human IFN-alpha, used clinically to treat certain states of neoplasia, is purified with a MAB against it, providing a highly purified lymphokine type therapeutic. IFN-beta and IFN-gamma are also purified by affinity methods (417,422–424,426) and in particular by their respective MABs. The availability of gamma-IFN receptors (427) may allow us in the future to purify IFN-gamma, the immune interferon, using RAC as has been done for IL-2 (6,7). Investigators should consult the original cited studies for specifics, but it is clear that MABs dominate the purification of IFNs, indicating the use of BAC for clinically used lymphokines.

2. Dehydrogenases

Equine liver alcohol dehydrogenase (ADH) has found use as a catalyst in organic synthesis (430,431). Large-scale purification of the enzyme was made possible by various BAC methods including Blue-Sepharose (431) and precipitation using a bifunctional NAD derivative (Bis-NAD) (432–434). These methods were used to purify ADH from kilogram quantities of liver efficiently and economically, prividing enzyme for industrial evaluation in various manufacturing processes as a catalyst.

3. Monoclonal Antibodies

To use MABs effectively for immunoaffinity purification, they must be highly purified. Protein A-Sepharose affinity chromatography has provided IgG-type MABs in highly purified form (84–87,287). The volume of the conditioned cell culture media that contain the MAB is reduced by a factor of 50–100 by ultrafiltration membranes (33), and then the affinity step is applied, followed by size exclusion HPLC, resulting in a highly purified MAB (84,287).

4. Human Factor VIII

Human Factor VIII has been purified on the large manufacturing scale using MAB against it and other steps, assuring limited presence of any virus (103).

5. Fibronectin

Gelatin-Sepharose CL-4B has been used to purify fibronectin in one step efficiently and economically (106). Gelatin is a substrate for fibronectin. Brandt et al. (393) demonstrated that gelatin immobilized in hollow fiber microporous membranes can be used to purify fibronectin efficiently and economically. Both methods can be used in manufacturing processes with reasonable economics to give highly purified fibronectin, a protein of utility in anchorage-dependent mammalian cell culture (435,436).

6. Antithrombin III

Heparin-Sepharose CL-6B has been used as the affinity step to purify antithrombin III for clinical use since 1972 (79,88,437). It is one of the few processes using BAC of which the actual manufacturing technology has been disclosed publicly.

7. Other Proteins and Enzymes

The large-scale purification of t-PA from human cell culture media (CM) that contained u-PA (urokinase) has been reported recently by our group (222,287). The two enzymes copurify because they are similar both structurally and chemically. Three affinity methods were used to separate them to try to obtain t-PA free of u-PA: (1) con A; (2) fibrin; and (3) MABs against t-PA. All three methods provided purified t-PA, but only the MABs provided t-PA that was free of u-PA, as measured by a Western blot method, an immunological and sensitive technique. The other two ligands, although very specific for t-PA, had some affinity also for u-PA. Zn-chelated Sepharose 6B was used to reduce the volume of the CM before using the other affinity methods. The metal ion affinity step isolated 100% of the t-PA and u-PA biological activities contained in the starting CM. BAC processes have been reported for several other proteins that can be used in large-scale purification efficiently and economically including calmodulin (102), penicillinases (104), beta-galactosidase (438,439), hepatic glucokinase (440), hepatitis B surface antigen (441), human insulin-like growth factor II (442), phosphoglycerate kinase (443), phosphofructokinase (444), nitrate reductase (445), glycerokinase (446), human pepsin, and gastricsin (447).

IX. PURIFICATION "ECONOMICS"

Table 5 shows the important parameters concerning the cost of purifying a protein or an enzyme from a complex biological stream. Each purification scheme for manufacturing a protein or enzyme will have special requirements and assumptions in the determination of cost as related to the selling price of the product. However, all purification schemes have the key elements as shown in Table 5, including the number of purification steps, biological activity percent recovery for each step, initial cost of the gel, and the number of times that the gel can be reused, which can be governed by sterility considerations. The amount of biological activity recovered in each step is the first issue in the determination of the purification cost to the product. Purification steps with less than 80% recovery of the biological activity start to contribute significantly to the overall cost. Purification schemes with more than three steps can have a significant impact on the overall cost. Biospecific affinity chromatography offers the possibility to recover nearly 100% of the activity and to minimize the number of purification steps to three or fewer. The cost contributed by the purification of the product can be minimal, if the previously stated conditions can be achieved with reasonable costs per step. A general cost analysis was made for a proprietary therapeutic enzyme, requiring about three major purification steps: (1) concentration, (2) BAC, and (3) size exclusion chromatography. The purification components could be used many times, but <100; the annual production was in kilogram quantities, and the cost of the complete plant was several million dollars but <$100 million. The analysis was made independently by the classical method of Aries and Newton for drugs (448,449) and by modern methods (448,450). Both analyses indicated that the contribution of the purification costs to the total cost of the product was not appreciable (448). It is obvious that purification costs can be a dominant factor in product cost, if the recovery of the biological activity is <50% for each step. The key elements for each purification step is to increase the *biological specific activity* of the purified protein with high recovery of the starting *biological activity*. The advice of Deutscher (451) to *rethink a purification procedure* should not be taken lightly.

Table 5   Purification "Economics"

Number of steps
Biological activity, % recovery
Cost of affinity column(s)
Actual cost
Number of times reused

X. FUTURE PROSPECTS

Michael S. Tswett, who coined the name *chromatography* for his successful methods of separating plant pigments in the early 1900s, made the profound statement that "every scientific advance is an advance in method" (452). Biospecific affinity chromatography is a major advance in method to purify proteins and enzymes. The method continues to advance rapidly, supported by basic studies on the hydrophobic effect (453–456), protein structure (168,171,273,350), thermodynamic and electrophoretic considerations (400,457,458), and separation of the Ag::Ab complex by very high pressures (111). High-performance affinity chromatography (26,27,366) is advancing very rapidly, capturing the imagination of chemical engineers, chemists, and other scientists. Receptor affinity chromatography (6,7) has the possibility to reduce purification of proteins and enzymes to one step, isolating only the biologically active molecules. The immobilization of artificial membranes on silica reported by Pigeon (459,460) offers possibilities for purification of proteins and enzymes similar to those used by the cell. The novel method developed by Haymore (274) and others (99,100,272,273) of introducing histidine residues, strategically placed in the protein via genetic engineering enhances significantly the economic potential of metal ion affinity chromatography. The method of introducing specific "tails," via genetic engineering, in the C-terminus of the protein, that have affinity properties has not been fully exploited for purification, although it was introduced in the early 1980s (461–464). A novel approach to the production of peptides has been to express the peptide fused to one or more proteins that can be affinity purified (442). Another recent genetic engineering approach is to use heat shock proteins as affinity ligands in appropriately designed systems for purification purposes (465–467). These approaches have the potential for a major reduction in purification costs for biotechnology based manufactured specialty chemicals, polymers, and fibers that require quantities in the millions of kilograms (471,472). The recent processing developments of using fluidized beds (108) and hollow fiber microporous membranes (393) with immobilized affinity ligands in the purification of proteins and enzymes potentially offer major reductions in purification costs. The commercial status of chromatography has been reported recently (468), and a much-needed "Guide to Protein Purification" (469) is available. Chicz and Regnier (470) discuss HPLC in terms of the varous chromatographic modes extensively and especially for *affinity*, which has the potential to solve major protein purification problems elegantly.

ACKNOWLEDGMENTS

The author wishes to express his thanks and sincere appreciation to the following, who generously provided publications in print, other material, and information for this chapter: Dr. Jerker Porath, Dr. Pedro Cuatrecasas, Dr.

Meir Wilchek, Dr. Fred E. Regnier, Dr. Jan-Christer Janson, Dr. Steven M. Cramer, Dr. Steve Brandt, Dr. Joseph K. Welply, Dr. Susan C. Howard, and Dr. Daniel T. Connolly. Drs. Porath and Janson were the students of the late Arne Tiselius, Uppsala University, Uppsala, Sweden. Also, special thanks are extended to Debbie Schaller, Sharon Hoss, and Carolyn O'Reilly for literature searches, and to Marilyn D. Reed for typing and formatting the manuscript.

REFERENCES

1. Cuatrecasas, P., Wilchek, M., and Anfinsen, C. B. (1968). Selective enzyme purification by affinity chromatography, *Proc. Natl. Acad. Sci. USA, 61*: 636.
2. Campbell, D. H., Leuscher, E., and Lerman, L. S. (1951). Immunologic adsorbents I. Isolation of antibody by means of a cellulose-protein antigen, *Proc. Natl. Acad. Sci. USA, 37*: 575.
3. Lerman, L. S. (1953). A biochemically specific method for enzyme isolation, *Proc. Natl. Acad. Sci. USA, 39*: 232.
4. Porath, J., Carlson, J., Olsson, I., and Belfrage, G. (1975). Metal chelate affinity chromatography: A new approach to protein fractionation, *Nature, 258*: 598.
5. Secher, D. S., and Burke, D. C. (1980). A monoclonal antibody for large-scale purification of human leukocyte interferon, *Nature, 285*: 446.
6. Bailon, P., Weber, D. V., Keeney, R. F., Fredericks, J. E., Smith, C., Familletti, P. C., and Smart, J. E. (1987). Receptor-affinity chromatography: A one-step purification for recombinant interleukin-2, *Bio/Technology, 5*:1195.
7. Bailon, P., and Weber, D. V. (1988). Receptor-affinity chromatography, *Nature, 335*: 839.
8. Tiselius, A. (1930). The moving boundary method of studying the electrophoresis of proteins, Dissertation, Uppsala University, Uppsala.
9. Tiselius, A. (1949). *Les Prix Nobel 1948*, Norstedt, Stockholm, pp. 60–61.
10. Tiselius, A., Porath, J., and Albertsson, P.-A. (1963). Separation and fractionation of macromolecules and particles, *Science, 141*:13.
11. Tiselius, A. (1968). Reflections from both sides of the counter, *Ann. Rev. Biochem., 37*: 1.
12. Sober, H. A., and Peterson, E. A. (1954). Chromatography of proteins on cellulose ion-exchangers, *J. Am. Chem. Soc., 76*: 1711.
13. Porath, J., and Flodin, P. (1959). Gel filtration: A method for desalting and group separation, *Nature, 183*: 1657.
14. Synge, R. L. M., and Tiselius A. (1950). Fractionation of hydrolysis products of amylose by electrokinetic ultrafiltration in an agar-agar jelly, *Biochemical J., 46*:xli.
15. Mould, D. L., and Synge, R. L. M. (1954). Separations of polysaccharides related to starch by electrokinetic ultrafiltration in collodion membranes, *Biochemical J., 58*: 571.
16. Mould, D. L. and Synge, R. L. M. (1954). The electrophoretic mobility and fractionation of complexes of hydrolysis products of amylose with iodine and potassium iodide, *Biochemical J., 58*: 585.

17. Tsuji, K., and Robertson, J. H. (1975). Improved high-performance liquid chromatographic method for polypeptide antibiotics and its application to study the effects of treatments to reduce microbial levels in bacitracin powder, *J. Chromatogr.*, *112*: 663.

18. Regnier, F. E., and Noel, R. (1976). Glycerolpropylsilane bonded phases in the steric exclusion chromatography of biological macromolecules, *J. Chromatogr. Sci.*, *14*: 316.

19. Regnier, F. E. (1976). Bonded carbohydrate stationary phases for chromatography, U.S. Patent 3,983,299, September 28.

20. Chang, S. H., Gooding, K. M., and Regnier, F. E. (1976). High-performance liquid chromatography of proteins, *J. Chromatogr.*, *125*: 103.

21. Martin, A. J. P., and Synge, R. L. M. (1941). A new form of chromatogram employing two liquid phases: 1) Theory of chromatography, 2) Application to the mirco-determination of the higher monoamino-acids of proteins, *Biochemical J.*, *35*: 1358.

22. Regnier, F. E., and Gooding, K. M. (1980). High-performance liquid chromatography of proteins: Review, *Anal. Biochem.*, *103*: 1.

23. Regnier, F. E. (1983). High-performance liquid chromatography of biopolymers, *Science*, *222* (4621): 245.

24. Regnier, F. E. (1987). HPLC of biological macromolecules: The first decade, *Chromatographia*, *24*: 241.

25. Ohlson, S., Hansson, L., Larsson, P.-O., and Mosbach, K. (1978). High Performance liquid affinity chromatography (HPLAC) and its application to the separation of enzymes and antigens, *FEBS Lett.*, *93*: 5.

26. Porath, J. (1988). High-performance immobilized-metal-ion affinity chromatography of peptides and proteins, *J. Chromatogr.*, *443*: 3.

27. Bergold, A. F., Muller, A. J., Hanggi, D. A., and Carr, P. W. (1988). High-performance affinity chromatography. *High-Performance Liquid Chromatography: Advances and Perspectives* (C. Horvath, ed.), Vol. 5, Academic Press, New York, pp. 95–209.

28. Harakas, N. K., and Builder, S. E. (1987). Industrial scale protein purification: A perspective, *Biotech. Progr.*, *3*: M2.

29. Shuler, M. L., ed. (1987). Symposium papers on protein purification at the 1986 Annual Meeting of A.I.Ch.E., *Biotech. Progr.*, *3*: 9.

30. Clark, W. M., and Harakas, N. K. (1989). Science and engineering for the purification of biomolecules, *Biotech. Progr.*, *5*: S3.

31. Schultz, J. S., ed. (1989). Symposium papers on protein purification at the 1988 Annual Meeting of A.I.Ch.E., *Biotech. Progr.*, *5*: 79.

32. Regnier, F. E. (1987). Chromatography of complex protein mixtures: Review, *J. Chromatogr.*, *418*: 115.

33. Harakas, N. K., Bentle, L. A., Mitchell, J. W., and Feder, J. (1982). Plant scale concentration/fractionation of biological streams via ultrafiltration, *Harnessing Theory for Practical Applications, Proceedings Third Wold Filtration Congress*, vol. 2, Uplands Press, Croydon, pp. 513–518.

34. Astrup, T., and Permin, P. M. (1947). Fibrinolysis in the animal organism, *Nature*, *159*: 681.

35. Astrup, T., Stage, A. (1952). Isolation of soluble fibrinolytic activator from animal tissue, *Nature*, *170*: 929.

36. Rijken, D. C., Wijngaards, G., Zaal-de Jong, M., and Welbergen, J. (1979). Purification and partial characterization of plasminogen activator from human uterine tissue, *Biochim. Biophys. Acta, 580*: 140.

37. Rijken, D. C. (1980). Plasminogen activator from human tissue, Ph.D. thesis, State University of Leiden.

38. Rijken, D. C., and Collen, D. (1981). Purification and characterization of the plasminogen activator secreted by human melanoma cells in culture, *J. Biol. Chem., 256*: 7035.

39. Sanzo, M. A., Marasa, J. C., Wittwer, A. J., Siegel, N. R., Harakas, N. K., and Feder, J. (1987). Purification and characterization of a tissue plasminogen activator-inhibitor complex from human umbilical vein endothelial cell conditioned medium, *Biochemistry, 26*: 7443.

40. Ny, T., Sawdey, M., Lawrence, D., Millan, J. L., and Loskutoff, D. J. (1986). Cloning and sequence of a cDNA coding for the human beta-migrating endothelial-cell-type plasminogen activator inhibitor, *Proc. Natl. Acad. Sci. USA, 83*: 6776.

41. Ginsburg, D., Zeheb, R., Yang, A. Y., Rafferty, U. M., Andearsen, P. A., Nielsen, L., Dano, K., Lebo, R. V., and Gelehrter, T. D. (1986). cDNA cloning of human plasminogen activator-inhibitor from endothelial cells, *J. Clin. Invest., 78*: 1683.

42. van Mourik, J. A., Lawrence, D. A., and Loskutoff, D. J. (1984). Purification of an inhibitor of plasminogen activator (antiactivator) synthesized by endothelial cells, *J. Biol. Chem., 259*: 14914.

43. Shing, Y., Folkman, J., Sullivan, R., Butterfield, C., Murray, J., and Klagsbrun, M. (1984). Heparin affinity: Purification of a tumor-derived capillary endothelial cell growth factor, *Science, 223*: 1296.

44. Bohlen, P., Baird, A., Esch, F., Ling, N., and Gospodarowicz, D. (1984). Isolation and partial molecular characterization of pituitary fibroblast growth factor, *Proc. Natl. Acad. Sci. USA, 81*: 5363.

45. Gospodarowicz, D., Cheng, J., Lui, G.-M., Baird, A., and Bohlen, P. (1984). Isolation of brain fibroblast growth factor by heparin-sepharose affinity chromatography: Identity with pituitary fibroblast growth factor, *Proc. Natl. Acad. Sci. USA, 81*: 6963.

46. Bohlen, P., Esch, F., Baird, A., Jones, K. L., and Gospodarowicz, D. (1985). Human brain fibroblast growth factor: Isolation and partial characterization, *FEBS Lett., 185*: 177.

47. Esch, F., Baird, A., Ling, N., Ueno, N., Hill, F., Denoroy, L., Klepper, R., Gospodarowicz, D., Bohlen, P., and Guillemin, R. (1985). Primary structure of bovine pituitary basic fibroblast growth factor (FGF) and comparison with the amino-terminal sequence of bovine brain acidic FGF, *Proc. Natl. Acad. Sci. USA, 82*: 6507.

48. Klagsbrun, M., Sasse, J., Sullivan, R., and Smith, J. A. (1986). Human tumor cells synthesize an endothelial cell growth factor that is structurally related to basic fibroblast growth factor, *Proc. Natl. Acad. Sci. USA, 83*: 2448.

49. Jaye, M., Howk, R., Burgess, W., Ricca, G. A., Chiu, I.-M., Ravera, M. W., O'Brien, S. J., Modi, W. S., Maciac, T., and Drohan, W. N. (1986). Human endothelial cell growth factor: Cloning, nucleotide sequence, and chromosome localization, *Science, 233*: 541.

50. Abraham, J. A., Whang, J. L., Tumolo, A., Mergia, A., Friedman, J., Gospoda- rowicz, D., and Fiddes, J. C. (1986). Human basic fibroblast growth factor: Nucleotide sequence and genomic organization, *EMBO J.*, *5*: 2325.

51. Lobb, R. R., Harper, J. W., and Fett, J. W. (1986). Purification of heparin- binding factors: A review, *Anal. Biochem.*, *154*: 1.

52. Folkman, J., and Klagsbrun, M. (1987). Angiogenic factors, *Science*, *235*: 442.

53. Thiersch, C. (1865). *Der Epitheliale Krebs, Namentlich der Haute—Eine Anatomisch-Klinische Untersuchung*, Verlag von Wilhelm Englemann, Leipzig, Germany, pp. 1–309.

54. Baird, A., Schubert, D., Ling, N., and Guillemin, R. (1988). Receptor- and heparin-binding domains of basic fibroblast growth factor, *Proc. Natl. Acad. Sci. USA*, *85*: 2324.

55. Jaques, L. B. (1979). Heparin: An old drug with a new paradigm, *Science*, *206*: 528.

56. Shing, Y. (1988). Heparin-copper bioaffinity chromatography of fibroblast growth factors, *J. Biol. Chem.*, *263*: 9059.

57. Connolly, D. T., Olander, J. V., Heuvelman, D. M., Nelson, R. L., Monsell, R., Siegel, N., Haymore, B., Leimgruber, R., and Feder, J. (1989). Human vascular permeability factor: Isolation from U937 cells, *J. Biol. Chem.*, *264*: 20017.

58. Keck, P. J., Hauser, S. D., Krivi, G., Sanzo, K., Warren, T., Feder, J., and Connolly, D. T. (1989). Vascular permeability factor, an endothelial cell mitogen, is related to platelet-derived growth factor, *Science 246*: 1309.

59. Janson, J.-C. (1989). Personal communication, May 23.

60. Jakoby, W. B., and Wilchek, M., eds. (1974). Affinity techniques, *Methods in Enzymology*, vol. 34, Academic Press, New York.

61. Sundaram, P. v., and Eckstein, F., eds. (1978). *Theory and Practice in Affinity Techniques*, Academic Press, New York.

62. Pharmacia LKB Biotechnology, Uppsala (1988). *Affinity Chromatography: Principles and Methods*.

63. Scouten, W. H. (1981). *Affinity Chromatography: Bioselective Adsorption on Inert Matrices*, John Wiley, New York.

64. Fiechter, A., ed. (1982). *Advances in Biochemical Engineering: Chromatography*, vol. 25, Springer-Verlag, New York.

65. Gribnau, T. C. J., Visser, J., and Nivard, R. J. F., eds. (1982). *Affinity Chromatography and Related Techniques*, Elsevier, New York.

66. Scopes, R. K. (1982). *Protein Purification: Principles and Practice*, Springer- Verlag, New York.

67. Chaiken, I. M., Wilchek, M., and Parikh, I., eds. (1983). *Affinity Chromatogra- phy and Biological Recognition*, Academic Press, New York.

68. Schott, H. (1984). *Affinity Chromatography: Template Chromatography of Nucleic Acids and Proteins*, Marcel Dekker, New York.

69. Dean, P. D. G., Johnson, W. S., and Middle, F. A., eds. (1985). *Affinity Chromatography: A Practical Approach*, IRL Press, Washington, DC.

70. Mohr, P., Pommerening, K. (1985). *Affinity Chromatography: Practical and Theoretical Aspects*, Marcel Dekker, New York.

71. Pharmacia Fine Chemicals, Uppsala (1980). *Cell Affinity Chromatography: Principles and Methods*.

72. Jennissen, H. P., Muller, W., eds. (1988). *Makromol. Macromol. Symp.*, *17* (Int. Symp. Affinity Chromatog. Interfacial Macromol. Interact. 1987).
73. Cuatrecasas, P., and Anfinsen, C. B. (1971). Affinity chromatography, *Ann. Rev. Biochem.*, *40*: 259.
74. Cuatrecasas, P., and Anfinsen, C. B. (1971). Affinity chromatography, *Meth. Enzymol.*, *22*: 345.
75. O'Carra, P., and Barry, S. (1972). Affinity chromatography of lactate dehydrogenase: Model studies demonstrating the potential of the technique in the mechanistic investigation as well as in the purification of multi-substrate enzymes, *FEBS Lett.*, *21*: 281.
76. Porath, J., and Kristiansen, T. (1975). Biospecific affinity chromatography and related methods, *The Proteins* (H. Neurath and R. L. Hill, eds.). Academic Press, New York, *1*: 95.
77. Sharma, S. K., and Mahendroo, P. P. (1980). Affinity chromatography of cells and cell membranes, *J. Chromatogr.*, *184*: 471.
78. Porath, J. (1981). Development of modern affinity chromatography (A review), *J. Chromatogr.*, *218*: 241.
79. Hill, E. A., and Hirtenstein, M. D. (1983). Affinity chromatography: Its application to industrial scale processes, *Advances in Biotechnology Processes*, *1*: 31.
80. Janson, J.-C. (1984). Large-scale affinity purification: State of the art and future prospects, *Trends Biotechnol.*, *2*: 1.
81. Wilchek, M., Miron, T., and Kohn, J. (1984). Affinity chromatography, *Methods Enzymol.*, *104*: 3.
82. Sulkowski, E. (1985). Purification of proteins by IMAC, *Trends Biotechnol.*, *3*: 1.
83. Parikh, I., and Cuatrecasas, P. (1985). Affinity chromatography, *Chem. Eng. News*, *63*(34): 17.
84. Scott, R. W., Duffy, S. A., Moellering, B. J., and Prior, C. (1987). Purification of monoclonal antibodies from large-scale mammalian cell culture perfusion systems, *Biotechnol. Prog.*, *3*: 49.
85. Oestlund, C. (1986). Large scale purification of monoclonal antibodies, *Trends Biotechnol.*, *4*: 288.
86. Kenney, A. C., and Chase, H. A. (1987). Automated production scale affinity purification of monoclonal antibodies, *J. Chem. Tech. Biotechnol.*, *39*: 173.
87. Malm, B. (1987). A method suitable for the isolation of monoclonal antibodies for large volumes of serum-containing hybridoma cell culture supernatants, *J. Immunolog. Methods*, *104*: 103.
88. Janson, J.-C. (1987). "Process Scale Purificiation of Biological Macromolecules," Proc. 4th European Congress on Biotechnology, *4*, pp. 121–133.
89. Falkenberg, C., Bjoerck, L., Aakerstroem, B., and Nilsson, S. (1987). Purification of Streptococcal protein G. Expressed by *Escherichia coli* by high performance liquid affinity chromatography using immobilized immunoglobulin G and albumin, *Biomed. Chromatogr.*, *2*: 221.
90. Thompson, J. A. (1987). A Review of high performance liquid chromatography in nucleic acids research, V. Nucleic acid affinity techniques in DNA and RNA research, *BioChromatography*, *2*: 68.

91. Topf, J. J., and Bailey, R. C. (1987). A Computer-controlled affinity purification system, *Adv. Instrum.*, *42*: 1461.
92. Clonis, Y. D. (1987). Large-scale affinity, *Bio/Technology*, *5*: 1290.
93. Porath, J. (1988). IMAC - immobilized metal ion affinity based chromatography, *Trends Anal. Chem.*, *7*: 254.
94. Sulkowski, E. (1988). Immobilized metal ion affinity chromatography of proteins on IDA-iron^{3+}, *Macromol. Macromol. Symp.*, *17* (Int. Symp. Affinity Chromatogr. Interfacial Macromol. Interact., 1987):pp. 335–348.
95. Huang, S. H., Roy, S., Hou, K. C., and Tsao, G. T. (1988). Scaling-up of affinity chromatography by radial-flow cartridges, *Biotechnolog. Progr.*, *4*: 159.
96. Arve, B. H., and Liapis, A. I. (1988). Biospecific adsorption in fixed and periodic countercurrent beds, *Biotechnol. Bioeng.*, *32*: 616.
97. Arve, B. H., and Liapis, A. I. (1987). Modeling and analysis of biospecific adsorption in a finite bath, *AIChE J.*, *33*: 179.
98. Arve, B. H., and Liapis, A. I. (1988). Modeling and analysis of elution stage of biospecific adsorption in finite bath, *Biotech. Bioeng.*, *31*: 240.
99. Smith, M. C., Furman, T. C., Ingolia, T. D., and Pidgeon, C. (1988). Chelating peptide-immobilized metal ion affinity chromatography: A new concept in affinity chromatography for recombinant proteins, *J. Biol. Chem.*, *263*: 7211.
100. Smith, M. C., Furman, T. C., and Pidgeon, C. (1987). Immobilized iminodiacetic acid metal peptide complexes. Identification of chelating peptide purification handles for recombinant proteins, *Inorg. Chem.*, *26*: 1965.
101. Anderson, L. (1988). Immobilized metal ion affinity chromatography, *ISI Atlas Sci.: Biochem.*, *1*: 318.
102. Rhoades, G. L., Tran, L., Key, S. R., Carrion, M. E., and Jarrett, H. W. (1988). Preparative high pressure affinity chromatography purification of calmodulin and S-100 from Brain, *BioChromatography*, *3*: 70.
103. Zimmerman, T. S. (1988). Purification of factor VIII by monoclonal antibody affinity chromatography, *Semin. Hematol.*, *25*: 25.
104. Kiss, L., Tar, A., Gal, S., Toth-Martinez, B. L., and Hernadi, F. J. (1988). Modified general affinity adsorbent for large-scale purification of penicillinases, *J. Chromatogr.*, *448*: 109.
105. Manabe, T., Higuchi, N., Okuyama, T., and Mukaiyama, Y. (1988). High-performance affinity chromatography of human serum concanavalin A binding proteins, *J. Chromatogr.*, *431*: 45.
106. Regnault, V., Rivalt, C., and Stoltz, J. F. (1988). Affinity purification of human plasma fibronectin on immobilized gelatin, *J. Chromatogr.*, *432*: 93.
107. Shibuya, N., Berry, J. E., and Goldstein, E. J. (1988). One-step purification of murine IgM and human alpha2-macroglobulin by affinity chromatography on immobilized snowdrop bulb lectin, *Arch. Biochem. Biophys.*, *267*: 676.
108. Somers, W., Van't Reit, K., Rozie, H., Rombouts, F. M., and Visser, J. (1989). Isolation and purification of endopolygalacturonase by affinity chromatography in a fluidized-bed reactor, *Chem. Eng. J.* (Lausanne), *40*: B7.
109. Burns, M. A. (1986). Continuous affinity chromatography using a magnetically stabilized fluidized bed, Ph.D. thesis, University of Pennsylvania, Philadelphia.
110. Burns, M. A., and Graves, D. J. (1987). Application of magnetically stabilized fluidized beds to bioseparations, *React. Polym.*, *6*: 45.

111. Olson, W., Leung, S. K., and Yarmuch, M. L. (1989). Recovery of antigens from immunoadsorbents using high pressure, *Bio/Technology*, 7: 369.

112. Vretblad, P. (1976). Purification of lectins by biospecific affinity chromatography, *Biochim. Biophys. Acta*, *434*: 169.

113. Lis, H., and Sharon, N. (1986). Lectins as molecules and as tools, *Ann. Rev. Biochem.*, *55*: 35.

114. Rademacher, T. W., Parekh, R. B., and Dwek, R. A. (1988). Glycobiology, *Ann. Rev. Biochem.*, *57*: 785.

115. Boyle, F. A., and Peters, T. J. (1988). Characterization of galactosyltransferase isoforms by ion-exchange and lectin affinity chromatography, *Clin. Chim. Acta*, *178*: 289.

116. Zwaagstra, J. C., Armstrong, G. D., and Leung, W. C. (1988). The use of lectin affinity columns for selection of precursor or fully glycosylated forms of glycoprotein gD1 of herpes simplex virus type 1, *J. Virol. Methods*, *20*: 21.

117. Einarsson, M., Brandt, J., and Kaplan, L. (1985). Large-scale purification of human tissue-type plasminogen activator using monoclonal antibodies, *Biochim. Biophys. Acta*, *830*: 1.

118. Parekh, R. B., Dwek, R. A., Thomas, J. R., Opdenakker, G., Rademacher, T. W., Wittwer, A. J., Howard, S. C., Nelson, R. L., Siegel, N. R., Jennings, M. G., Harakas, N. K., and Feder, J. (1989). Cell type-specific and site-specific *N*-glycosylation of type I and type II human tissue plasminogen activator, *Biochemistry*, *28*: 7644.

119. Wittwer, A. J., Howard, S. C., Carr, L. S., Harakas, N. K., Feder, J., Parekh, R. B., Dwek, R. A., and Rademacher, T. W. (1989). Effects of *N*-glycosylation on *in vitro* activity of bowes melanoma and human colon fibroblast tissue plasminogen activator, *Biochemistry*, *28*: 7662.

120. Weply, J. (1991). Protein glycosylation: Factors that regulate oligosaccharide structure, *Animal Cell Bioreactors* (C. S. Ho and D. I. C. Wang, eds.), Butterworth-Heinemann, Boston, pp. 59–72.

121. Farach-Carson, M. C., and Carson, D. D. (1989). Extraction and isolation of glycoproteins and proteoglycans, *BioTechniques*, 7: 482.

122. Axen, R., Porath, J., and Ernback, S. (1967). Chemical coupling of peptides and proteins to polysaccharides by means of cyanogen halides, *Nature*, *214*: 1302.

123. Porath, J., Axe, R., and Ernback, S. (1967). Chemical coupling of proteins to agarose, *Nature*, *215*: 1491.

124. Porath, J. (1968). Molecular sieving and adsorption, *Nature*, *218*: 834.

125. Cuatrecasas, P. (1970). Protein purification by affinity chromatography: Derivatizations of agarose and polyacrylamide beads, *J. Biol. Chem.*, *245*: 3059.

126. Cuatrecasas, P. (1970). Agarose derivatives for purification of protein by affinity chromatography, *Nature*, *228*: 1327.

127. Cuatrecasas, P. (1970). Topography of the active site of staphylococcal nuclease: Affinity labeling with diazonium substrate analogues, *J. Biol. Chem.*, *245*: 574.

128. Steers, E. Jr., Cuatrecasas, P., and Pollard, H. B. (1971). The Purification of beta-galactosidase from *Escherichia coli* by Affinity chromatography, *J. Biol. Chem.*, *246*: 196.

129. Kohler, G., and Milstein, C. (1975). Continuous cultures of fused cells secreting antibody of predefined specificity, *Nature, 256*: 495.
130. Milstein, C. (1980). Monoclonal antibodies, *Sci. Am., 243*(4): 66.
131. Milstein, C. (1986). From antibody structure to immunological diversification of immune response, *Science, 231*: 1261.
132. Kohler, G. (1986). Derivation and diversification of monoclonal antibodies, *Science, 233*: 1281.
133. Porath, J., Aspberg, K., Drevin, H., and Axen, R. (1973). Preparation of cyanogen bromide-activated agarose gels, *J. of Chromatography, 86*: 53.
134. March, S. C., Parikh, I., and Cuatrecasas, P. (1973). A simplified method for cyanogen bromide activation of agarose for affinity chromatography, *Anal. Biochem., 60*: 149.
135. Cuatrecasas, P., and Parikh, I. (1972). Adsorbents for affinity chromatography: Use of *N*-hydroxysuccinimide esters of agarose, *Biochemistry, 11*: 2291.
136. Bio-Rad, Richmond, Calif. (1989). *Activated Immunoaffinity Supports*, pp. 1–38.
137. Wong, K. Y., Hawley, D., Vigneri, R., and Goldfine, I. D. (1988). Comparison of solubilized and purified plasma membrane and nuclear insulin receptors, *Biochemistry, 27*: 375.
138. Rehm, H., and Lazdunski, M. (1988). Purification and subunit structure of a putative K^+-channel protein identified by its binding properties for dendrotoxin I, *Proc. Natl. Acad. Sci. USA, 85*: 4919.
139. Baumbach, G. A., and Hammond, D. J. (1992). Protein purification using affinity ligands deduced from peptide libraries, *BioPharm, 5*(4): 24.
140. Sundberg, L., and Porath, J. (1974). Preparation of adsorbents for biospecific affinity chromatography I. Attachment of group-containing ligands to insoluble polymers by means of bifunctional oxiranes, *J. Chromatography, 90*: 87.
141. Brandt, J., Andersson, L.-O., and Porath, J. (1975). Covalent attachment of proteins to polysaccharide carriers by means of benjoquinone, *Biochim. Biophys. Acta, 386*: 196.
142. Nilsson, K. and Mosbach, K. (1980). *p*-Toluenesulfonyl chloride as an activating agent of agarose for the preparation of immobilized affinity ligands and proteins, *Eur. J. Biochem., 112*: 397.
143. Nilsson, K., and Mosbach, K. (1981). Immobilization of enzymes and affinity ligands to various hydroxyl group carrying supports using highly reactive sulfonyl chlorides, *Biochem. Biophys, Res. Commun., 102*: 449.
144. Nilsson, K., and Mosbach, K. (1981). Immobilization of ligands with organic sulfonyl chlorides, *Methods in Enzymology, 104*: 56.
145. Kohn, J., and Wilchek, M. (1983). 1-Cyano-4-dimethylamino pyridinium tetrafluoroborate as a cyanylating agent for the covalent attachment of ligand to polysaccharide resins, *FEBS Lett., 154*: 209.
146. Jost, R., Miron, T., and Wilchek, M. (1974). The mode of adsorption of proteins to aliphatic and aromatic amines coupled to cyanogen bromide-activated agarose, *Biochim. Biophys. Acta, 362*: 75.
147. Kohn, J., and Wilchek, M. (1981). Procedures for the analysis of cyanogen bromide-activated Sepharose or Sephadex by quantitative determination of cyanate esters and imidocarbonates, *Anal. Biochem., 115*: 375.
148. Kohn, J., and Wilchek, M. (1981). Mechanism of activation of Sepharose and Sephadex by cyanogen bromide, *Enzyme Microb. Technol., 4*: 161.

149. Kohn, J., and Wilchek, M. (1982). A new approach (cyano-transfer) for cyanogen bromide activation of Sepharose at neutral pH, which yields activated resins, free of interfering nitrogen derivatives, *Biochem. Biophys. Res. Commun.*, *107*: 878.

150. Kohn, J., Lenger, R., and Wilchek, M. (1983). *p*-Nitrophenylcyanate—An efficient, convenient, and nonhazardous substitute for cyanogen bromide as an activating agent for Sepharose, *Applied Biochem. Biotech.*, *8*: 227.

151. Axen, R., Drevin, H., and Carlsson, J. (1975). Preparation of modified agarose gels containing thiol groups, *Acta Chemica Scandinavica*, *B 29*: 471.

152. Kincaid, R. I., and Vaughan, M. (1983). Affinity chromatography of brain cyclic nucleotide phosphodiesterase using 3-(2-pyridyldithio)propionyl-substituted calmodulin linked to thiol-Sepharose, *Biochemistry*, *22*: 826.

153. Buettner, W., Becker, M., Rupprich, C., Boeden, H. F., Henklein, P., Loth, F., and Dautzenberg,, H. (1989). A novel carbonochloridate for activation of supports containing hydroxyl groups, *Biotechnol. Bioeng.*, *33*: 26.

154. Holton, O. D., III, and Vicalvi, J. J., Jr. (1991). Optimization of monoclonal antibody immobilization on hydrazide-preactivated hollow fiber membrane, *BioTechniques*, *11*: 662.

155. O'Shannessy, D. J. (1990). Hydrazido-derivatized supports in affinity chromatography, *J. Chromatography*, *510*: 13.

156. O'Shannessy, D. J., and Hoffman, W. L. (1987). Site-directed immobilization of glycoproteins on hydrazide-containing solid supports, *Biotechnol. Appl. Biochem.*, *9*: 488.

157. Pierce, Inc., Rockford, Ill. (1991). *Immuno Technology: Catalog and Handbook*, p. B10.

158. Nachman, M., Azad, A. R. M., and Bailon, P. (1992). Membrane-based receptor affinity chromatography, *J. Chromatography*, *597*: 229.

159. Bethel, G. S., Ayers, J. S., Hearn, M. T. W., and Hancock, W. S. (1981). Investigation of the activation of various insoluble polysaccharides with 1,1'-carbonyldiimidazole and of the properties of the activated matrices, *J. Chromatography*, *219*: 361.

160. Newman, J. D., and Harrison, L. C. (1985). Homogeneous bivalent insulin receptor: Purification using insulin coupled to 1,1'-carbonyldiimidazole activated-agarose, *Biochem. Biophys. Res. Commun.*, *132*: 1059.

161. Pierce, Rockford, Ill. (1991). *Immuno Technology: Catalog and Handbook*, p. B14.

162. Hill, M., and Ario, B. (1992). Activation of matrices by 4,6-diphenylthieno[3,4-*d*]-1,3-dioxol-2-one-5,5-dioxide: High-performance liquid affinity chromatographic separations, *J. Chromatography*, *589*: 101.

163. Fuglistaller, P. (1989). Comparison of immunoglobulin binding capacities and ligand leakage using eight different protein A affinity chromatography matrices, *J. Immunol. Methods*, *124*: 171.

164. Johansson, B.-L. (1992). Determination of leakage products from chromatographic media aimed for protein purification, *BioPharm*, *5*(3): 34.

165. Antonsen, K. P., Colton, C. K., and Yarmush, M. L. (1991). elution conditions and degradation mechanisms in long-term immunoadsorbent use, *Biotechnol. Progr.*, *7*: 159.

166. Porath, J. (1978). The discovery of Sephadex, *Trends Biol. Sciences*, *3*: N100.

167. Hjerten, S. (1962). Chromatographic separation according to size of macro-molecules and cell particles on columns of agarose suspensions, *Arch. Biochem. Biophys.*, *99*: 466.
168. Regnier, F. E. (1987). The role of protein structure in chromatographic behavior, *Science*, *238*: 319.
169. Cohen, S. A., Benedek, K., Tapuhi, Y., Ford, J. C., and Karger, B. L. (1985). Conformational effects in the reversed-phase liquid chromatography of ribonuclease A, *Anal. Biochem.*, *144*: 275.
170. Silman, I. H., and Katchalski, E. (1966). Water-insoluble derivatives of enzymes, antigens, and antibodies, *Ann. Rev. Biochem.*, *35*: 873.
171. Chothia, C. (1976). the nature of the accessible and buried surfaces in proteins, *J. Mol. Biol.*, *105*: 1.
172. Helfferich, F. (1961). 'Ligand exchange': A novel separation technique, *Nature*, *100*: 1001.
173. Porath, J., and Fryklund, L. (1970). Chromatography of proteins on dipolar ion adsorbants, *Nature*, *226*: 1169.
174. Gabel, D., and Porath, J. (1972). Molecular properties of immobilized proteins, *Biochemical J.*, *127*: 13P.
175. O'Carra, P., Barry, S., and Griffin, T. (1973). Spacer-arms in affinity chromatography: The need for a more rigorous approach, *Biochem. Soc. Trans.*, *1*: 289.
176. Lowe, C. R. (1977). The synthesis of several 8-substituted derivatives of adenosine 5'-monophosphate to study the effect of the nature of the spacer arm in affinity chromatography, *Eur. J. Biochem.*, *73*: 265.
177. Jaulmes, A., and Vidal-Madjar, C. (1989). Theoretical Aspects of quantitative chromatography: An overview, *Advances in Chromatography, vol. 28* (J. Calvin Giddings, Eli Grushka, and Phyllis R. Brown, eds.), Marcel Dekker, New York, pp. 1–64.
178. Belew, M., Porath, J., Fohlman, J., and Janson, J.-C. (1978). Adsorption phenomena on sephacryl® S-200 superfine, *J. Chromatography*, *147*: 205.
179. Janson, J.-C., and Hedman, P. (1982). Large-scale chromatography of proteins, *Advances Biochemical Engineering*, *25*: 43.
180. Porath, J., Laas, T., and Janson, J.-C. (1975). Agar derivatives for chromatography, electrophoresis and gel-bound enzymes III. Rigid agarose gels cross-linked with divinyl sulphone (DVS), *J. Chromatography*, *103*: 49.
181. Miron, T., and Wilchek, M. (1981). Polyacrylhydrazido-agarose: Preparation via periodate oxidation and use for enzyme immobilization and affinity chromatography, *J. Chromatography*, *215*: 53.
182. Arcangioli, B., Pochet, S., Sousa, R., and Huynh, D. T. (1989). Preparation and use of a universal primed Sepharose for the purification of DNA-binding proteins, *Eur. J. Biochem.*, *179*: 359.
183. Ngo, T. T. (1988). Polymeric matrix for affinity chromatography and immobilization of ligands, U.S. Patent 4,753,983, June 28 (Assignee: BioProbe International).
184. Moriguchi, S., Suzuki, H., Watanabe, H., Sato, M., Abe, M., and Iwata, Y. (1988). Porous chitosan granules as adsorbents and their use in chromatography, *Ger. Offen. DE 3,727,707 A1*, February 25 (Applicant: Kawasumi Laboratories, Inc.).
185. Hood, L. E. (1989). Personal communication, July 5.

186. Kopperschlager, G., Freyer, R., Diezel, W., and Hofmann, E. (1968). Some kinetic and molecular properties of yeast phosphofructonkinase, *FEBS Lett.*, *1*: 137.

187. Haff, L. A., and Easterday, R. L. (1978). Cibacron-blue-Sepharose: A tool for general ligand affinity chromatography, *Theory and Practice in Affinity-Techniques* (P. V. Sundaram and F. Eckstein, eds.), Academic Press, New York pp. 23-44.

188. Lowe, C. R., Small, D. A. P., and Atkinson, A. (1981). Minireview—Some preparative and analytical applications of triazine dyes, *Int. J. Biochem.*, *13*: 33.

189. Kopperschlager, G., Bohme, H.-J., and Hofmann, E. (1982). Cibacron Blue F3G-A and related dyes as ligands in affinity chromatography, *Advances Biochemical Engineering*, *25*: 101.

190. Lowe, C. R., and Pearson, J. C. (1984). Affinity chromatography on immobilized dyes, *Meth. Enzym.*, *104*: 97.

191. Lowe, C. R., Burton, S. J., Pearson, J. C., Clonis, Y. D., and Stead, V. (1986). Design and application of biomimetic dyes in biotechnology, *J. Chromatography*, *376*: 121.

192. Miribel, L., Gianazza, E., and Arnaud, P. (1988). The use of dye-ligand affinity chromatography for the purification of nonenzymic human plasma proteins, *J. Biochem. Biophys. Methods*, *16*: 1.

193. Anspach, B., Unger, K. K., Davies, J., and Hearn, M. T. W. (1988). Affinity chromatography with triazine dyes immobilized onto activated non-porous monodisperse silicas, *J. Chromatogr.*, *457*: 195.

194. Kroviarski, Y., Chochet, S., Vadon, C., Truskolaski, A., Boivin, P., and Bertrand, O. (1988). New strategies for the screening of a large number of immobilized dyes for the purification of enzymes from human hemolysate, *J. Chromatogr.*, *449*: 403.

195. Viatakis, G., Skarpelis, G., Stratidaki, I., Bouriotis, V., and Clonis, Y. D. (1987). Dye-ligand chromatography for the resolution and purification of restriction endonucleases, *Appl. Biochem. Biotechnol.*, *15*: 201.

196. Pharmacia, Inc., Piscataway, New Jersey (1983). Gels for ligand immobilization, Pharmacia Data Sheet.

197. Pierce, Inc., Rockford, Illinois (1988). Affinity chromatography and gel permeation, Pierce Handbook and General Catalog.

198. Pharmacia, Inc., Piscataway, New Jersey (1984). Tresyl-activated Sepharose 4B, Pharmacia Data Sheet.

199. Pharmacia, Inc., Piscataway, New Jersey (1987). EAH and ECH Sepharose 4B, Pharmacia Data Sheet.

200. Pharmacia Inc., Piscataway, New Jersey (1975). Con A-Sepharose 4B, Pharmacia.

201. Pharmacia, Inc., Piscataway, New Jersey (1982). Arginine-Sepharose 4B for affinity chromatography, Pharmacia Data Sheet.

202. Pharmacia LKB Biotechnology, Piscataway, New Jersey (1988). Lysine-Sepharose 4B for affinity chromatography, Data Sheet.

203. Pharmacia, Inc., (1986). Heparin-Sepharose CL-6B, Pharmacia Data Sheet.

204. Pharmacia, Inc., Piscataway, New Jersey (1983). Calmodulin-Sepharose 4B and calmodulin, Pharmacia Data Sheet.

205. Morin, L. G., Austin, G. E., and Mullins, R. H. (1988). Capacity related characteristics of Glyco-Gel affinity chromatographic support, *Clin. Biochem.*, *21*(4): 225.

206. Pierce, Inc., Rockford, Illinois (1989). Glyco-Gel, Pierce Data Sheet.

207. Arsenis, C., and McCormick, D. B. (1964). Purification of liver flavokinase by column chromatography on flavin-cellulose compounds, *J. Biol. Chem.*, *239*: 3093.

208. Arsenis, C., and McCormick, D. B. (1966). Purification of flavin mononucleotide-dependent enzymes by column chromatography on flavin phosphate cellulose compounds, *241*: 330.

209. Cuatrecasas, P., and Wilchek, M. (1968). Single-step purification of avidin from egg white by affinity chromatography on biocytin-sepharose columns, *Biochem. Biophys. Res. Commun.*, *33*: 235.

210. Deutsch, D. G., and Mertz, E. T. (1970). Plasminogen: Purification from human plasma by affinity chromatography, *Science*, *170*: 1095.

211. Sundberg, L., Porath, J., and Aspberg, K. (1970). Simultaneous isolation of trypsin inhibitor and anti-A phytohemaglutinin from *Vicia cracca* by means of biospecific adsorption, *Biochim. Biophys. Acta*, *221*: 384.

212. Allen, R. H., and Majerus, P. W. (1973). Isolation of vitamin B_{12}-binding proteins using affinity chromatography I. Preparation and properties of vitamin B_{12}-Sepharose, *J. Biol. Chem.*, *267*: 7695.

213. Allen, R. H., and Majerus, P. W. (1972). Isolation of vitamin B_{12}-binding proteins using affinity chromatography II. Purification and properties of a human granulocyte vitamin B_{12}-binding protein, *J. Biol. Chem.*, *247*: 7702.

214. Allen, R. H., and Majerus, P. W. (1972). Isolation of viatamin B_{12}-binding proteins using affinity chromatography III. Purification and properties of human plasma transcobalamin II, *J. Biol. Chem.*, *247*: 7709.

215. Sundberg, L., and Porath, J. (1972). Affinity chromatography of carbonic anhydrase, *FEBS Lett.*, *24*(2): 229.

216. Brodelius, P., and Mosbach, K. (1973). Separation of the isoenzymes of lactate dehydrogenase by affinity chromatography using an immobilized AMP-analogue, *FEBS Lett.*, *35*: 223.

217. Letarte-Muirhaed, M., Barclay, A. N., and Williams, A. F. (1975). Purification of the Thy-1 molecule, a major cell-surface glycoprotein of rat thymocytes, *Biochem. J.*, *151*: 685.

218. Jankowski, W. J., von Muenchhausen, W., Sulkowski, E., and Carter, W. A. (1976). Binding of human interferons to immobilized cibacron blue F3GA: The nature of molecular interaction, *Biochemistry*, *15*: 5182.

219. Knight, E., Jr., and Fahey, D. (1981). Human fibroblast interferon, *J. Biol. Chem.*, *256*: 3609.

220. Allen, G. K., and Rosenquist, B. D. (1988). Beaded agarose affinity chromatography of bovine fibroblast interferon, *Am. J. Vet. Res.*, *49*: 762.

221. Wittwer, A. J., Elmes, R. J., and Harakas, N. K. (1985). Unpublished work.

222. Harakas, N. K., Schaumann, J. P., Connolly, D. T., Wittwer, A. J., Olander, J. V., and Feder, J. (1988). Large-scale purification of tissue type plasminogen activator from cultured human cells, *Biotechnology Progress*, *4*: 149

223. Stevens, A., and Augusteyn, R. C. (1988). Isolation of α-crystallin and its subunits by affinity chromatography on immobilized monoclonal antibodies, *Exp. Eye Res.*, *46*(4): 499.

224. Freitag, N., and McEntee, K. (1988). Affinity chromatography of RecA protein and RecA nucleoprotein complexes on RecA protein-agarose columns, *J. Biol. Chem.*, *263*: 19525.

225. Subbaramaiah, K., and Sharma, R. (1988). Affinity binding of higher plant β-amylases to starch. A rapid purification method, *Starch/Staerke*, *40*: 182.

226. Lecommandeur, D., MacGregor, A. W., and Daussant, J. (1988). Purification of germinated barley α-amylase isozymes and limit-dextrinase by chromato-focusing and affinity chromatography, *J. Chromatogr.*, *441*: 436.

227. Pusztai, A., Grant, G., Stewart, J. C., and Watt, W. B. (1988). Isolation of soybean trypsin inhibitors by affinity chromatography on anhydrotrypsin-Sepharose 4B, *Anal. Biochem.*, *172*: 108.

228. Kelleher, F. M., Dubbs, S. B., and Bhavanandan, V. P. (1988). Purification of galactose oxidase from Dactylium dendroides by affinity chromatography on melibiose-polyacrylamide, *Arch. Biochem. Biophys.*, *263*: 349.

229. Kang, S., and Niemetz, J. (1988). Purification of human brain tissue factor, *Thromb. Haemostasis*, *59*: 400.

230. Dakour, J., Lundblad, A., and Zopf, D. (1988). Detection and isolation of oligosaccharides with Le[a] and Le[b] blood group activities by affinity chromatography using monoclonal antibodies, *Arch. Biochem. Biophys.*, *264*: 203.

231. Poole, R. C., and Halestrap, A. P. (1988). Purification of a 55 kDa mitochondrial protein by α-cyanocinnamate affinity chromatography, *Biochem. Soc. Trans.*, *16*: 602.

232. Al-Mashikhi, S. A., and Nakai, S. (1988). Separation of immunoglobulin and transferrin from blood serum and plasma by metal chelate interaction chromatography, *J. Dairy Sci.*, *71*: 1756.

233. Perrino, F. W., Meyer, R. R., Bobst, A. M., and Rein, D. C. (1988). Interaction of a folded chromosome-associated protein with single-stranded DNA-binding protein of *Escherichia coli*, identified by affinity chromatography, *J. Biol. Chem.*, *263*: 11833.

234. Sundquist, A. R., and Fahey, R. C. (1988). The novel disulfide reductase bis-γ-glutamylcystine reductase and dihydrolipoamide dehydrogenase from Halobacterium halobium: Purification by immobilized-metal-ion affinity chromatography and properties of the enzymes, *J. Bacteriol.*, *170*: 3459.

235. Yatohgo, T., Izumi, M., Kashiwagi, H., and Hayashi, M. (1988). Novel purification of vitronectin from human plasma by heparin affinity chromatography, *Cell Struct. Funct.*, *13*: 281.

236. Ikeda, S., Swenson, R. P., and Ives, D. H. (1988). Amino-terminal nucleotide-binding sequences of a Lactobacillus deoxynucleoside kinase complex isolated by novel affinity chromatography, *Biochemistry*, *27*: 8648.

237. Tomme, P., McCrae, S., Wood, T. M., and Claeyssens, M. (1988). Chromatographic separation of cellulolytic enzymes, *Meth. Enzym.*, *160* (Biomass, Pt. A): 187.

238. Kazama, M., Tahara, C., Abe, T., and Kasai, K. (1988). Quantitative analysis of fibrin-binding affinity of fibrinolytic components by frontal affinity chromatography, *Thromb. Res.* (Suppl. 8): 81.

239. Jones, L. R., Wegener, A. D., and Simmerman, H. K. B. (1988). Purification of phospholamban from canine cardiac sarcoplasmic reticulum vesicles by use of sulfhydryl group affinity chromatography, *Meth. Enzym.*, *157* (Biomembranes, Pt. Q): 360.

240. Brooks, S. P. J., and Storey, K. B. (1988). Purification of phosphofructokinase using transition-state analog affinity chromatography, *J. Chromatogr.*, *455*: 291.

241. Lindberg, U., Schutt, C. E., Hellsten, E., Tjaeder, A. C., and Hult, T. (1988). The use of poly(*L*-proline)-Sepharose in the isolation of profilin and profilactin complexes, *Biochim. Biophys. Acta*, *967*: 391.

242. Gascon, F., and Molina, E. (1989). Precision of measurement of glycated hemoglobin by affinity chromatography on regenerated columns, *Clin. Chem.* (Winston-Salem, N.C.), *35*: 191.

243. Waheed, A., and Shadduck, R. K. (1989). Purification of human urine colony-stimulating factor by affinity chromatography, *Exp. Hematol.* (N.Y.), *17*: 61.

244. Schlosshauer, B. (1989). Purification of neuronal cell surface proteins and generation of epitope-specific monoclonal antibodies against cell adhesion molecules, *J. Neurochem.*, *52*: 82.

245. Kamihira, M., Taniguchi, M., Iijima, S., and Kobayashi, T. (1988). Purification of recombinant α-amylase with immunoaffinity chromatography using monoclonal antibody, *J. Ferment. Technol.*, *66*: 625.

246. Boegli, C., Hofer, A., and Furlan, M. (1988). Isolation of fibrinogen Aα-chain by affinity chromatography on concanavalin A-Sepharose, *Thromb. Haemostasis*, *60*: 308.

247. Wilson, H. M., Griffin, B. A., and Skinner, E. R. (1989). A novel procedure for the separation of high-density lipoprotein subspecies by affinity chromatography, *Biochem. Soc. Trans.*, *17*: 152.

248. Ono, K., and Oka, S. (1988). Immobilized glucoamylase inhibitors and their properties and application, *Bio Ind.*, *5*: 691.

249. Brown, J. E., and Cowgill, C. A. (1989). Phospholipid affinity purification of factor VII:C, U.S. Patent 4,795,806, January 3 (Assignee: Miles Laboratories, Inc.).

250. Dasch, J. R., Pace, D. R., Waegell, W., Inenaga, D., and Ellingsworth, L. (1989). Monoclonal antibodies recognizing transforming growth factor-β: Bioactivity neutralization and transforming growth factor β2 affinity purification, *J. Immunology*, *142*: 1536.

251. Lebreton, J. P. (1977). Purification of the human plasma alpha$_2$-SH glycoprotein by zinc chelate affinity chromatography, *FEBS Lett.*, *80*: 351.

252. Edy, V. G., Billiau, a., and De Somer, P. (1977). Purification of human fibroblast interferon by zinc chelate affinity chromatography, *J. Biol. Chem.*, *252*: 5934.

253. Weselake, R. J., Chesney, S. L., Petkau, A., and Friesen, A. D. (1986). Purification of human copper, zinc superoxide dismutase by copper chelate affinity chromatography, *Analytical Biochemistry*, *155*: 193.

254. Miyata-Asano, M., Ito K., Ikeda, H., Sekiguchi, S. Arai, K., and Taniguchi, N. (1986). Purification of copper-zinc-superoxide and catalase from human erythrocytes by copper-chelate affinity chromatography, *J. Chromatography*, *370*: 501.

255. Electricwala, A., and Atkinson, T. (1988). Rapid tandem purification of tissue plasminogen activator by metal chelate and affinity chromatography, *Chim. Oggi, 6*: 63.

256. Hubert, P., and Porath, J. (1980). Metal chelate affinity chromatography I. Influence of various parameters on the retention of nucleotides and related compounds, *J. Chromatography., 198*: 247.

257. Hubert, P., and Porath, J. (1981). Metal chelate affinity chromatography II. Group separation of mono- and dinucleotides, *J. Chromatography, 206*: 164.

258. Lonnerdal, B., and Keen, C. L. (1982). Metal chelate affinity chromatography of proteins, *J. Applied Biochem., 4*: 203.

259. Porath, J., and Olin, B. (1983). Immobilized metal ion affinity adsorption and immobilized metal ion affinity chromatography of biomaterials. Serum protein affinities for gel-immobilized iron and nickel ions, *Biochemistry, 22*: 1621.

260. Ramadan, N., and Porath, J. (1985). Fe^{3+}-hydroxamate as immobilized metal affinity-adsorbent for protein chromatography, *J. Chromatography, 321*: 93.

261. Ramadan, N., and Porath, J. (1985). Separation of serum proteins on a Fe^{3+}-monohydroxamate adsorbent, *J. Chromatography, 321*: 105.

262. Hemdan, E. S., and Porath, J. (1985). Development of immobilized metal affinity chromatography I.   Comparison of two iminodiacetate gels, *J. Chromatography, 323*: 247.

263. Hemdan, E. S., and Porath, J. (1985). Development of immobilized metal affinity chromatography II. Interaction of amino acids with immobilized nickel iminodiacetate, *J. Chromatography, 323*: 255.

264. Hemdan, E. S., and Porath, J. (1985). Development of immobilized metal affinity chromatography III.   Interaction of oligopeptides with immobilized nickel iminodiacetate, *J. Chromatography, 323*: 265.

265. Muszyfiska, G., Andersson, L., and Porath, J. (1986). Selective adsorption of phosphoproteins on gel-immobilized ferric chelate, *Biochemistry, 25*: 6850.

266. Andersson, L., and Porath, J. (1986).   Isolation of phosphoproteins by immobilized metal (Fe^{3+}) affinity chromatography, *Analytical Biochemistry, 154*: 250.

267. Coppenhaver, D. H. (1986). Nickel chelate chromatography of human immune interferon, *Meth. Enzym., 119*: 199.

268. Belew, M., Yip, T.-T., Andersson, L. and Porath, J. (1987).   Interaction of proteins with immobilized Cu^{2+}—Quantitation of adsorption capacity, adsorption isotherms and equilibrium constants by frontal analysis, *J. Chromatography, 403*: 197.

269. Hutchens, T. W., Yip, T.-T., and Porath, J. (1988).   Protein interaction with immobilized ligands: Quantitative analyses of equilibrium partition data and comparison with Analytical chromatographic approaches using immobilized metal affinity adsorbents, *Analytical Biochemistry, 170*: 168.

270. Andersson, L., Sulkowski, E., and Porath, J. (1987). Purification of commercial human albumin on immobilized $IDA-Ni^{2+}$, *J. Chromatography, 421*: 141.

271. Nakagawa, Y., Yip, T.-T., Belew, M., and Porath, J. (1988). High-performance immobilized metal ion affinity chromatography of peptides: Analytical separation of biologically active synthetic peptides, *Anal. Biochem., 168*: 75.

272. Hochuli, E., Bannwarth, W., Doebeli, H., Gentz, R., and Stueber, D. (1988). Genetic approach to facilitate purification of recombinant proteins with a novel metal chelate adsorbent, *Bio/Technology, 6*: 1321.

273. Hemdan, E. S., Zhao, Y.-J., Sulkowski, E., and Porath J. (1989). Surface topography of histidine residues: A facile probe by immobilized metal ion affinity chromatography, *Proc. Natl. Acad. Sci. USA, 86*: 1811.

274. Haymore, B. L., Bild, G. S., Salsgiver, W. J., Staten, N. R., and Krivi, G. G. (1992). Introducing strong metal-binding sites onto surfaces of proteins for facile and efficient metal-affinity purifications, *Methods: A Companion to Methods of Enzymology, 4*: 25.

275. Pharmacia, Inc., Piscataway, New Jersey (1986). Chelating Sepharose (R) fast flow, *Pharmacia Data Sheet*.

276. Pharmacia LKB Biotechnology, Piscataway, New Jersey (1988). Chelating Superose, *Pharmacia LKB Biotechnology Data File FPLC*.

277. Mirlas, B., and Lonngren, J. (1988). Analytical specifications and quality control test methods for chelating Sepharose 6B, *Pharmacia LKB Biotechnology, data Sheet*, Pharmacia LKB Biotechnology, Piscataway, New Jersey.

278. Sairam, M. R., Clarke, W. C., Chug, D., Porath, J., and Li, C. H. (1974). Purification of antibodies to protein hormones by affinity chromatography on divinylsulfonyl Sepharose, *Biol. Biophys. Res. Commun., 61*: 355.

279. Anfinsen, C. B., Bose, S., Corley, L., and Gurari-Rotman, D. (1974). Partial purification of human interferon by affinity chromatography, *Proc. Nat. Acad. Sci, USA, 71*: 3139.

280. Staehelin, T., Hobbe, D. S., Kung, H.-F., Lai, C.-Y., and Pestka, S. (1981). Purification and characterization of recombinant human leukocyte interferon (IFLrA) with monoclonal antibodies, *J. Biol. Chem., 296*: 9750.

281. Staehelin, T., Durrer, B., Schmidt, J., Takacs, B., Stocker, J., Miggiano, V., Stahli, C., Rubinstein, M., Levy, W. P., Hershberg, R., and Pestka, S. (1981). Production of hybridomas secreting monoclonal antibodies to the human leukocyte interferons, *Proc. Natl. Acad. Sci. USA, 78*: 1848.

282. Krivi, G. G., Bittner, M. L., Rowold, E., Jr., Wong, E. Y., Glenn, K. C., Rose, K. S., and Tiemeier, D. C. (1985). Purification of *rec*A-based fusion proteins by immunoadsorbent chromatography, *J. Biol. Chem., 260*: 10263.

283. Civalleri, L., Federico, R., and Pini, C. (1986). Single-step purification of superoxide dismutase from bovine erythrocytes by immunosorbent column, *Biotechnology and Applied Biochem., 8*:387.

284. Carlton, G. J. (1984). Immunosorbent separations, *Meth. Enzym., 104*: 381.

285. Bruck, C., Drebin, J. A., Glineu, C., and Portetelle, D. (1986). Purification of mouse monoclonal antibodies from ascitic fluid by DEAE Affi-Gel Blue Chromatography, *Meth. Enzym., 121*: 587.

286. Burchel, S. W. (1986). Purification and analysis of monoclonal antibodies by high-performance liquid chromatography, *Meth. Enzym., 121*: 596.

287. Schaumann, J. P., Olander, J. V., Harakas, N. K., and Feder, J. (1989). Monoclonal antibody specific for human colon fibroblast-derived t-PA, U.S. Patent 4,833,085, May 23 (Assignee: Monsanto Company).

288. Schwumaan, L. (1987). Affinity purification of monoclonal antibody from tissue culture supernatant using protein A-Sepharose CL-4B, *Bioprocess Technol., 2*: 199.

289. Danielsson, A., Ljunglof, A., and Lindblom, H. (1988). One-step purification of monoclonal IgG antibodies from mouse ascites, *J. Immunolog. Methods, 115*: 79.

290. Shibuya, N., Berry, J. E., and Goldstein, I. J. (1988). One-step purification of purine IgM and human α_2-Macroglobulin by affinity chromatography on immobilized snowdrop bulb lectin, *Arch. Biochem. Biophys., 267*: 676.

291. Davie, J. M. (1982). Hybridomas: A revolution in reagent production, *Pharmacological Reviews, 34*: 115.

292. Bott, R., and Sarma, R. (1976). Crystal Structure of turkey egg-white lysozyme: Results of the molecular replacement method at 5 Å resolution, *J. Mol. Biol., 106*: 1037.

293. Atassi, M. Z., and Lee, C.-L. (1978). Boundary refinement of the lysozyme antigenic site around the disulphide bond 6-127 (Sitel) by 'surface-simulation' synthesis, *Biochem. J., 171*: 419.

294. Smith-Gill, S. J., Wilson, A. C., Potter, M., Prager, E. M., Feldmann, R. J., and Mainhart, C. R. (1982). Mapping the antigenic epitope for a monoclonal antibody against lysozyme, *J. Immunology, 128*: 314.

295. Smith-Gill, S. J., Lavoie, t. B., and Mainhart, C. R. (1984). Antigenetic regions defined by monoclonal antibodies correspond to structural domains of avian lysozyme, *133*: 384.

296. Janis, L. J., Grott, A., and Regnier, F. E. (1989). Immunological chromatographic analysis of lysozyme variants, *J. Chromatography, 476*: 235.

297. MacGregor, I. R., Micklem, L. R., James, K., and Pepper, D. S. (1985). Characterization of epitopes on human tissue plasminogen activator recognized by a group of monoclonal antibodies, *Thromb. Haemostasis, 53*: 45.

298. Bachmann, F., and Kruithof, I. R., E. K. O. (1984). Tissue plasminogen activator: Chemical and physiological aspects, *Sem. Thromb. Hemost., 10*: 6.

299. Prickett, K. S., Amberg, D. C., and Hopp, T. P. (1989). A calcium-dependent antibody for identification and purification of recombinant proteins, *Biotechniques, 7*: 580.

300. Janis, L. J., and Regnier, R. E. (1988). Immunological-chromatographic analysis, *J. Chromatography, 444*: 1.

301. Morgan, M. R. A., Brown, P. J., Leyland, M. J., and Dean, P. D. G. (1978). Electrophoresis: A new preparative desorption technique in affinity chromatography (and immunoadsorption), *FEBS Lett., 87*: 239.

302. Van, C. J., Good, R. J., and Chaudhury, M. K. (1986). Nature of the antigen-antibody interaction, primary and secondary bonds: Optimal conditions for association and dissociation, *J. Chromatography, 376*: 111.

303. Pharmacia LKB Biotechnology, Piscataway, New Jersey (1988). Protein A Sepharose CL-4B, Pharmacia LKB Biotechnology Data Sheet.

304. Pharmacia LKB Biotechnology, Piscataway, New Jersey (1988). Protein G and protein G Sepharose 4 fast flow, Pharmacia LKB Biotechnology Data Sheet.

305. Pharmacia LKB Biotechnology, Piscataway, New Jersey (1988). MAbTrap™G, Pharmacia LKB Biotechnology Data File Affinity Media.

306. Pharmacia, Inc., Piscataway, New Jersey (1987). Protein A Superose, Pharmacia FPLC: Data File.

307. Pharmacia LKB Biotechnology, Piscataway, New Jersey (1988). FPLC for monoclonal antibody purification.

308. Beckman Instruments, Inc., San Ramos, California (1986). Antibody purification by rProtein A, Beckman Information Sheet No. 5012.

309. Beckman Instruments, Inc. San Ramos, California (1986). rProtein A* purification kit, Beckman Information Sheet No. 5014.

310. Robb, R. F. (1988). Structure-function relations for the interleukin-2 receptor, *Cellular and Molecular Aspects of Inflammation* (George Poste and Stanley T. Crooke, eds.), Plenum Press, New York/London, pp. 97–122.

311. Weber, D. V., Keeney, R. F., Familletti, P. C., and Bailon, P. (1988). Medium-scale ligand-affinity purification of two soluble forms of human interleukin-2 receptor, *J. Chromatography, 431*: 55.

312. Hakimi, J., Seals, C., Anderson, L. E., Podlaski, F. J., Lin, P., Danho, W., Jenson, J. C., Perkins, A., Donadio, P. E., Familletti, P. C., Pan, Y.-C. E., T. W.-H., Chizzonite, R. A., Casabo, L., Nelson, D. L., and Cullen, B. R. (1987). Biochemical and functional analysis of soluble human interleukin-2 receptor produced in rodent cells, *J. Biol. Chem., 262*: 17336.

313. Bailon, P., Weber, D. V., Gately, M., Smart, J. E., Lorberboum-Galski, H., Fitzgerald, D., and Pastan, I. (1988). Purification and partial characterization of interleukin 2-pseudomonas exotoxin fusion protein, *Bio/Technology, 7*: 1326.

314. Lorberboum-Galski, H., FitzGerald, D., Chaudhary, V., Adhya, S., and Pastan, I. (1988). Cytotoxic activity of an interleukin 2-*pseudomonas* exotoxin chimeric protein produced in *Escherichia coli, Proc. Natl. Acad. Sci. USA, 85*: 1922.

315. Honjo, T., and Shimizu, A. (1989). Interleukin 2 receptor and a method for production thereof, U.S. Patent No. 4,816,565, March 28.

316. Phares, C. K. (1988). Use of receptor affinity chromatography in purification of the growth hormone-like factor produced by plerocercoids of the tapeworm Spirometra mansonoides, *J. Recept. Res., 8*: 645.

317. Williams, W. V., Weiner, D. B., Cohen, J. C., and Greene, M. I., (1989). Development and use of receptor binding peptides derived from antireceptor antibodies, *Bio/Technology, 7*: 471.

318. Kinet, J.-P. (1989). Antibody-cell interactions: Fc receptors, *Cell, 57*: 351.

319. Tedesco, J. L., Pearsall, K. M., Thompson, M., and Krull, U. J. (1988). Affinity purification of the mammalian β-2-adrenergic receptor, *J. Biochem. Biophys. Methods, 17*:215.

320. Fournier, A., Zhang, Z. Q., and Tan, Y. H. (1988). Preparation and characterization of biotinylated probes for the β-interferon receptor, *Int. J. Biochem., 20*: 1151.

321. Urdal, D. L., Call, S. M., Jackson, J. L., and Dower, S. K. (1988). Affinity purification and chemical analysis of the interleukin-1 receptor, *J. Biol. Chem., 263*: 2870.

322. Sims, J. E., March, C. J., Cosman, D., Widmer, M. B., MacDonald, H. R., McMahan, C. J., Grubin, C. E., Wignall, J. M., Jackson, J. L., Call, S. M., Friend, D., Alpert, A. R., Gillis, S., Urdal, D. L., and Dower, S. K. (1988). cDNA expression cloning of the IL-1 receptor, a member of the immunoglobulin superfamily, *Science, 241*: 585.

323. Blank, U., Ra, C., Miller, L., White, K., Metzger, H., and Kinet, J.-P. (1989). Complete structure and expression in transfected cells of high affinity IgE receptor, *Nature, 337*: 187.

324. Mita, S., Tominaga, A., Hitoshi, Y., Sakamoto, K., Honjo, T., Akagi, M., Kikuchi, Y., Yamaguchi, N., and Takatsu, K. (1989). Characterization of high-affinity receptors for interleukin 5 on interleukin 5-dependent cell lines, *Proc. Natl. Acad. Sci. USA*, *86*: 2311.

325. Strominger, J. L. (1989). Developmental biology of T cell receptors, *Science*, *244*: 943.

326. Strominger, J. L. (1989). The $\tau\delta$ T cell receptor and class 1b MHC-related proteins: Enigmatic molecules of immune recognition, *Cell*, *57*: 895.

327. Brown, G. L., Nanney, L. B., Griffen, J., Cramer, A. B., Yancey, J. M., Cutsinger, L. J., Holtzin, L., Schultz, G. S., Jurkiewicz, M. J., and Lynch. J. B. (1989). Enhancement of wound healing by topical treatment with epidermal growth factor, *N. Engl. J. Med.*, *321*: 76.

328. Clementi, M., Festa, A., Testa, I., Bagnarelli, P., Devescovi, G., and Carloni, G. (1989). Expression of high- and low-affinity epidermal growth factor receptors in human hepatoma cell lines, *FEBS Lett.*, *249*: 297.

329. Goldstein, I. M. (1989). Personal communication, March 9.

330. Ersson, B., Aspberg, K., and Porath, J. (1973). The phytohemagglutinin from sun hemp seeds (Crotalaria juncea): Purification by biospecific affinity chromatography, *Biochim. Biophys. Acta*, *310*: 446.

331. Howard, S. C., Wittwer, A. J., Carr, L. S., Harakas, N. K., and Feder, J. (1989). Effect of proportion of type I and type II t-PA glycoforms on secreted t-PA activity, *J. Cell Biol.*, *107*: 584a.

332. Ashford, D., Dwek, R. A., Welply, J. K., Amatayakul, S., Homans, S. W., Lis, H., Taylor, G. N., Sharon, N., and Rademacher, T. W. (1987). The $\beta1\rightarrow$D-xylose and α1-3-L-fucose substituted *N*-linked oligosaccharides from *Erythrina cristagalli* lectin, *Eur. J. Biochem.*, *166*: 311.

333. Welply, J. K. (1989). Sequencing methods for carbohydrates and their biological applications, *Trends Biotechnol.*, *7*: 5.

334. Welply, J. K. (1988). Oligosaccharides: Sequencing and applications, *Newsletter: Technical Community of Monsanto*, *14*(11): 1.

335. Castellino, F. J. (1984). Biochemistry of human plasminogen, *Sem. Thromb. Hemost.*, *10*: 18.

336. Lloyd, K. O. (1970). The preparation of two insoluble forms of the phytohemagglutinin, concanavalin A, and their interactions with polysaccharides and glycoproteins, *Arch. of Biochem. Biophys.*, *137*: 460.

337. Aspberg, K., and Porath, J. (1970). Group-specific adsorption of glycoproteins, *Acta Chem. Scand.*, *24*: 1839.

338. Lotan, R., and Nicolson, G. L. (1979). Purification of cell membrane glycoproteins by lectin affinity chromatography, *Biochim. Biophys. Acta*, *559*: 329.

339. Brewer, C. F., and Bhattacharyya, L. (1986). Specificity of concanavalin A binding to asparagine-linked glycopeptides, *J. Biol. Chem.*, *261*: 7306.

340. Nishikawa, Y., Pegg, W., Paulsen, H., and Schachter, H. (1988). Control of glycoprotein synthesis. Purification and characterization of rabbit liver UDP-*N*-acetylglucosamine:β-1,2-*N*-acetylglucosaminyltransferase I, *J. Biol. Chem.*, *263*: 8270.

341. Sueyoshi, S., Tsuji, T., and Osawa, T. (1988). Carbohydrate-binding specificities of five lectins that bind to *O*-glycosyl-linked carbohydrate chains. Quantitative analysis by frontal-affinity chromatography, *Carbohydr. Res., 178.* 213.

342. Reading, C. L., Hickey, C. M., and Yong, W. (1988). Analysis of cell surface glycoprotein changes related to hematopoietic differentiation, *J. Cell. Biochem., 37*: 21.

343. Wang, W. C., Clark, G. F., Smith, D. F., and Cummings, R. D. (1988). Separation of oligosaccharides containing terminal α-linked galactose residues by affinity chromatography on *Griffonia simplicifolia I* bound to concanavalin A-Sepharose, *Anal. Biochem, 175*: 390.

344. Thompson, S., and Turner, G. A. (1988). A new method for the analysis of blood serum glycoproteins using Sepharose coupled lectins and its application in human disease, *Lectins: Biol., Biochem., Clin. Biochem., 6*: 453.

345 Hase, S., and Ikenaka, T. (1986). Separation of sugar chains from glycoproteins using fast affinity chromatography, *Chromatogram, 7*: 2.

346. Osawa, T., and Tsuji, T. (1987). Fractionation and structural assessment of oligosaccharides and glycopeptides by use of immobilized lectins, *Ann. Rev. Biochem. 56*: 21.

347. Porath, J., Sundberg, L., Fornstedt, N., and Olsson, I. (1973). Salting-out in amphiphilic gels as a new approach to hydrophobic adsorption, *Nature, 245*: 465.

348. Hutchens, T. W., and Porath, J. (1986). Thiophilic adsorption of immunoglobulins—Analysis of conditions optimal for selective immobilization and purification, *Anal. Biochem., 159*: 217.

349. Porath, J. (1986). Salt-promoted adsorption: Recent developments, *J. Chromatography, 376*: 331.

350. Porath, J. (1987). Metal ion-hydrophobic, thiophilic and π-electron governed interactions and their application to salt-promoted protein adsorption chromatography, *Biotechnol. Progr., 3*: 14.

351. Hutchens, T. W., and Porath, J. (1987). Thiophilic adsorption: A comparison of model protein behavior, *Biochemistry, 26*: 7199.

352. Belew, M., Juntti, N., Larsson, A., and Porath, J. (1987). A one-step purification method for monoclonal antibodies based on salt-promoted adsorption chromatography on a 'thiophilic' adsorbent, *J. Immunolog. Methods, 102*: 173.

353. Porath, J. (1987). Salting-out adsorption techniques for protein purification, *Biopolymers, 26*: S193.

354. Porath, J., and Belew, M. (1987). 'Thiophilic' interaction and the selective adsorption of proteins, *Trends Biotechnol., 5*: 225.

355. Tiselius, A. (1948). *Ark. Kem. Min. Geol., 26B*: 1.

356. Hofmeister, H. (1888). Zur Lehre von der Wirkung der Saltze. Sweite Mittheilung, *Arch. Exp. Pharmakol., 24*: 247.

357. Frenz, J., and Horvath, C. (1988). High-performance displacement chromatography, *High-Performance Liquid Chromatography: Advances and Perspectives* (C. Horvath, ed.), Academic Press, New York, *5*: 212.

358. Cramer, S. M., and Subramanian, G. (1990). Recent advances in the theory and practice of displacement chromatography, *Separation and Purification Methods, 19*: 31.

359. Subramanian, G., Jayaraman, G., and Cramer, S. M. (1989). "Displacement chromatography of biopolymers: Extension to group specific affinity systems and development of novel displacer compounds," 1989 Annual Meeting of the American Institute of Chemical Engineers, San Francisco, California.

360. Berkowitz, S. (1987). Silica-based chromatography products, *Bio/Technology*, *5*: 611.

361. Borchert, A., Larsson, P.-O., and Mosbach, K. (1982). High-performance liquid affinity chromatography on silica-bound concanavalin A, *J. Chromatography*, *244*: 49.

362. Larsson, P.-O. (1984). High-performance liquid affinity chromatography, *Meth. Enzym.*, *104*: 212.

363. Nahum, A., and Horvath, C. (1981). Surface silanols in silica-bonded hydrocarbonaceous stationary phases I. Dual retention mechanism in reversed-phase chromatography, *J. Chromatography*, *203*: 53.

364. Ernst-Cabrera, K., and Wilchek, M. (1988). Polymeric supports for affinity chromatography and high-performance affinity chromatography, *Makromol. Chem. Macromol. Symp.*, *19*: 145.

365. Rassi, Z. E., and Horvath, C. (1986). Metal chelate-interaction chromatography of proteins with iminodiacetic acid-bonded stationary phases on silica support, *J. Chromatography*, *359*: 241.

366. Chicz, R. M., and Regnier, F. E. (1989). Immobilized-metal affinity and hydroxyapatite chromatography of genetically engineered subtilisin, *Anal. Chem.*, *61*: 1742.

367. Fassina, G., Swaisgood, H. E., and Chaiken, I. M. (1986). Quantitative high-performance affinity chromatography: Evaluation of use for analyzing peptide and protein interactions, *J. Chromatography*, *376*: 87.

368. Caliceti, P., Fassina, G., and Chaiken, I. M. (1987). Direct analysis of Glu-analytical immuno-high-performance liquid affinity chromatography, *Appl. Biochem. Biotechnol.*, *16*: 119.

369. Ito, N., Noguchi, K., Kazama, M., and Kasai, K. (1987). Direct analysis of Glu-plasminogen and Lys-plasminogen in human plasma with high-performance affinity chromatography, *Ketsueki Myakkan*, *18*: 602.

370. Reid, T. S., and Gisch, D. J. (1988). Applications for group specific ligands in fast, high performance affinity chromatography, *BioChromatography*, *3*: 201.

371. Boyle, D. M., and Van der Walt, L. A. (1988). High-performance affinity chromatography of human progesterone receptor, *J. Chromatogr.*, *455*: 434.

372. Torres, J. L., Guzman, R., Carbonell, R. G., and Kilpatrick, P. K. (1988). Affinity surfactants as reversibly bound ligands for high-performance affinity chromatography, *Anal. Biochem.*, *171*: 411.

373. Varady, L., Kalghatgi, K. and Horvath, C. (1988). Rapid high-performance affinity chromatography on micropellicular sorbents, *J. Chromatogr.*, *485*: 207.

374. Ohlson, S., Nilsson, R., Niss, U., Kjellberg, B. M., and Freiburghaus, C. (1988). A novel approach to monoclonal antibody separation using high performance liquid affinity chromatography (HPLAC) with SelectiSpher-10 protein G, *J. Immunol. Methods*, *114*: 175.

375. Ohlson, S., Gudmundsson, B. M., Wikstroem, P., and Larsson, P. O. (1988). High-performance liquid affinity chromatography: Rapid immunoanalysis of transferrin in serum, *Clin. Chem.* (Winston-Salem, N.C.), *34*: 2039.

376. Nakamura, K., Toyoda, K., and Kato, Y. (1988). High-performance affinity chromatography of proteins on TSKgel Heparin-5PW, *J. Chromatogr.*, *445*: 234.

377. Josic, D., Hofmann, W., Habermann, R., and Reutter, W. (1988). High-performance concanavalin A affinity chromatography of liver and hepatoma membrane proteins, *J. Chromatogr.*, *44*: 29.

378. Honda, S., Suzuki, S., Nitta, T., and Kakehi, K. (1988). Analytical high-performance affinity chromatography of ovalbumin-derived glycopeptides on columns of concanavalin A- and wheat germ agglutinin-immobilized gels, *J. Chromatogr.*, *438*: 73.

379. Vidal-Madjar, C., Jaulmes, A., Racine, M., and Sebille, B. (1988). Determination of binding equilibrium constants by numerical simulation in zonal high-performance affinity chromatography, *J. Chromatogr.*, *458*: 13.

380. Sten, O. (1988). Low-affinity adsorbent for affinity chromatography useful for biochemical applications, *EP290,406 Al*, November 9 (Applicant: Perstorp Biolytica AB).

381. Yang, C.-M., and Tsao, G. T. (1982). Affinity chromatography, *Advances Biochemical Engineering*, *25*: 19.

382. Larsson, P.-O., and Mosbach, K. (1979). Affinity precipitation of enzymes, *FEBS Lett.*, *98*: 333.

383. Johansson, G. (1984). Affinity partitioning, *Meth. Enzym.*, *104*: 356.

384. Senstad, C., and Mattiasson, B. (1989). Affinity-precipitation using chitosan as ligand carrier, *Biotechnol. Bioeng.*, *33*: 216.

385. Schneider, M. (1978). Process for extracting a polypeptide from an aqueous solution, U.S. Patent 4,066,505.

386. Hariri, M. H., Ely, J. F., and Mansoori, G. A. (1989). Bioseparations: Design and engineering of partitioning systems, *Bio/Technology*, *7*: 686.

387. Yang, C.-M., and Tsao, G. T. (1982). Packed-bed adsorption theories and their applications to affinity chromatography, *Adv. Biochem. Eng.*, *25*: 1

388. Ugelstad, J., Soderberg, L., Berge, A., and Bergstrom, J. (1983). Monodisperse polymer particles—A step forward for chromatography, *Nature*, *309*: 95.

389. Margel, S. (1989). Affinity separation with polyaldehyde microsphere beads, *J. Chromatogr.*, *462*: 177.

390. Harakas, N. K. (1962). *Moving bed heat transfer*, Ph.D. thesis, North carolina State University, Raleigh, N.C.

391. Harakas, N. K., and Beatty, K. O., Jr. (1963). Moving bed heat transfer I. Effect of interstitial gas with fine particles, *Chem. Eng. Symp. Ser.*, *59*: 122.

392. Herak, D. C., and Merrill, E. W. (1989). Affinity cross-flow filtration: Experimental and modeling work using the system of HSA and Cibacron Blue-agarose, *Biotechnol. Progr.*, *5*: 9.

393. Brandt, S., Goffe, R. A., Kessler, S. B., O'Connor, J. L., and Zale, S. E. (1988). Membrane-based affinity technology for commercial scale purifications, *Bio/Technology*, *6*: 779.

394. Sepracor, Inc., Marlborough, Mass. (1989). Affinity-15 membrane chromatography system: Advanced hollow fiber membrane-based protein purification, *Sepracor Information Sheet*.

395. Mattiasson, B., and Ramstorp, M. (1984). Ultrafiltration affinity purification: Isolation of concanavalin A from seeds of *Canavalia ensiformis*, *J. Chromatogr.*, *283*: 323.

396. Chose, T. B., Masse, P., and Verdier, A. (1986). Separation of trypsin from trypsin α-chymotrypsin mixture by affinity—ultrafiltration, *Biotech. Lett.*, *8*: 163.

397. Luong, J. H. T., Nguyen, A.-L., and Male, K. B. (1987). Affinity cross-flow filtration for purifying biomolecules, *Bio/Technology*, *5*: 564.

398. Pungor, E., Jr., Afeyan, N. B., Gordon, N. F., and Cooney, C. L. (1987). Continuous affinity-recycle extraction: A novel protein separation technique, *Bio/Technology*, *5*: 604.

399. Boucher, D. F., and Alves, G. E. (1959). Dimensionless numbers, *Chem. Eng. Prog.*, *55*: 55.

400. Olson, W. C., and Yarmush, M. L. (1987). Electrophoretic elution from monoclonal antibody immunoadsorbents: A theoretical and experimental investigation of controlling parameters, *Biotechnol. Prog.*, *3*: 177.

401. Powers, J. D., Kilpatrick, P. L., and Carbonell, R. G. (1989). Protein purification by affinity binding to unilamellar vesicles, *Biotechnol. Bioeng.*, *33*: 173.

402. Woll, J. M., Hatton,, T. A., and Yarmush, M. L. (1989). Bioaffinity separations using reversed micellar extraction, *Biotechnol. Prog.*, *5*: 57.

403. Mosbach, K., and Andersson, L. (1977). Magnetic ferrofluids for preparation of magnetic polymers and their application in affinity chromatography, *Nature*, *270*: 259.

404. Hirschbein, B. L., and Whitesides, G. M. (1982). Affinity separation of enzymes from mixtures containing suspended solids: Comparisons of magnetic and nonmagnetic techniques, *Applied Biochem. and Biotech.*, *7*: 157.

405. Halling, P. J., and Dunnill, P. (1980). Magnetic supports for immobilized enzymes and bioaffinity adsorbents, *Enzyme Microbial Technol.*, *2*: 2.

406. Menz, E. T., Havelick, J., Groman, E. V., and Josephson, L. (1986). Magnetic affinity chromatography: An emerging technique, *Am. Biotechnol. Lab.*, *4*: 46.

407. Tice, P. A., Mazsaroff, I., Lin, N. T., and Regnier, F. E. (1987). Effects of large sample loads on column lifetime in preparative-scale liquid chromatography, *J. Chromatography*, *410*: 43.

408. Mazsaroff, I., Bischoff, R., Tice, P. A., and Regnier, F. E. (1988). Influence of mobile phase pH on high-performance liquid chromatographic column loading capacity: Implications for the design of preparative protein separations, *J. Chromatography*, *437*: 429.

409. Chase, H. A. (1988). Optimization and scale-up of affinity chromatography, *Makromol. Macromol. Symp.*, *17* (Int.Symp. Affinity Chromatogr. Interfacial Macromol. Interact., 1987): 467.

410. Bite, M. G., Berezenko, S., Reed, F. J. S., and Derry, L. (1988). Macrosorb kieselguhr-agarose composite adsorbents: New tools for downstream process design and scale up, *Appl. Biochem. Biotechnol.*, *18*: 275.

411. Hubble, J. (1987). Cooperative binding interactions in affinity chromatography: Theoretical considerations, *Biotechnol. Bioeng.*, *30*: 208.

412. Doulah, M. S. (1987). Prediction of mass transfer parameters of affinity chromatography through breakthrough data analysis, *Process Technol. Proc.*, *4*: 499.

413. Arve, B. H. (1986). The modeling and analysis of multicomponent, multivalent biospecific adsorption, Ph.D. thesis, University of Missouri, Rolla, Mo.

414. Anderson, D. J. (1986). Determination of equilibrium and rate constants for concanavalin A and various sugars using high-performance affinity chromatography, Ph.D. thesis, Iowa State Univ, Ames, Iowa.

415. Carlsson, R., and Glad, C. (1989). Monoclonal antibodies into the '90s: The all-purpose tool, *Bio/Technology*, 7: 567.

416. Pestka, S. (1983). The human interferons—From protein purification and sequence to cloning and expression in bacteria: Before, between, and beyond, *Arch. Biochem. Biophys.*, *221*: 1.

417. Pestka, S. (1986). Interferon from 1981 to 1986, *Meth. Enzym.*, *119.*: 3.

418. Berg, K., Heron, I., and Hamilton, R. (1978). Purification of human interferon by antibody affinity chromatography, using highly absorbed anti-interferon, *Scand. J. Immunol.*, 8: 429.

419. Mikulski, A. J., Heine, J. W., Le, H. V., and Sulkowski, E. (1980). Large scale purification of human fibroblast interferon, *Preparative Biochem.*, *10*: 103.

420. Tarnowski, S. J., Roy, S. K., Liptak, R. A., Lee, D. K., and Ning, R. Y. (1986). Large-scale purification of recombinant human leukocyte interferons, *Meth. Enzym.*, *119*: 153.

421. Thatcher, D. R., and Panayotatos, N. (1986). Purification of recombinant human IFN-α2, *Meth. Enzym.*, *119*: 166.

422. Moschera, J. A., Woehle, D., Tsai, K. P., Chen, C.-H., and Tarnowski, S. J. (1986). Purification of recombinant human fibroblast interferon produced in *Escherichia coli*, *Meth. Enzym.*, *119*: 177.

423. Lin. L. S., Yamamoto, R., and Drummond, R. J. (1986). Purification of recombinant human interferon β expressed in *Escherichia coli*, *Meth. Enzym.*, *119*: 183.

424. Sugi, M., Kato, H., Fujimoto, M., Utsumi, J., Hosoi, K., Shimizu, H., and Kobayashi, S. (1987). Monoclonal antibody to human β interferon: Characterization and application, *Hybridoma*, 6: 313.

425. Braude, I. A. (1986). Purification of natural human immune interferon induced by A-23187 and mezerein, *Meth. Enzym.*, *119*: 193.

426. Rung, H.-F., Pan, Y.-C. E., Moschera, J., Tsai, K., Bekesi, E., Chang, M., Sugino, H., and Honda, S. (1986). Purification of recombinant human immune interferon, *Meth. Enzym.*, *119*: 204.

427. Aguet, M., and Merlin, G. (1987). Purification of human γ interferon receptors by sequential affinity chromatography on immobilized monoclonal antireceptor antibodies and human γ interferon, *J. Exp. Med.*, *165*(4): 988.

428. Ahl, R., and Gottschalk M. (1986). Production and purification of bovine interferon β, *Meth. Enzym.*, *119*: 211.

429. van der Meide, P. H., Wubben, J., Vuverberg, K., and Schellekens, H. (1986). Production, purification, and characterization of rat interferon from transformed rat cells, *Meth. Enzym.*, *119*: 220.

430. Andersson, L., and Mosbach, K. (1979). The use of biochemical solid-phase techniques in the study of alcohol dehydrogenase 2. Selective carboxymethylation of bioaffinity-bound alcohol dehydrogenase, *Eur. J. Biochem.*, *94*: 565.

431. Roy, S. K., and Nishikawa, A. H. (1979). Large-scale isolation of equine liver alcohol dehydrogenase on a blue agarose gel, *Biotechnol. Bioeng.*, *21*: 775.

432. Flygare, S., Griffin, T., Larsson, P. O., and Mosbach, K. (1983). Affinity precipitation of dehydrogenases, *Anal. Biochem.*, *133*: 409.

433. Larsson, P. O., Flygare, S., and Mosbach, K. (1984). Affinity precipitation of dehydrogenases, *Meth. Enzym.*, *104*: 364.
434. Andersson, L., and Mosbach, K. (1982). Alcohol dehydrogenase from horse liver by affinity chromatography, *Meth. Enzym.*, *89*: 435.
435. Harakas, N. K. (1984). Industrial mammalian cell culture: Physiology-technology-products, *Annual Reports on Fermentation*, vol. 7 (G. T. Tsao, ed.), Academic Press, New York, p. 159–211.
436. Feder, J., and Tolbert, W. R. (1983). The large scale cultivation of mammalian cells, *Sci. Am.*, *248*(1): 36.
437. Wickerhauser, M., Williams, C., and Mercer, J. (1979). Development of large scale fractionation methods VII. Preparation of antithrombin III concentrate, *Vox Sang*, *36*: 281.
438. Robinson, P. J., Dunnill, P., and Lilly, M. D. (1972). Factors affecting scale-up of affinity chromatography of β-galactosidase, *Biochim. Biophys. Acta*, *285*: 28.
439. Robinson, P. J., Wheatley, M. A., Janson, J.-C., Dunnill, P., and Lilly, M. D. (1974). Pilot scale affinity chromatography: Purification of β-galactosidase, *Biotechnol. Bioeng.*, *26*: 1103.
440. Holroyde, M. J., Chesher, J. M. E., Trayer, I. P., and Walker, D. G. (1976). Studies on the use of Sepharose-*N*-(6-aminohexanoyl)-2-amino-2-deoxy-D-glucopyranose for the large-scale purification of hepatic glucokinase, *Biochem. J.*, *153*: 351.
441. Neurath, A. R., Prince, A. M., and Giacalone, J. (1977). Large-scale purification of hepatitis B surface antigen using affinity chromatography, *Experientia*, *34*: 414.
442. Hammarberg, B., Nygren, P.-A., Holmgren, E., Elmblad, A., Tally, M., Hellman, U., Moks, T., and Uhlen, M. (1989). Dual affinity fusion approach and its use to express recombinant human insulin-like growth factor II, *Proc. Natl. Acad. Sci. USA*, *86*: 4367.
443. Kulbe, K. D., and Schuer, R. (1979). Large-scale preparation of phosphoglycerate kinase from *Saccharomyces cerevisiae* using cibacron blue-Sepharose 4 B pseudoaffinity chromatography, *Anal. Biochem.*, *93*:46.
444. Kopperschlager, G., and Johansson, G. (1982). Affinity partitioning with polymer-bound cibacron blue F3G-A for rapid, large-scale purification of phosphofructokinase from baker's yeast, *Anal. Biochem.*, *124*: 117.
445. Ramadoss, C. S., Steczko, J., Uhlig, J. W., and Axelrod, B. (1983). Effect of albumin on binding and recovery of enzymes in affinity chromatography on cibacron blue, *Anal. Biochem.*, *130*: 481.
446. Scawen, M. D., Hammond, P. M., Comer, M. J., and Atkinson, T. (1983). The application of triazine dye affinity chromatography to the large-scale purification of glycerokinase from *Bacillus stearothermophilus*, *Anal. Biochem.*, *132*: 413.
447. Kucerova, Z., Pohl, J., and Korbova, L. (1986). Separation of human pepsin and gastricsin by affinity chromatography with an immobilized synthetic inhibitor, *J. Chromatography*, *376*: 409.
448. Allman, J., and Harakas, N. K. (1988). Unpublished work.
449. Aries, R. S., and Newton, R. D. (1955). *Chemical Cost Estimates*, McGraw-Hill, New York.
450. Monsanto Co. (1978). Manufacturing cost estimate and ROI Monsanto Standards, unpublished work.

451. Deutscher, M. P. (1990). Rethinking your purification procedure, *Meth. Enzym., 182:779.*

452. Horvath, C. ed. (1988). *High-Performance Liquid Chromatography: Advances and Perspectives,* vol. 5, Academic Press, New York.

453. Tanford, C. (1978). The hydrophobic effect and the organization of living matter, *Science, 200:* 1012.

454. Fausnaugh, J. L., and Regnier, F. E. (1986). Solute and mobile phase contributions to retention in hydrophobic interaction chromatography of proteins, *J. Chromatogr., 359:* 131.

455. Wu, S.-L., Figueroa, A., and Karger, B. L. (1986). Protein conformational effects in hydrophobic interaction chromatography: Retention characterization and the role of mobile phase additives and stationary phase hydrophobicity, *J. Chromatogr., 371:* 3.

456. Chicz, R. M. and Regnier, F. E. (1990). Microenvironmental contributions to the chromatographic behavior of subtilisin in hydrophobic-interaction and reversed-phase chromatography, *J. Chromatogr., 500:* 503.

457. Mazaroff, I., Varady, L., and Regnier, F. E. (1989). A thermodynamic model for electrostatic interaction chromatography of proteins, *J. Chromatogr., 499:* 63.

458. Chicz, R. M., and Regnier, F. E. (1990). Single amino acid contributions to protein retention in cation-exchange chromatography: Resolution of genetically engineered subtilisin variants, *Anal. Chem., 61:* 2059.

459. Worthy, W. (1988). Chromatography columns mimic cell membranes, *Chem. Eng. News, 66*(50): 23.

460. Pidgeon, C., and Venkataram, U. V. (1988). Immobilized artificial membrane chromatography: Supports composed of membrane lipids, *Anal. Biochem., 176:* 36.

461. Tiemeier, D. C., Krivi, G. G., and Glover, G. I. (1982). Personal communication, unpublished work.

462. Brewer, S. J., and Sassenfeld, H. M. (1985). The purification of recombinant proteins using C-terminal polyarginine fusions, *Trends Biotech., 3:* 119.

463. Persson, M., Bergstrand, M. G., Bulow, L., and Mosbach, K. (1988). Enzyme purification by genetically attached polycysteine and polyphenylalanine affinity tails, *Anal. Biochem., 172:* 330.

464. Mosbach, K. (1988). Novel approaches to affinity chromatography, *Makromol. Macromol. Symp., 17* (Int. Symp. affinity Chromatogr. Interfacial Macromol. Interact., 1987), pp. 325–333.

465. Knight, P. (1989). Downstream processing, *Bio/Technology, 7:* 777.

466. Goloubinoff, P., Gatenby, A. A., and Lorimer, G. H. (1989). GroE heat-shock proteins promote assembly of foreign prokaryotic ribulose bisphosphate carboxylase oligomers in *Escherichia coli, Nature, 337:* 44.

467. Mitraki, A., and King J. (1989). Protein folding intermediates and inclusion body formation, *Bio/Technology, 7:* 690.

468. Knight, P. (1989). Chromatography: 1989 report, *Bio/Technology, 7:* 243.

469. Deutscher, M. P., ed. (1990). *Guide to Protein Purification Techniques, Methods in Enzymology,* vol. 182, Academic Press, Orlando.

470. Chicz, R. M., and Regnier, F. E. (1990). High-performance liquid chromato-
      graphy: Effective protein purification by various chromatographic modes, *Meth.
      Enzym.*, *182*: 392.
471. Hill, J. C., and Harakas, N. K. (1990). Production of specialty chemicals,
      polymers, and fibers using recombinant DNA, *Biotechnol. Progr.*, *6*: 169.
472. Schultz, J. C., ed. (1990). Symposium papers on the production of nonclinical
      products by recombinant DNA and other biological methodologies at the 1989
      Annual Meeting of A.I.Ch.E., *Biotechnol. Progr.*, *6*: 171.

9

Freeze Drying: A Practical Overview

Larry A. Gatlin
Glaxo Research Institute, Research Triangle Park, North Carolina

Steven L. Nail
Purdue University, West Lafayette, Indiana

I. INTRODUCTION

Freeze drying, or lyophilization, is an important pharmaceutical process that allows for the preservation of heat-sensitive drugs and biologicals. This process uses low temperature and pressure to remove a solvent, typically water, by the process of sublimation, which is a change in phase from solid to vapor without passing through the liquid phase. The most common application of freeze drying in the pharmaceutical industry is in the manufacture of injectable products. The process is also used, however, in the manufacture of diagnostics and infrequently for oral solid dosage forms where very rapid dissolution rates are required.

Products that are freeze dried can possess several characteristics that provide significant advantages over products dried by alternative methods. First, since drying takes place at low temperature, chemical decomposition is minimized. Second, a freeze dried product has a very high specific surface area, promoting fast, complete product dissolution. Third, freeze drying is more compatible than dry powder filling in a sterile operation. Since in the freeze drying process the vials are filled with filtered solution, the fill weight control is more precise than for powder filling; the absence of powder during filling minimizes problems with particulate contamination in a clean, aseptic environment.

Freeze drying was introduced as a practical commercial process about the time of World War II for the preservation of blood plasma. This was followed by the freeze drying of antibiotics such as penicillin. Application of freeze drying continued to increase as vaccines, steroids, vitamins, and many diagnostics were developed. The relative importance of pharmaceutical freeze drying will expand as the next generation of therapeutic agents is developed. Many of these new products are expected to be proteins, peptides, and other macromolecules that are chemically or physically unstable in aqueous solution. This instability may be related to the secondary, tertiary, and even quaternary structures needed for biological activity. The formulation and manufacture of these products will present a challenge to the formulation scientist, and freeze drying will be a necessary tool for the development of these products.

A. Process Overview

The liquid product to be freeze dried is aseptically placed into vials. The vials are usually partially stoppered with a special slotted rubber closure that allows water vapor to escape. The vials are then aseptically transferred, usually in metal trays, to the freeze dryer. The trays holding the filled, partially stoppered vials may be placed directly on the freeze dryer shelf or, to reduce resistance to heat transfer, the trays may have removable bottoms that allow the vials to rest directly on the shelf.

The shelves of the freeze dryer contain internal channels with circulating silicone oil or another suitable heat transfer fluid. Prechilling of the shelves may be necessary for certain products that are particularly unstable. A temperature-measuring device is placed in several different vials spaced throughout the freeze dryer chamber prior to freezing. These devices can be

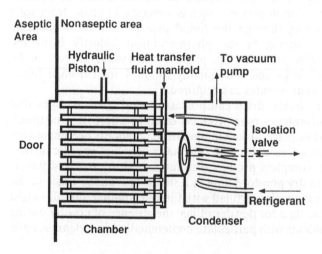

Figure 1 Schematic diagram of freeze dryer.

used to monitor the process or for sequencing of the freeze dry cycle. A schematic of a pharmaceutical freeze dryer is shown in Fig. 1.

The product is first cooled to a sufficiently low temperature to allow complete solidification of the vial contents. The chamber pressure is then reduced to below the vapor pressure of ice corresponding to the temperature of the product. Once this pressure is reached, the temperature of the shelves is increased to provide energy for sublimation. During the drying a receding boundary is observed in the vial as the frozen layer decreases in thickness and the thickness of the partially dried solids increases (Fig. 2). This drying phase, where most of the water is removed, is called primary drying. When most of the water is gone, additional drying time is required to remove water adsorbed to, or trapped within, the solid matrix. This is called secondary drying. A representative plot of product temperature, shelf temperature, and chamber pressure during the freezing, primary drying, and secondary drying is shown in Fig. 3. Once the product is sufficiently dry, the chamber pressure may be increased with a gas, usually an inert gas such as nitrogen, or kept under vacuum while the partially inserted stoppers are completely seated into the vials within the dryer by hydraulic compression of the shelf stack.

The most important objective in developing a freeze dried product is to assure that the product quality is maintained throughout the shelf life. Critical requirements include recovery of the original chemical or biological potency after reconstitution, rapid and complete dissolution, appropriate residual moisture level, and acceptable cake appearance. Additionally, drying conditions are chosen for optimal processing, since the drying process is costly. In fact, drying contributes most of the manufacturing cost of the final dosage form, and of the drying processes used freeze drying is the most

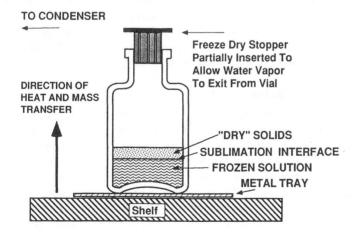

Figure 2 Schematic of a vial during primary freeze drying.

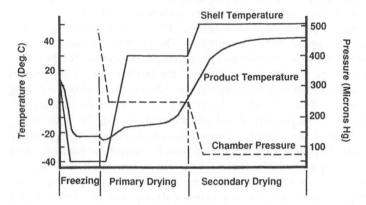

Figure 3   Process variables during the freeze dry cycle.

expensive in both capital investment and operating expense. The challenge is to understand the physical chemistry of "frozen" solutions, the heat and mass transfer characteristics of the freeze drying process, temperature and pressure measurement, process monitoring, and considerations of freeze dry system design. Some of these topics are discussed below. Additional details can be found in cited references.

II. THE FREEZING PROCESS

Freezing is a critical step in the freeze drying process. The microstructure of both the ice and the solute formed during freezing determines both the quality of the final product and its processing characteristics, such as the rates of primary and secondary drying. Below is a discussion of the physical events associated with the freezing process: supercooling, ice crystallization, concentration of solutes, and crystallization of the solute.

A. Phase Diagram of Water

The phase diagram of water is given in Fig. 4. At the triple point, ice, water, and water vapor coexist in equilibrium (0.0098°C and 4.58 mm Hg). Freeze drying takes place below this triple point, where the water passes directly from a solid to a gas. The 4.58 mm Hg pressure is the vapor pressure of water and not the total pressure of the system. Thus sublimation does occur at atmospheric pressure as long as the water vapor pressure is below 4.58 mm Hg. The phenomenon of "freezer burn" is testimony to this process at atmospheric pressure. The Eskimos once used atmospheric freeze drying to preserve meat.

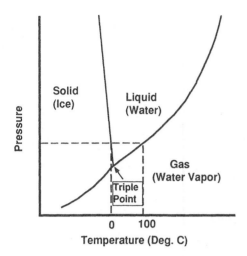

Figure 4 Phase diagram of water.

B. Freezing of Aqueous Solutions

A plot of a freezing process for a simple aqueous solution of sodium chloride is shown in Fig. 5. In the segment ab, the product temperature decreases to well below the equilibrium freezing point T_f of the product. At point b, nucleation of ice crystals occurs.

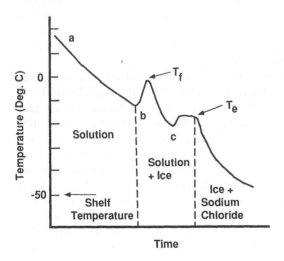

Figure 5 Temperature vs. time for freezing of sodium chloride/water.

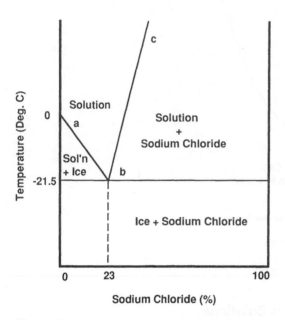

Figure 6   Phase diagram for a sodium chloride/water system.

Nucleation may be either heterogeneous, caused by suspended impurities or by the walls of the container, or homogeneous, caused by spontaneous ordering of water molecules to initiate crystallization. Typically nucleation is heterogeneous since homogeneous nucleation of pure water occurs at about -40°C. However, since injectable dosage forms are filtered and relatively free of suspended impurities, supercooling usually occurs and is often in the range of 10 to 15°C below the equilibrium freezing point.

As nucleation and crystal growth of ice begins at point b, the latent heat of fusion is released and the temperature increases to the equilibrium freezing point T_f. As cooling continues along segment $T_f\text{-}c$, the ice crystals grow and the interstitial fluid becomes more concentrated. At point c, crystallization of the concentrated interstitial fluid occurs, which for this case is a eutectic mixture of crystalline sodium chloride and ice. A eutectic, for this discussion, is defined as an intimate physical mixture of two or more crystalline solids that melt as if they were a single pure compound. After eutectic crystallization is complete at point T_e, there is no remaining liquid. Thus no further changes in the microstructure of the frozen system occurs as the temperature is decreased. As the product continues to cool below the eutectic temperature, the temperature decrease is more rapid because ice has a lower heat capacity than water.

The phase diagram of the sodium-chloride–water system is given in Fig. 6. The line ab represents the equilibrium freezing temperature of the solution T_f as a function of sodium chloride concentration. The line bc is the solubility of sodium chloride in water. The intersection of the lines at point b is -21.5°C, which is the the eutectic temperature for an aqueous sodium chloride system. The concentration of sodium chloride in the eutectic mixture is about 23%. This phase diagram is for a simple binary eutectic system. Other phase diagrams can be very complex (1,2). Knowledge of the system's phase diagram is of great benefit in the development of a freeze drying cycle for a product.

The eutectic temperature is important in the freeze drying process because it represents the maximum allowable product temperature during primary drying. If the product temperature exceeds the eutectic temperature while ice is present, then drying takes place from the liquid state instead of the solid state; and the desirable properties of a freeze dried product may be lost. Eutectic behavior, however, is only observed for crystalline systems. In many cases the solute does not readily crystallize during freezing. A representative freezing curve for such a noncrystalline product is shown in Fig. 7. The initial segment of the freezing is similar to that seen in Fig. 5. As the temperature continues to be decreased, however, the secondary or eutectic crystallization does not occur. Instead, a slight slope change is seen in the temperature vs. time curve at the glass transition temperature T_g. The glass transition concept is used with amorphous systems and in this context corresponds to a change in the viscosity of the system from a viscous liquid to a glass.

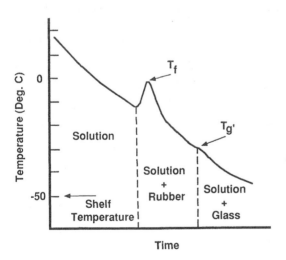

Figure 7   Temperature vs. time for freezing of an amorphous solute.

The importance of the glass transition for amorphous systems is similar to the eutectic of a crystalline system and represents the maximum allowable product temperature during the primary drying of the product. Although the glass transition temperature may be equated to the collapse temperature, they are not actually equivalent. The glass transition temperature is measured in a closed system of constant composition, whereas collapse is a dynamic process that can occur during the drying process (3). If the product temperature exceeds either the glass transition or the eutectic temperature of the corresponding system, then the product can "collapse." This collapse, which is explained in more detail below, can at best be an aesthetic problem and at worst result in rejection of the product.

The desirable properties of a freeze dried product result from the microstructure formed during the freezing process, which must be retained during the removal of ice. Fig. 8 is a sketch showing the microstructure of a frozen solution containing a crystalline or amorphous solute. The interstitial material in the crystalline system is a mixture of eutectic ice and crystalline solute. When both the ice and the preeutectic ice are sublimed, a crystalline solid containing very little water remains. In an amorphous system, the glassy interstitial material must be sufficiently rigid to support its own weight after the ice is removed. This rigidity is found at temperatures below the product glass transition temperature where viscosity is sufficiently high to prevent flow during the drying process. It is estimated that the viscosity is greater than 10^{14} poise in systems below the glass transition temperature. Above the glass transition, however, the solute can flow, resulting in collapse of the product. The rate of this flow depends on temperature and residual water content.

Solution freezing behavior in sterile filtered products does not typically follow equilibrium phase diagrams. The behavior of these systems has been represented by "supplemented phase diagrams" as described by MacKenzie

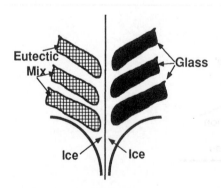

Figure 8 Schematic of microstructure for a crystalline or amorphous solute.

(4) or as "state diagrams" as described by Franks (5). The value observed as a collapse temperature is greatly affected by the measurement method and the residual water content; thus a wider temperature range is typically reported for amorphous systems than for eutectic systems.

C. Thermal Treatments

Solutes such as sodium chloride readily crystallize from solution during freezing. Many other solutes, however, do not crystallize so easily. Since most aseptically filled solutions supercool, which leads to a rapid freezing rate once the ice has nucleated, a metastable amorphous solute phase may be formed. It is possible thermally to treat some systems to induce crystallization of the solute by warming them to a temperature above the glass transition temperature but below the melting temperature of the system. Three cephalosporins that all freeze in the amorphous form were investigated by Gatlin and DeLuca (6); without being thermally treated before drying, they remained in the less desirable amorphous form. The amorphous phase for some products has an adverse affect on the product stability, and for many cephalosporins the crystalline form is at least an order of magnitude more stable than the amorphous form (7,8). Other product characteristics such as reconstitution time and cake appearance can also be affected by crystallinity of the solutes.

D. Characterization of Freezing Behavior

Characterization of the frozen formulation is an important step in the development of a product. Data appropriately gathered can provide information that can help to determine whether constituents crystallize upon freezing and how this modifies the freezing behavior. These data also provide a good estimation of the maximum allowable product temperature during primary drying. The collapse temperatures of various compounds are collated in Ref. 9.

The three common methods of obtaining these data—thermal analysis, thermoelectric (or electrokinetic) analysis, and freeze dry microscopy—are briefly described below.

1. Thermal Analysis

Materials that undergo a physical or chemical change as a function of temperature typically release or absorb energy in the form of heat. Differential thermal analysis (DTA) measures the temperature of both a sample and a thermally inert reference material as a function of temperature. Sample transitions result in energy changes, which cause temperature differences ΔT between the sample and the reference. Plotting this differential temperature against the programmed temperature of the system provides information on the temperature at which a transition occurs and whether the transition is exothermic (heat released) or endothermic (heat adsorbed). A technique closely related to DTA is differential scanning calorimetry (DSC). In DSC the system temperature is also carefully controlled; however, when a transition occurs the energy provided to maintain the sample and the reference at the same temperature is modulated. The energy necessary to maintain these temperatures is measured and recorded; this energy is equal to the energy absorbed or evolved in the sample transition.

Typical thermal transitions seen using DSC to characterize frozen systems are shown in Fig. 9. The heat capacity of a sample is proportional to the displacement from the "blank" baseline. A baseline shift toward higher heat capacity is typically seen for glass transitions and denotes a decrease in the order within the system. Increased rotational energy at the molecular level at temperatures above the glass transition temperature allows flexibility and elastomeric properties in polymeric materials. Endotherms typically indicate physical changes, such as melting, and if the endotherm is sharp the compound typically is more pure. Exothermic behavior is associated with increased molecular order such as in crystallization of metastable compounds.

Characterization of a thermal event as reversible or irreversible provides insight into its nature. For a reversible event, the transition recurs as the sample is cooled and rewarmed such as would be seen with the melting of ice at zero degrees. An irreversible event such as an excipient crystallization exotherm will not be observed a second time if the sample is not melted before it is cooled and rewarmed over the same temperature range.

Typically a thermal analysis experiment is begun by placing a small amount of sample in an aluminum sample pan and placing the pan in the thermal cell of the instrument. A thermally inert reference material such as

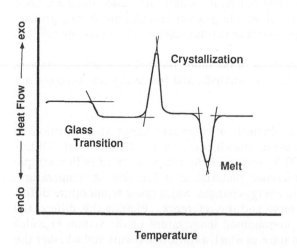

Figure 9 Thermal transitions relevant to frozen solutions.

an empty pan is also appropriately placed in the instrument thermal cell. A continuous small stream of dry nitrogen is used to flush the sample cell to prevent condensation of moisture within the cell. The sample is then cooled to a predetermined temperature of approximately -50°C and slowly warmed at 1 to 5°C per minute to a temperature above the freezing point of the sample. The analysis is carried out during sample warming because transitions observed during cooling tend to be inaccurate due to sample super-cooling. Typical thermograms of sodium chloride, mannitol, and cefazolin sodium are given in Fig. 10; they are representative of eutectic melt, crystallization, and glass transition, respectively, followed by a crystallization.

The thermogram of sodium chloride in water shows two endotherms; a eutectic melting endotherm at -21.5°C and a melting endotherm for the preeutectic ice at about -0.3°C.

Thermograms of formulations intended for freeze drying are seldom so well defined. Eutectic melting, when it occurs, generally takes place at higher temperatures for most compounds and may be obscured by the melting endotherm of preeutectic ice. The thermogram of sodium-chloride–water is also easily interpreted because the sodium chloride crystallizes readily during the freezing process. Other solutes may crystallize more slowly, incompletely, or not at all. The thermogram of mannitol, a commonly used

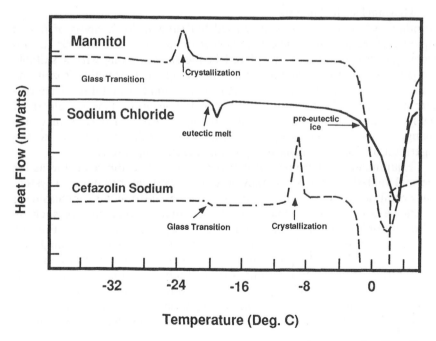

Figure 10 DSC thermograms of mannitol, sodium chloride, and cefazolin sodium.

excipient in freeze drying, is shown in Fig. 10. When a solution of 5% mannitol is frozen rapidly, a metastable phase is initially formed. As the solution is warmed and the glass transition temperature T_g of the amorphous system is exceeded, the decreased viscosity allows greater freedom of movement of both water and mannitol, and a phase change occurs toward a more thermodynamically stable state—crystallization of both the solute and the amorphous ice. This is seen as a crystallization exotherm at about -25°C. Once the solute crystallizes, the solute exhibits eutectic behavior. A separate eutectic melting endotherm is not seen in this system because of the high melting endotherm of the mannitol-water eutectic.

For cefazolin sodium, shown in Fig. 10 (10) a glass transition occurs at about -20°C, a crystallization exotherm at about -11°C, followed by a melting endotherm at about -4°C.

The glass transition of a frozen amorphous system is an important characteristic because, as discussed above, it represents the maximum allowable operating temperature during primary drying. However, detection of glass transitions by thermal analysis can be difficult because of the low energy involved in the transition. For example, in the sorbitol thermogram a glass transition occurs at about -51°C but is barely resolved. Use of more concentrated sample solutions can improve sensitivity, as can use of expanded scales to "blow up" selected portions of a thermogram.

2. Thermoelectric Analysis

Another technique, not as widely used but suitable for analysis of frozen aqueous systems, is thermoelectric analysis, or electrokinetic analysis. In this technique, two electrodes are placed in the sample along with a suitable temperature-measuring device. When the sample is thoroughly frozen, the resistance to electrical current is high due to limited mobility of charge-carrying species. As the sample is warmed and begins to thaw, the electrical resistance drops dramatically as ionic mobility increases. The resistance may change as melting begins by three orders of magnitude or more, so the logarithm of resistance is usually plotted against temperature.

Equipment for thermoelectric analysis is not as readily available as for thermal analysis, and it is generally up to the investigator to devise a system using components from several sources. However, instruments for measuring resistance are available from some freeze dryer manufacturers such as Edwards High Vacuum (Tonawanda, New York) or Usifroid (Paris, France) and from other suppliers such as Heironetics, Inc. (Wallingford, Pennsylvania). Typical equipment used for thermoelectric analysis consists of a controlled temperature system capable of subambient temperatures such as a mechanical bath or chamber cooled by controlled introduction of liquid nitrogen, a suitable temperature-measuring device, electrodes for resistance measurement, a log resistance amplifier with power supply, and appropriate analog or digital equipment for recording electrical resistance as a function of product temperature.

The log resistance amplifier measures the bulk electrical resistance of a sample by measuring the current that results when a voltage of known amplitude is impressed across two electrodes immersed in a conducting substance. To overcome the effects of electrode polarization at the surfaces, alternating current is used. The electrode may take a variety of shapes; L-shaped electrodes arranged in a parallel configuration and "sandwich" electrodes consisting of two gold-surfaced electrodes rigidly separated by a hydrophobic insulating material are typical.

In the thermoelectric analysis experiment a small sample of 1 to 2 mL is placed in a vial along with an electrode and a temperature-measuring device. The vial is placed in a low temperature bath and frozen to below -50°C. The bath temperature is then increased at a rate of 1 to 2°C/min. As with thermal analysis, it is important to collect data during the warming phase as opposed to freezing because of the effects of supercooling. Temperature and log resistance data are collected until the sample is thawed. This may be done by computer or by an analog x–y recorder. Use of a computer has the advantage of facilitating digital smoothing and differentiation of the resistance vs. temperature data (11).

The log resistance vs. temperature curve for sodium chloride in water is shown in Fig. 11. The resistance drops sharply at the eutectic point, and no significant change is seen at the melting point of the preeutectic ice, since melting of the ice has little effect on the mobility of the charge-carrying species. This is an advantage for eutectic point determination for compounds with very high eutectic temperatures, such as sodium sulfate. In ther-

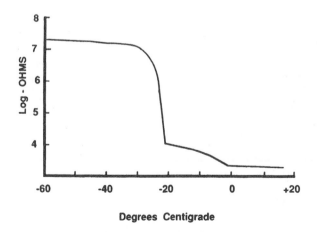

Figure 11 Log resistance vs. temperature for sodium chloride (0.9%).

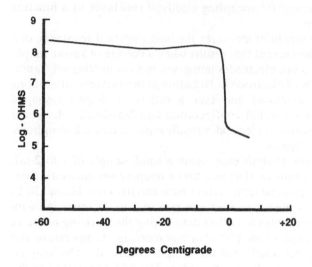

Figure 12   Log resistance vs. temperature for mannitol.

mal analysis, the eutectic melting endotherm would be hidden by the melting endotherm of ice.

Examination of the electrical resistance vs. temperature behavior of simple binary mixtures illustrates dramatic potential interactions, although the significance of this is not fully understood. The log resistance vs. tem-

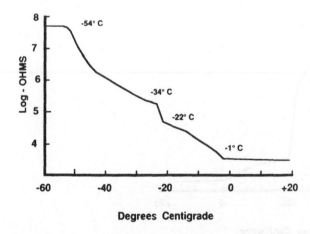

Figure 13   Log resistance vs. temperature for sodium chloride/mannitol mixture (mola-ratio 1.25:1).

perature profile of mannitol is shown in Fig. 12. The resistance remains high and nearly independent of temperature above approximately -2°C. At the eutectic temperature, the resistance drops sharply by over two orders of magnitude. If the experiment is repeated for a mixture of sodium chloride and mannitol in a molar ratio of 1.25:1, the curve shown in Fig. 13 is obtained. There is roughly a four log decrease in resistance between -50°C and -1°C, but the rate of decrease is even more gradual. While there is an inflection point at -34°C, the log resistance vs. temperature relationship does not suggest any temperature that represents a clear eutectic melt.

While resistance vs. temperature data are unambiguous for simple eutectic systems, the data become more difficult to interpret as the complexity of the system increases. There are no published data, for example, to support the idea that thermoelectric analysis can be used to measure glass transition temperatures in amorphous systems. Further research is needed to draw well-supported conclusions regarding the general utility of thermoelectric analysis as a tool for characterizing formulations.

3. Freeze Dry Microscopy

The most visual method for characterizing the freezing and freeze drying behavior of a formulation is by direct observation under a microscope. Equipment for microscopic observation of freezing and freeze drying has been described by McCrone (12), MacKenzie (13), Freedman et al. (14), Flink et al. (15), Flink and Gejl-Hansen (16), Pikal et al. (17), and Kochs et al. (18). The systems described by these investigators comprise a microscope, a freeze drying stage, a cooling system, a probe for sample temperature measurement, and a vacuum system.

The freeze drying stage is the most critical part of the system. Designs vary widely, but most stages consist of a metal or Plexiglass block with windows on each side to allow light transmission through the sample. A microscope slide that supports the sample is usually placed on a metal block containing channels for circulation of a cooling or heating fluid. The fluid may be either a gas, such as dry nitrogen, which passes through a cooling coil, or a liquid such as alcohol. Heating of the sample is accomplished either by increasing the temperature of the incoming fluid stream (14–17), using a resistance heater between the cooled block and the sample (12), or by placing a conductive coating on a glass slide as a compensatory heater (13,18). In the system described by MacKenzie, the sample cell is immersed in a controlled temperature alcohol bath, and the freezing/drying process is observed through the bath.

Most freeze drying microscope stages are designed such that the temperature is nearly constant across the sample. This minimizes uncertainty in sample temperature arising from placement of the thermocouple. However, the stages described by Freedman et al. and Kochs et al. are designed such that a temperature gradient exists across the sample. This mimics the situation encountered in actual freezing and drying but does present a problem in determining the precise sample temperature at a given time. The working distance, or the distance between the sample and the top of the stage cover, is a critical design feature of the stage. If the working distance is more than about 7 mm, a special long working distance (LWD) microscope objective may be required.

Since ice crystals are birefringent, a polarized light microscope is useful for observing phase transitions during freezing and during freeze drying. The crystallinity of the freeze dried solid can then also be observed directly.

Experimentally, a few microliters of sample is placed on a microscope slide, a cover slip is placed over the sample, and the slide is placed on the controlled temperature block. The stage is then covered with a metal lid containing a viewing window. The vacuum seal between the lid and the body of the stage is generally accomplished by an O-ring. A stream of dry nitrogen or air is usually blown across the windows to prevent condensation of atmospheric moisture on the windows. After the sample is frozen to a predetermined temperature, the stage is evacuated to less than about 0.5 torr, and the sample is heated. A distinct drying front can be seen moving across the sample as drying proceeds, and changes in sample morphology can be observed as a function of temperature and time.

The main advantage of microscopy as an analytical tool is the easy observability of collapse as compared with both thermal analysis and thermo-electric analysis. In thermal analysis, the glass transition involves very low energy; thus it can be difficult to detect. For thermoelectric analysis, the applicability to detection of glass transitions has not been established. While the collapse temperature is easy to observe, the observed temperature of this transition is more dependent on the experimental conditions used during its measurement than a eutectic temperature (3). In particular, the observed collapse temperature increases with increased sublimation rate. After the sublimation interface passes a particular volume element of the sample, water is removed from the amorphous phase. This increases the concentration of solute, thereby increasing the viscosity and retarding collapse. This effect is more pronounced at faster sublimation rates, since water is also removed from the amorphous phase faster. In general, a product freeze drying in a vial will collapse at a slightly higher temperature than the collapse temperature as measured by the microscopic method (3).

III. THE PRIMARY DRYING PROCESS

Primary drying is characterized by a receding boundary layer of ice in the vial (Fig. 2). The driving force for sublimation of ice during primary drying is the difference between the vapor pressure of ice at the sublimation front and the partial pressure of water vapor in the freeze dry chamber. Since the driving force is determined only by differences in vapor pressure of water within the system, and not by the total system pressure, it is a misconception that freeze drying can take place only under high vacuum. However, freeze drying at atmospheric pressure must take place by *molecular diffusion* of water against a pressure gradient (air), which is a slow process. It was not until advances in vacuum pump technology allowed the freeze dry chamber to be rapidly pumped down to a total pressure of less than the vapor pressure of ice in the product that freeze drying became a commercially practical process. For example, the vapor pressure of ice at -35°C is 0.168 mm Hg (168 μm Hg). Reducing the system pressure below this value allows drying to take place by *bulk flow* of water vapor, which is the transfer of vapor in the same direction as the pressure difference.

Since the vapor pressure increases by roughly 70% for every 5°C increase in temperature, maximum process efficiency requires that the product temperature be maintained as high as possible without exceeding the maximum allowable product temperature during drying. As discussed above, the maximum allowable product temperature is determined either by the eutectic melting temperature or by the collapse temperature of the product. In either case, exceeding the maximum allowable product temperature results in an unacceptable product.

A. Sublimation of Ice

Sublimation of ice is not an inherently slow process, and in theory 2 g of ice can sublimate in 0.9 minutes. In practice, however, the time required to freeze dry a of product in a vial with 2 g of water may be in the range of 4 to 8 hours. This difference is due to the limitations in the rate of transfer of heat from the shelf to the sublimation front, limitations in the rate of transfer of water vapor from the product to the condenser, or both.

B. Transfer Operations in Primary Drying

Transfer operations such as heat and mass transfer are conceptually described as a flow rate, or flux (flow rate per unit area). This is determined by dividing a driving force by a resistance (or, reciprocally, a driving force multiplied by a conductance). The overall drying rate is determined by driving forces (temperature differences or pressure differences) divided by the sum of a series of resistances to either heat or mass transfer. In order to maximize process efficiency it is necessary first to determine whether the process is heat transfer-limited or mass transfer-limited. Once this is determined then the *limiting resistance* is identified and steps are taken to minimize this resistance.

Understanding heat and mass transfer in freeze drying requires an understanding that gases behave differently at the low pressures encountered in freeze drying than at the moderate vacuums used in other pharmaceutical unit operations. For example, at atmospheric pressure and at modest vacuum (above about 100 mm Hg), thermal conductivity of a gas is nearly independent of pressure. This does not apply at the pressures used for freeze drying, which has important implications for heat transfer. The flow characteristics of gas at freeze dry pressures may also be much different than flow at higher pressures. This is important when dealing with mass transfer in freeze drying, where the flow of vapor through the bed of "dried" solids is often simplified by picturing the solid phase as a bundle of capillaries that increase in length as drying proceeds. For an in-depth treatment, the reader is referred to Ref. 9 or the excellent book by Dushman and Lafferty (19).

C. Behavior of Gases at Low Pressure

Units of pressure commonly used in freeze drying are the following:

1 standard atmosphere = 760 mm Hg at 0°C
1 mm Hg = 1 torr = 1.33 millibar
1 μm = 10^{-3} mm Hg = 1.33 microbars

Pressure is usually expressed as micrometers of mercury (μm Hg) in the United States. In Europe, it is more common to express pressure as a decimal fraction of 1 millibar. The normal operating pressure range for freeze drying is from 10 μm Hg to about 0.5 torr.

The transport properties of gases in evacuated systems are usually divided into three categories according to the range of values of a dimensionless number called the *Knudsen number*. The Knudsen number is defined as the ratio of the mean free path L of a molecule to a characteristic dimension a of the system containing the gas. For example, for gas flowing in a tube, the characteristic dimension of this system is the diameter of the tube. For water vapor flowing through a matrix of partially dried solids during freeze drying, the characteristic dimension is the average diameter of the channels created by the removal of ice. The mean free path or the average distance traveled by a gas molecule between collisions, for example, at a vacuum of 26 in. Hg (typical of a vacuum dryer operating at modest vacuum) is about 3×10^{-5} cm.

At modest vacuums, where the mean free path is very short, collisions between molecules occur much more frequently than collisions of molecules with the boundaries of the system. These collisions between molecules determine the viscosity of the gas, and the flow is viscous. At low pressures, the mean free path may be large compared with the characteristic dimension of the system. For the example above of water vapor flowing through a porous cake of partially dried solids at a pressure of 50 μm, the mean free path is 0.06 cm, and the average pore diameter may be about 0.005 cm. In this case, collisions of molecules with the channel walls are much more frequent than collisions between molecules, and the flow of vapor is limited by collisions with the channel walls rather than by collisions between molecules. This behavior is called *molecular* or *Knudsen flow*.

A third flow regime lies between viscous flow and molecular flow and, depending on the pressure, exhibits some properties of both. This range is called *transition flow*. Limits to the Knudsen number that delineate these flow regimes are as follows: when $Kn = \bar{L}/a < 0.01$, the flow is viscous; when $Kn > 1.0$, the flow is molecular; and when $0.01 < Kn < 1.0$, the flow is transitional. Viscous flow is described by the Poiseuille equation. It should be noted that the conductance of the tube is directly related to the average pressure in the tube.

For *molecular flow* through a tube of constant cross-sectional area A, perimeter H, and length L, the conductance of the tube is independent of pressure. This makes sense, since the flow properties are determined by collisions of gas molecules with the boundaries of the system, and not by collisions between gas molecules. For a given gas at a constant temperature, the conductance depends only on the geometry of the tube. Conductance increases with the square of the cross-sectional area and is inversely proportional to the length of the tube. For these reasons, it is best to design freeze dryers with short, large diameter piping, particularly between the chamber and the condenser.

The conductance of an orifice is considerably less under molecular flow conditions than under viscous flow conditions. For example, consider a cylindrical tube with a radius of 1 cm and a length of 100 cm. For water vapor at an average pressure of 4 mm Hg and a temperature of -20°C, the mean free path L is 1.25×10^{-3} cms which is in the viscous flow range. The conductance of the tube is equal to 101.3 liter/s. However, for the same tube at a system pressure of 1 μm Hg, the mean free path is about 3 cm, and since molecular flow conditions apply, the conductance of the tube at this pressure is 1.14 liter/s. For additional information on how to calculate the viscosity of a gas see Ref. 19.

Several practical lessons about freeze drying can be gleaned from this information. First, the flow regime, which is determined by both the pressure and the effective diameter of the pores in the plug of dried solids, has a dramatic influence on resistance of the dried matrix to the flow of vapor. If the dried matrix is pictured as a bundle of parallel capillaries, the above example shows that the resistance of a capillary is two orders of magnitude higher under molecular flow conditions than under viscous flow conditions. Second, conductance of a capillary is independent of pressure under molecular flow conditions but is directly proportional to pressure under viscous flow conditions. Third, the conductance of a capillary under molecular flow conditions is directly proportional to the third power of the effective radius of the orifice, since the conductance is directly proportional to the square of the area (fourth power of the radius) but is inversely proportional to the surface area of the orifice (HL). Under viscous flow conditions the conductance is proportional to the fourth power of the radius.

An assumption inherent in the Poiseuille equation is that the flow velocity at the wall of the tube is zero. As the pressure decreases below the range where viscous flow conditions apply, the assumption of zero velocity at the wall no longer applies, as "slipping" of the gas over the walls of the tube becomes appreciable. As pressure is further reduced, the flow characteristics gradually change from viscous slip flow to molecular flow. The conductance of a tube in the transition range is described by adding a "slip" term to the Poiseuille equation. For further discussion of slip and flow characteristics of gases in the transition range, the reader is referred to Ref. 18.

Application of these concepts is included below in the discussion of heat and mass transfer.

D. Heat Transfer in Primary Drying

Transfer of heat from the heat source—usually a heated shelf—to the product is often the rate-limiting step in the freeze drying process. This is explained by the high heat input (670 cal g^{-1}) required and by the difficulty of transferring heat in systems under high vacuum.

There are three basic mechanisms for heat transfer: conduction, convection, and radiation. *Conduction* is the transfer of heat by molecular motion between differential volume elements of a material. *Convection* is the transfer of heat by bulk flow of a fluid, either from density differences (natural convection) or because an external force is applied (forced convection). Heat transfer by natural convection has been shown to be negligible at the low pressures encountered in freeze drying (9). Heat transfer by *thermal radiation* arises when a substance, because of thermal excitation, emits radiation in an amount determined by its absolute temperature.

In the earlier example, the maximum rate of sublimation was calculated for 2 g of ice in a vial without regard to heat or mass transfer limitations. Now consider the same vial (radius = 0.9 cm, wall thickness = 0.2 cm) on an aluminum tray (thickness = 0.4 cm) in contact with a heated shelf. Assume for now that the bottom of the glass vial is flat and in complete contact with the shelf. Similarly, assume that the metal tray is in complete contact with the heated shelf, so that the thermal resistance at the interface between materials is negligible. The thickness L of the ice layer in the vial is 2 cm^3/π (0.9 cm)^2 = 0.79 cm, which represents the maximum resistance to heat transfer and occurs at the beginning of drying. Also assume a shelf temperature of 0°C and temperature at the sublimation front of -18°C. Since heat transfer and mass transfer are related by the heat of sublimation, this leads to a sublimation rate of approximately 1 g/h.

Inspection, however, of the bottom of any glass vial shows that good thermal contact between the glass and the shelf is not a good assumption. The concave shape of the vial bottom results in poor thermal contact. In fact, the actual contact area between a typical vial and the shelf is only about 5% of the total surface of the vial bottom. Heat transfer is worse when vials are placed in metal trays, since trays can warp considerably and contribute further to poor thermal contact. The interfacial resistance due to lack of good thermal contact between the product and the heat source is amplified by the high vacuum present in the chamber during drying. Estimating the magnitude of this resistance requires an understanding of the nature of thermal conductivity of gases at low pressure; a detailed description is given in Refs. 9 and 19.

To illustrate this point, the example discussed above is used to analyze heat transfer under actual process conditions. Vials of the same dimensions and fill volume as described above are placed on an aluminum tray and freeze dried in a pilot freeze dryer equipped with a thief to remove pre-weighed samples during primary drying, thereby allowing measurement of the drying rate (20). Instead of water, the vials contain a formulation (methylprednisolone sodium succinate in phosphate buffer) to be freeze dried. In this study, the primary drying rate was measured at a constant shelf temperature (45°C) as a function of chamber pressure. Weight loss vs. time during primary drying for several pressures is shown in Fig. 14. At a chamber pressure of 40 μm Hg, the slope of the weight loss vs. time plot indicates an average drying rate of 0.081 g^{-1} cm^{-2} h^{-1}. The average product temperature during primary drying is about -18°C. It has been shown that over 90% of the total resistance to heat transfer is accounted for by the vapor phase between materials.

Assuming that the composition of the vapor phase is entirely water vapor during primary drying—a good assumption—and using the value for

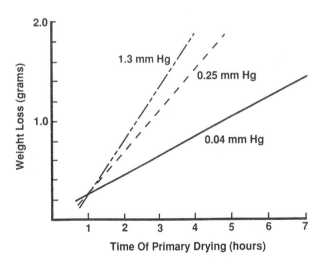

Figure 14 Weight loss vs. time during primary drying for methylprednisolone sodium succinate formulation.

the free molecular conductance of water vapor at 40 μm Hg, the predicted thermal conductance is 0.908 cal $°C^{-1}$ h^{-1} cm^{-2}. The resistance is the reciprocal of this value, or 1.10 cal^{-1} °C h cm^2, which is very close to the experimentally derived value above. Note that, unlike the other materials, the resistance of the gas phase does not depend on the thickness of the gaps in the system as long as molecular flow conditions apply. As the transition range is reached at higher drying pressures, deviations between resistance calculated using free molecular conductance values and experimentally derived resistance become larger.

The linearity of the weight loss vs. time plots in Figure 14 means that the controlling resistance is something other than the frozen product. If thermal resistance of the frozen product were controlling, the rate of weight loss would be expected to increase with drying time, since the thickness of the frozen layer decreases with time.

1. Effect of Chamber Pressure

a. Heat Transfer by Conduction. The effect of chamber pressure on primary drying rate for the system described above is illustrated in Fig. 15. The drying rate increases sharply, and nearly linearly, at chamber pressures below about 200 μm. Above this value, the drying rate vs. pressure profile levels off and increases only slightly with continued increase in pressure above about 400 μm. This is again consistent with a *heat transfer-limited* process, where the *controlling resistance* is the vapor phase present at the interfaces between several materials in series between the heat source and the sublimation interface. At low pressures, which are at or near free molecular flow

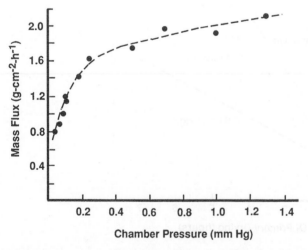

Figure 15 Effect of chamber pressure on primary drying for methylprednisolone sodium succinate formulation.

conditions, this limiting resistance increases linearly with pressure. At higher pressures, where the flow is transitional, the limiting resistance becomes less dependent on system pressure.

Of course, these observations are valid only for the formulation studied. In this case, the drug crystallizes during freezing and has a high (about -8°C) eutectic point. For amorphous solutes, the tendency to collapse may result in a mass transfer-limited process, which would result in an entirely different relationship between chamber pressure and drying rate.

b. Heat Transfer by Thermal Radiation. Heat transfer by thermal radiation is different from heat transfer by either conduction or convection. Unlike conduction or convection, matter is not required for heat transfer by thermal radiation. In fact, the presence of any material between bodies exchanging heat by radiation impedes heat transfer. In conduction and convection, the amount of heat transfer depends on the temperature difference. In radiation, the amount of heat transfer depends not only on the temperature difference between bodies but also on the absolute temperature. The quality of the radiation (the wavelength, or frequency) also depends on the absolute temperature. When thermal radiation strikes a surface, it may be absorbed, reflected, or transmitted.

It has been calculated that thermal radiation could account for about 5% of the measured heat transfer in the freeze drying process under the conditions described above. This is consistent with the above discussion, where free molecular conductance of water vapor alone accounts for nearly all of the total heat transfer, irrespective of other competing mechanisms.

The above examples show that the surface emissivity of materials is a critical factor in radiative heat transfer. Introducing an aluminum tray reduces heat transfer by a factor of about 5. It can be shown that replacing the aluminum tray with a stainless steel tray significantly increases the potential contribution of radiative heat transfer.

In summary, heat transfer by thermal radiation can contribute a small fraction of the total heat transfer, depending on the configuration of the system (e.g., tray vs. vials directly on the shelf) and the materials used. However, in conventional freeze drying of pharmaceuticals, conduction is the dominant heat transfer mechanism, and the limiting resistance is usually the interfacial resistance caused by poor thermal contact between materials. The resistance of this interface is determined by water vapor during primary drying, and at the low end of the operating pressure range in freeze drying this resistance can be estimated using the free molecular conductance of water vapor.

E. Mass Transfer in Primary Drying

Mass transfer in primary drying refers to the transfer of water vapor from the product through open channels, remaining after the sublimation of ice, to the condenser. The sublimation rate is expressed as

$$\text{Sublimation rate} = \frac{\text{pressure difference}}{\text{resistance}} \tag{1}$$

Thus the rate of transfer is the ratio of a driving force (pressure difference) to a resistance. Resistance is used here instead of permeability (the reciprocal of resistance) because resistances in series are additive. Referring to Fig. 16, the total resistance to mass transfer is the sum of several resistances in series—the "dried" product, the vial (usually including a partially inserted stopper), and the chamber. Analysis of mass transfer resistance follows the same form as analysis of the series of resistances to heat transfer discussed above. For heat transfer, individual resistances are analyzed by measuring temperature differences. In mass transfer, resistances are analyzed by measuring pressure differences.

Excellent basic work on heat and mass transfer in freeze drying has been done by M. J. Pikal and coworkers (17,21,22). Vial freeze drying experiments were carried out by attaching a glass tube to the head space of a vial that was connected to an external pressure sensor, allowing continuous monitoring of partial pressure of water vapor in the head space of the vial. Based on calculations of resistance from such experiments, the relative resistance values shown in Fig. 16 were obtained. As might be expected, the resistance of the dried product is usually the limiting resistance to water vapor transfer during primary drying. This assumes that the stopper is properly oriented. If the stopper is inserted too far into the neck of the vial, the permeability of the stopper approaches zero.

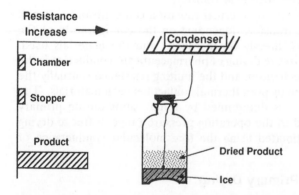

Figure 16 Relative resistance to mass transfer in freeze drying. (Redrawn from Ref. 24.)

1. Vapor Flow in the "Dry" Cake

Mass transfer within the dry layer may occur by two mechanisms: *bulk flow*, the movement of material in the direction of a pressure gradient, or *diffusive flow*, the movement of material by molecular motion from higher concentration to lower concentration (or partial pressure). Bulk flow through the porous bed of dried solute may be either molecular or viscous, depending on the average pressure and the effective pore diameter in the dried matrix. Simatos (23) reports that the range of effective pore diameters in the dried layer is 15 to 600 μm. For example, at a sublimation interface temperature of -20°C, a vial headspace pressure of 100 μm, and an average pore diameter of 50 μm, the mean free path of a water molecule is 90 μm and the Knudsen number is 1.8, corresponding to a molecular flow mechanism in the dried cake. The conductance F, or permeability, is independent of pressure and is inversely proportional to the thickness of the dried layer. Permeability is also directly proportional to the square root of temperature.

For viscous flow of water vapor through the dry layer, the Poiseuille equation, discussed above, applies. It can be shown that the permeability of the product is directly dependent on the average pressure in the system and inversely related to the viscosity of the gas. The flow regime during primary drying is frequently in the transition range, where the flow characteristics change from approximating viscous flow at low Knudsen numbers to those of molecular flow at Knudsen numbers approaching 1; and it can be shown that, regardless of the flow regime during primary drying, the resistance to mass transfer increases as the depth of the dry layer increases.

Pikal (17) reports several types of dependence of dried product resistance on the thickness, none of which corresponds to a simple proportionality to the thickness. For Type I behavior, resistance increases linearly but has a positive value. Type II behavior demonstrates the same linear increase with thickness of the dry layer, but a very high initial resistance is observed, which may correspond to a relatively impermeable skin on the surface of the product that is disrupted after a short time. Types III and IV behaviors both show a diminishing effect of thickness on product resistance.

Regardless of the quantitative relationship it is important to minimize the depth of product in a vial when freeze drying is mass transfer-limited. A cake thickness of less than half the height of the vial is a useful general rule.

Based on the governing equations (9), it is expected that, at least to the extent that vapor flow through the dry layer is viscous, the product resistance should *decrease* with increased average pressure across the cake. Simatos (23) reported that the resistance of freeze dried meat decreases linearly with total pressure in the viscous and transitional flow regimes. Pikal, however, using a microbalance technique, observed increased product resistance with increasing system pressure (17). In addition, the product resistance should decrease with increased temperature. This has been verified experimentally by Pikal and coworkers (21). In general, the resistance of the dry layer increases with concentration of solute. The increase in resistance is roughly proportional to volume percent solid for KCl, while for polyvinylpyrolidone, product resistance is nearly independent of solution concentration between 10% and 23% (21).

The method of freezing can have a substantial effect on the resistance of the dried cake to mass transfer during primary drying. Quast and Karel, studying freeze dried coffee extract, observed a fivefold difference in permeability of dried material to water vapor between fast freezing and very slow freezing, with higher permeability associated with slow freezing (24). In general, the faster the freezing rate, the smaller the ice crystals formed, and the smaller the average pore size created by sublimation of ice. If the dry layer can be represented as a bundle of capillaries, the permeability is expected to increase proportionally to the third power of the average pore diameter for molecular flow and to the fourth power for viscous flow. Moreover, the freezing rate can determine the flow regime, since, for a given pressure, very small pore sizes favor the predominance of molecular flow conditions. As discussed earlier, the resistance of any channel is much higher under molecular flow conditions than under viscous flow conditions.

For shelf freezing, a slow rate of decrease in shelf temperature does not necessarily mean a slow rate of freezing. The effect of supercooling is to promote fast freezing, since, once nucleation starts, the process proceeds rapidly.

Thermal treatment, discussed above, sometimes can be used to offset the effects of fast freezing. After the product is frozen, the temperature is increased to a temperature lower than the melting point, then recooled to a lower temperature. This may result in continuation of ice crystal growth, so that isolated ice crystals can become interconnected, resulting in a continuous channel. Ice crystals can also increase in diameter, which decreases the resistance to the flow of water vapor.

2. Diffusive Flow
Diffusion is mass transfer by molecular motion driven by concentration (or partial pressure) differences in a multicomponent system. In freeze drying, water vapor is usually the only component being transported, so diffusion is not usually relevant as a mass transfer mechanism in freeze drying. Many times, however, transport of water vapor cannot take place by flow through open channels. Sometimes, especially during fast freezing, isolated ice crystals are formed, surrounded by a glassy phase consisting of "unfrozen" water and solute. If the solute collapses at the sublimation front, channels for bulk flow of water vapor may be sealed off by the flow of solute. In either case, the drying rate is determined by the removal of water from the glassy matrix. This is analogous to Knudsen flow through capillaries of molecular dimensions. Based on the discussion above, the rate of drying in

such systems would be expected to be, and is, very slow. For this reason, product collapse and freezing conditions that result in isolated ice crystals should be avoided.

3. Drying Rate for a Mass Transfer-Controlled Process

For the earlier example of a heat transfer-controlled process with the limiting resistance being the intervening gas phase between materials in series, the observed primary drying rate is, as predicted by theory, nearly constant at pressures near the low end of the operating range for freeze drying. When mass transfer is the controlling resistance and the product resistance is limiting, the drying rate would be expected to decrease with time as the thickness of the "dried" product increases. Quantitatively, the drying rate is proportional to the square root of time during primary drying. The reader is referred to Ref. 25 for mathematical details.

IV. SECONDARY DRYING

When ice crystals have been removed from the product by direct sublimation, the product temperature increases sharply (Fig. 3), since the heat of sublimation is no longer required and heat continues to be applied to the product. This abrupt increase in product temperature signals the beginning of secondary drying.

Secondary drying is the removal of unfrozen water. It follows that the amount of residual water to be removed during secondary drying depends mostly on whether the solute, or solutes, crystallize before primary drying. For a crystalline solute, essentially all of the water is present as either eutectic ice or preeutectic ice (Fig. 8). When all ice has sublimed, the only water remaining is water adsorbed to the surface of the solute crystals, unless water of hydration is present within the matrix. In this case, the product is essentially dry when primary drying is complete, and secondary drying is brief.

For an amorphous solute, however, the solute is present in a glassy matrix containing perhaps as much as 40% water. Since there are few, if any, open channels for mass transfer from the interior of the glass phase to the surface, this process must take place by molecular diffusion. Because of the large amount of water to be removed and the slow mechanism of transfer, secondary drying can be the most time-consuming phase of freeze drying for an amorphous solute.

The general practice in freeze drying is to increase the shelf temperature somewhat during secondary drying and to decrease chamber pressure to the lowest attainable level (26,27). This practice is based on the idea that since ice is no longer present and there is no concern about "meltback," the product can withstand higher heat input. Also, the water remaining during secondary drying is more strongly bound, thus requiring more energy for its removal. Decreasing the chamber pressure to the maximum attainable vacuum has traditionally been thought to favor desorption of water.

The approach to establishing optimum process conditions during secondary drying is the same as described in the discussion of primary drying above, i.e., identify the limiting resistance and use conditions that minimize this resistance. Possible resistances include (1) heat transfer to the evaporation zone, (2) diffusion of water within the solid to the surface, (3) evaporation at the surface, (4) transport of water vapor within the porous plug of solids, or (5) transport of water vapor from the head space of the vial to the condenser. At this writing, the only published data dealing with the kinetics of secondary drying in a pharmaceutically relevant system have been those of Pikal and coworkers (28). The rate of drying was studied using a micro-balance and by "quenching" the process by stoppering individual vials at various times during secondary drying in a pilot freeze dryer.

The findings of this study by Pikal et al. were as follows: (1) water content decreased rapidly during the first few hours of secondary drying, reaching a plateau level of residual moisture; (2) this plateau moisture level decreased significantly as drying temperature was increased; (3) chamber pressure had no measurable influence on secondary drying rate at pressures below 200 μm Hg; (4) depth of the freeze dried cake had no measurable effect on secondary drying rate; and (5) drying rate increases significantly as the specific surface area of solids increases. Pikal concluded that the rate-limiting mass transfer process for drying an amorphous solid is either evaporation at the solid-vapor interface or diffusion of water within the solid, probably the former.

The strong dependency of secondary drying rate on specific surface area of solids suggests that the rate of freezing should have a significant impact on the rate of secondary drying. As discussed above, slow freezing is expected to produce relatively large ice crystals and interstitial solid material of low specific surface area: hence a lower rate of secondary drying. Conversely, fast freezing produces small ice crystals and a relatively high specific surface area of solids: thus a faster secondary drying rate. The effect of freezing on drying rate would be expected to be different for primary and secondary drying, fast primary drying being promoted by slow freezing.

Of course, the concept of collapse for an amorphous solute still applies during secondary drying, and if the temperature is raised too soon after the onset of secondary drying, the product temperature may exceed the collapse temperature. As secondary drying proceeds and water is removed from the amorphous system, the viscosity increases, raising the collapse temperature.

A. Role of Residual Water in Stability of Freeze Dried Products

Residual water content is frequently a critical product characteristic with respect to stability of freeze dried products, particularly for proteins (29–31).

The release of "bound," or unfrozen, water during secondary drying is generally described by sorption-desorption isotherms. Weight percent water is usually plotted against partial pressure of water or relative humidity. Sorption-desorption isotherms usually exhibit hysteresis, where the amount of water associated with the solid is greater for the desorption isotherm than for the adsorption isotherm for a given relative humidity. The thermodynamic state of water associated with pharmaceutical systems is a matter of general interest to pharmaceutical scientists (32,33) and has been proposed to exist in three different states: (1) tightly or "irrotationally bound" water, usually existing in a definite stoichiometry with the solid; (2) unbound or bulk water; and (3) an intermediate form, with rotational frequencies reduced relative to liquid water by a factor of 10^4 to 10^5.

There is a critical difference between the water uptake properties of an amorphous solid and the same solid in crystalline form. For crystalline materials, the amount of water adsorbed depends on the available surface area. For amorphous solids, it is possible for water to dissolve in the solid, acting as a plasticizer to reduce the glass transition temperature of the solid T_g. In the frozen amorphous system, where the content of unfrozen water is high, the solute is present in a solution of amorphous water, whereas during secondary drying water exists in a solution of amorphous solid. Glass transitions are important to the properties of the system. If the product temperature is above T_g for the frozen system, collapse occurs. What is less frequently recognized is that the temperature of the "dried" product relative to T_g of the solid also affects the viscosity of the system. If the dried product temperature is 20°C above T_g of the solid, the viscosity decreases from about 10^{13} poise at T_g to 10^8 poise (33), causing a significant increase in the molecular mobility of the solid and the water. This can promote a variety of "solid state" interactions leading to instability of the final product. A small amount of residual moisture in an amorphous system can have a dramatic effect on the glass transition temperature of the solid. Given the large depression of the glass transition temperatures by small amounts of water, it is not surprising that substantial differences in stability are seen for small differences in residual moisture.

V. PROCESS MONITORING

The previous sections all point to the importance of maintaining the appropriate product temperature during freeze drying. Exceeding the maximum allowable product temperature results in loss of the desirable properties of a freeze dried product, and drying at temperatures well below the maximum allowable temperature results in loss of process efficiency and poor utilization of capacity, ultimately requiring unnecessary investment in very expensive facilities and equipment.

The high cost per production lot of many therapeutic agents demands careful attention to process monitoring. One freeze dryer load of some of the newer biotechnology-derived therapeutic agents may represent millions of dollars in sales. This cost may not be recoverable if product is damaged during freeze drying.

Product temperature during freeze drying is determined by the relative rates of heat and mass transfer, which are governed by both the shelf temperature and the chamber pressure. Thus both shelf temperature and chamber pressure are critical process variables. The observed value of these variables depends on the method used for measurement. This is particularly true for pressure measurement.

The first two parts of this section deal with some fundamental and practical aspects of temperature and pressure measurement methods that are relevant to the freeze drying process. The last section presents some techniques to monitor the status of the product during the process, with emphasis on methods that do not depend on monitoring of individual vials.

A. Temperature Measurement

The choice of a thermometer for a particular application depends on the temperature range to be measured (about -80°C to about 120°C for freeze drying) and on sensitivity, accuracy, reproducibility, and cost. For example, a mercury-in-glass thermometer is useless for freeze drying, since mercury freezes at about -38°C. In addition, an electrical output is needed for recording and controlling temperature. The most common temperature measurement methods in freeze drying are resistance thermometers, thermocouples, and, less frequently, thermistors.

1. Resistance Thermometers

Resistance thermometry uses changes in the electrical resistance of metals with temperature to measure temperature. Resistance thermometers, or resistance temperature detectors (RTDs), are commonly available with sensing elements of platinum, nickel, 70% nickel/30% iron (Balco), or copper. Platinum is the most common element because of its commercial availability in very pure form and its linear resistance vs. temperature profile over a range from less than -200°C to around 600°C. Because of its excellent stability and repeatability, the platinum resistance thermometer is the international standard for temperature measurements between the triple point of hydrogen at 13.81K and the freezing point of antimony at 630.75K.

In a typical design of an RTD probe, the platinum wire (diameter 0.025 mm or less) is generally wound around a ceramic tube, followed by another ceramic layer such that the sensing element is completely embedded. This assembly may then be encapsulated within a glass or stainless steel sheath to give maximum protection to the element. Like any thermometer, the RTD senses its own temperature. Since the temperature of interest is that of the surrounding medium, the accuracy of the RTD depends on the ability of the probe to conduct heat from the surrounding medium to the sensing element. The lag time required to conduct heat from the medium being measured to the sensing element is expressed quantitatively as the *time constant* of a particular sensor. The time constant is the time required for the sensor to reach 64% of a step change in temperature. For example, if the sensor is quickly removed from an ice bath at 0°C and placed in boiling water at 100°C, the time constant is the time required for the output of the sensor to reach 64°C. Time constants for RTDs may vary from about 0.1 s for unencapsulated platinum/ceramic elements to 10–20 s for stainless steel encapsulated probes. Since freeze drying is a slow process relative to many other industrial operations, fast response of the RTD is not important.

Because the measuring current heats the element wire, errors in temperature measurement may occur due to self-heating of the probe (34). The magnitude of this error depends on the design of the probe. Choice of the best sensor involves a trade-off between fast response and low self-heating. A small probe with minimum encasing gives fast response but has low surface area to dissipate heat. Encasing the probe to provide a large surface area helps to dissipate heat but slows response. Of course, the magnitude of the self-heating error depends on the heat transfer characteristics of the medium being measured. Given that the sublimation rate will probably be on the order of 0.5 g/h, the self-heating effect only accounts for perhaps a 0.02% error. For reasons discussed below, it is true that monitored vials are somewhat nonrepresentative of the entire batch, and this must be kept in mind when using individual vials to monitor the process. However, the nonrepresentative nature of these vials does not arise from the RTD self-heating effect.

Because of the construction of a resistance temperature detector, the temperature sensed is an average temperature over the surface of the probe. Where this is not desired, the effect can be minimized by using tip-sensitive probes, where temperature is sensed through a copper-alloy tip. Many configurations of RTD are available for specialized applications. Ribbon-type RTDs are useful in freeze drying for determination of shelf surface temperature or for measuring the temperature of the surface of a pipe.

Resistance of the sensing element is typically measured by a Wheatstone bridge circuit to compare the potential drop across the sensing element with the drop across a standard resistor carrying the same current. The measured resistance includes not only the sensing element but also the wire leads. The leads, unless of very low resistance, can be a significant source of error. The error will be proportionately larger at low temperatures because of the decreasing resistance of the sensing element with temperature. For this reason, the three-wire circuit is the most widely used method in industrial applications. The circuit is configured such that the third lead compensates for lead wire resistance by dividing the resistance of the two lead wires equally between both arms of the Wheatstone bridge circuit.

In summary, resistance temperature detectors are well suited to monitoring temperatures in the freeze dry process. RTDs are sensitive, accurate, and reproducible over the range of temperatures encountered in the process. Two limitations of RTDs—relatively slow response time and the self-heating effect—are not significant drawbacks for freeze drying applications.

2. Thermocouples

The thermocouple is based on the principle that when a circuit is formed by joining the ends of two wires made from different metals, and the junction is exposed to different temperatures, an electrical potential (emf) develops between the two wires that is directly related to the temperature difference, and a current flow in the circuit. The thermocouple is the most widely used temperature-measuring device for industrial applications. Since the voltage produced by the thermocouple is a function of the difference in temperature between the hot (or measuring) and cold junctions, the temperature of the cold junction must be known. For laboratory measurements, an ice bath is generally used. For industrial applications, an electronic bridge circuit is used, which makes it appear that the thermocouple has been referenced to some fixed temperature. While any two dissimilar conductors will develop an emf when their junctions are at different temperatures, only a few combinations have been put to practical use. The most widely used thermocouple types are as follows:

Type	Materials
S	Platinum-platinum 10% rhodium
R	Platinum-platinum 13% rhodium
J	Iron-constantan
T	Cooper-constantan
K	Chromel-Alumel
E	Chromel-constantan

The type J thermocouple is not recommended for use below 0°C because of possible rusting and embrittlement of the iron. Type T thermocouples are recommended for low-temperature work. Type E is also suitable for subzero temperatures, since chromel-constantan has the highest emf output of any standard thermocouple. Types T and E can be used at temperatures as low as 50K. Thermocouples have several advantages over RTDs: (1) faster response—using very thin wires, time constants of a few milliseconds can be obtained; (2) ruggedness—thermocouples are well suited to applications requiring resistance to mechanical shock; (3) high temperature capability—

thermocouples with noble metal junctions may be rated as high as 1800°C; (4) point sensing—by using thin wires, temperatures can be measured at very precise locations; (5) cost—thermocouple probes are inexpensive; however, for long lead runs, cost will escalate considerably; (6) no self-heating error—because of the very low voltage developed by a thermocouple circuit, self-heating error is negligible.

Limitations of thermocouples include (1) repeatability and stability-thermocouples are less repeatable and less stable than RTDs; (2) nonlinearity—since the emf vs. temperature plot is nonlinear, careful attention to calibration is necessary; (3) accuracy—limits of error are wider for thermocouples than for RTDs; (4) leads—only thermocouple wire may be used. For remote location measurements, this can add significantly to the system cost.

As with RTDs, a large variety of configurations, including surface probes, are available.

3. Thermistors

Thermistors belong to a class of solids known as semiconductors and are generally made from nickel, cobalt, and manganese oxides. The resistance of thermistors varies sharply with temperature and, in comparison with resistance thermometers and thermocouples, thermistors have the following advantages: (1) they have a temperature coefficient of resistance about 10 times that of metals, with correspondingly greater sensitivity; (2) they have a much higher resistance than metals, eliminating any measurement errors due to resistance of lead wires; (3) no cold junction compensation is necessary with thermistors; (4) they have a negative coefficient of resistance, which means that resistance increases with decreasing temperature. Thus sensitivity increases with decreasing temperature.

Thus over a limited temperature range, thermistors would seem to offer all the best features of resistance thermometers and thermocouples, with better sensitivity than either. However, thermistors have some disadvantages and limitations: (1) the temperature-resistance relationship is nonlinear, with the resistance varying exponentially with temperature; (2) relatively high variation in resistance between thermistors of a given type (+20%), which means that thermistors of a given type cannot always be used interchangeably with a common calibration; (3) thermistors have a narrow temperature range over which the calibration is stable. Thermistors are not widely used in industrial freeze drying applications.

B. Pressure Measurement

Accurate measurement of pressure is critical in freeze drying, since pressure affects both heat and mass transfer. The methods discussed here are the mercury manometer, the mechanical manometer, the thermal conductivity manometer, and the capacitance manometer.

1. Mercury Manometer

The mercury manometer provides a direct measurement of pressure and is considered a primary standard for such measurements. A common type of mercury manometer is the McLeod gauge. Since this type of gauge is not accurate when water vapor is present (19), and because of the mercury used in the system, these gauges are not typically used for monitoring in the manufacture of pharmaceuticals.

2. Thermal Conductivity Gauges

As discussed in the heat transfer section above, energy is dissipated from a heated surface in a gas at low pressure by radiation and by conduction. The sensitivity of the conductivity method for determination of pressure depends on the following: (1) energy loss from the filament by radiation being small relative to energy loss by conduction; (2) free molecular flow, i.e., pressure below about 100 μm; (3) constant gas phase composition.

The energy loss by thermal radiation for a perfect radiator is about 100 times that due to conduction by a gas (19). For this reason, the filament used should have as low a value of emissivity as possible. Platinum is commonly used, which has an emissivity in the range of 0.03 to 0.10. The response is nearly linear in the range of 10^{-2} to 10^{-1} mm Hg (10 to 100 μm). Above 100 μm, the sensitivity decreases rapidly and vanishes at about 1 mm (1000 μm), as the flow regime changes from molecular to transition.

In summary, thermal conductivity gauges are subject to several sources of error: (1) As the filament becomes oxidized or otherwise contaminated with foreign material, the emissivity of the surface increases. This leads to significant energy loss by radiation, thus leading to errors in measuring an unknown pressure. (2) The sensitivity decreases markedly above about 100 μm. Also, the output signal becomes nonlinear. In the case of an analog meter, this nonlinearity can be compensated for by a nonlinear scale. In the case of digital readout, the output must be linearized by appropriate analog or digital circuitry. (3) As the composition of gas in the system of interest changes, errors are introduced because the functional relationship between rate of energy loss from the filament and pressure depends on the gas present. Strictly speaking, the gauge is accurate only for the gas used when the instrument is calibrated, generally nitrogen.

Another type of thermal conductivity gauge is the Pirani gauge. The principle is the same; however, the change in resistance is monitored as a function of pressure, using a Wheatstone bridge circuit, when the current is held constant.

3. Mechanical Manometers

Mechanical manometers depend on the measurement of mechanical deformation of a thin wall or diaphragm under pressure. Measurement is done by admitting the unknown pressure to a hermetically sealed instrument case, where it exerts a pressure on a flat evacuated capsule that has been permanently sealed. Movement of the capsule is transmitted by a lever system to the pointer that registers pressure on the dial.

Mechanical manometers have the advantage of simplicity, low cost, no need for auxiliary electrical equipment, and measurement of pressure independent of the nature of the gas. Disadvantages are a lower limit of about 0.2 mm Hg and no electrical signal to use for recording or controlling pressure. Mechanical manometers are useful instruments for freeze dryers, particularly as troubleshooting aids.

4. Capacitance Manometer

The capacitance of any capacitor is directly proportional to the dielectric constant of the medium relative to that of air, and to a geometry factor. All capacitance transducers operate either by varying the dielectric constant while holding the geometry constant or by varying the geometry with a constant dielectric constant. A flexible metal diaphragm (usually made of Inconel) is placed between two fixed electrodes. The reference side of the diaphragm is evacuated to 10^{-7} torr and sealed to provide a zero reference pressure. A change in the output voltage due to a change in capacitance of the parallel plate capacitor is directly proportional to the applied pressure. The diaphragm deflection is a measure of the force per unit area; thus it represents a true total pressure independent of gas phase composition.

Capacitance manometers used in freeze drying have a range of 0.1 to 1000 μm or 1 μm to 10 torr, and accuracy ranging from 0.05% to 3% of reading, depending on the model chosen (35). Sources of error in pressure measurement with the capacitance manometer include temperature effects and hysteresis effects arising from over-pressurization of the sensor (35). In recent years, capacitance manometers have become widely used for measurement and control of pressure in the freeze drying process.

C. Process Monitoring Techniques

The traditional method of process monitoring is to place thermocouples or RTDs in several vials of product and record product temperature throughout the freeze dry cycle (Fig. 3). Freezing, primary drying, and secondary drying are easily identifiable, making product temperature monitoring a valuable tool for cycle development and scale-up. However, there are several aspects of product temperature monitoring that should be kept in mind by the development scientist. Most importantly, the presence of a temperature probe in a vial acts as a site for heterogeneous nucleation of ice, thereby reducing the extent of supercooling relative to nonmonitored vials (36). Since monitored vials freeze first, "soak times" are generally used as a process control strategy for automated cycle sequencing in order to assure that all vials are frozen prior to evacuating the system. A soak timer generally is started when all monitored vials reach a programmed temperature, indicative of complete solidification of the product. After the predetermined soak time elapses, the process continues.

Because monitored vials supercool less and freeze sooner, they also freeze more slowly and have larger ice crystals (thus larger pores in the dried matrix), less resistance to mass transfer, and a faster drying rate than nonmonitored vials. Thus the nonrepresentative nature of monitored vials arising from differences in supercooling characteristics carries over from the freezing process to the drying process. Analysis of production data by Pikal (36) shows that for every 10°C increase in supercooling, the resistance of the dried product to mass transfer increases by 33%, the mean product temperature increases by 0.9°C, and the drying time increases by about 10%. This means that in order to assure product dryness at the nominal end of a freeze dry cycle, a second soak time should be used.

There are other drawbacks to product temperature monitoring as a routine process-monitoring technique. The trend in the parenteral products industry is to move toward better assurance of product sterility by developing technology that places absolute barriers between operators and product, preventing accidental introduction of microorganisms into the product via the operator. Placement of temperature probes in individual vials of product requires an operator to come into close proximity with trays of sterile product. Because of edge effects and tray warpage, the most meaningful location for a monitored vial is the center of the tray, since the center vials are usually the last to freeze and the last to dry. Placement of temperature measurement probes in the center of a tray requires reaching over vials, thereby compromising sterility. Also, any automated system that sequences the freeze dry cycle based on product temperature data must have a way of dealing with erroneous temperature data arising from vials that tip over after probe placement, vials for which the temperature probe is not in contact with product, and probes with faulty lead wires or bad connections to the external circuitry. For these reasons, the development scientist should look for opportunities to improve process monitoring by using techniques that are not dependent on data from individual vials. Some of these techniques, mostly applicable to detecting the end point of drying, are reviewed below.

Product electrical resistance can also be used to monitor and control the freeze dry cycle (11). Since this technique also involves introduction of a probe into individual vials, the same considerations apply as with product temperature measurement.

1. Comparative Pressure Measurement

In the discussion above, it was shown that thermal conductivity pressure gauges are sensitive to gas phase composition due to differences in thermal conductivity. Since the free molecular conductivity of water vapor is considerably higher than that of nitrogen or air, this gauge is preferentially sensitive to water vapor. The capacitance manometer, on the other hand, measures

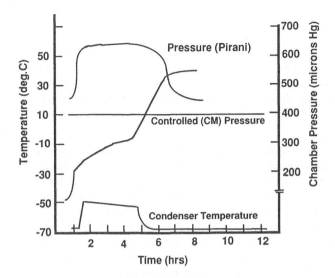

Figure 17   Detection of process end point by comparative pressure measurement. CM = capacitance manometer.

force per unit area, independent of gas phase composition. If pressure is controlled at a constant value using a capacitance manometer in a pressure control loop, and chamber pressure is simultaneously monitored by a thermal conductivity-type gauge, an output similar to that shown in Fig. 17 is observed (37). The output of the thermal conductivity gauge increases relative to that of the capacitance manometer at the beginning of drying, reaches a steady-state value during primary drying, and decreases to a new steady-state value as the end of drying is reached. In this way, the thermal conductivity gauge gives information about the status of the drying cycle without the need to place probes in individual vials. Note that the absolute value of the pressure as measured by the thermal conductivity gauge is not important, only the change in response as the partial pressure of water vapor decreases.

2. Pressure Rise

A feature offered on some commercial freeze dry automation packages is the ability to close the main valve intermittently between the chamber and the condenser for a short period of time as the drying cycle approaches the end point. When water vapor is still being released from the product, the pressure rises quickly. As the product dries, the pressure rise decreases. When the pressure rise reaches the background leak rate of the chamber, no additional water is being removed from the product (37).

Successful application of the pressure rise method of cycle end point detection requires a low, and constant, leak rate of the freeze dry chamber, since the method assumes that the increase in pressure with the main valve closed is entirely due to water vapor. It is necessary to test frequently the leak rate of the chamber to establish a baseline leak rate. Frequent leak rate testing is even more important after the system is steam sterilized, since it is common for the high temperature of steam sterilization to cause leaks in the system.

3. Trap Method

A process-monitoring technique reported by Pikal and coworkers (38) uses a capacitance manometer along with an in-line cold trap and a valve between the trap and the freeze dry chamber. The vapor composition in the chamber is determined by first measuring the total pressure in the chamber with the isolation valve open and the cold trap at ambient temperature. Then the isolation valve is closed, trapping a sample of the vapor phase from the process, and the cold finger is cooled to -78°C with dry ice. Since the vapor pressure of ice at this temperature is negligible, the capacitance manometer reading, after allowing time for equilibration, is the pressure of noncondensable gases in the sample. Partial pressure of water vapor is determined by the difference between the initial and the final reading. Since this method requires operator intervention and equilibration times, it is probably better suited to laboratory or pilot studies than to production process monitoring.

4. Electronic Hygrometer

Electronic hygrometers measure dew point, or frost point, by one of two types of sensors: (1) optical measurement of condensation of water on a mirror where the surface temperature is carefully controlled, or (2) measurement of capacitance of an aluminum oxide capacitor where the capacitance is a function of the extent of water vapor adsorption to the capacitor. While not widely applied to freeze drying, such sensors have been shown to detect the end point of freeze drying (39).

5. Residual Gas Analysis

A residual gas analyzer (RGA) is a small quadrapole mass spectrometer, generally limited to mass-to-charge ratios (m/e) of 200 or less. Mass spectrometers operate at pressures of 10^{-6} torr or less, requiring a diffusion pump. Since freeze dryers operate at much higher pressures, the vapor phase inside the freeze dryer is analyzed by a small bleed stream from the freeze dryer to the RGA. The simplest form of residual gas analyzer is the helium leak detector, for which the analyzer senses a single m/e signal of 2. Leaks in the system are located by trial and error with helium at a likely point of leakage with the operator watching for a signal from the detector.

With the ability to obtain a mass spectrum of the vapor phase within the freeze dryer, the RGA gives more information than detection of leaks. Measurement of water vapor partial pressure can provide an accurate measurement of cycle end point. Backstreaming of fractionated pump oil can be detected for process validation purposes (40), as well as outgassing of elastomeric closures (41) and sublimation of low molecular weight volatile components of a formulation.

6. Sequential Stoppering

While sequential stoppering is not a technique for routine process monitoring, it should be mentioned as a tool for cycle development, particularly for scale-up from pilot freeze dryers to production equipment. Sequential stoppering is used in freeze dryers with hydraulically movable shelves for internal stoppering, where vials on one shelf at a time are stoppered to "quench" the freeze dry process at various times as the process approaches the end point. In this way, a number of points on the moisture content vs. drying time curve (depending on the number of shelves in the dryer) can be obtained with a single run. This allows more efficient definition of the appropriate cycle end point.

7. Sample Thief

Most manufacturers of commercial freeze dry equipment offer some type of sample thief, which allows removal of vials during the cycle without disturbing process conditions. Such thieves come in a variety of configurations, but all consist of a movable arm with an externally activated mechanism to grip the neck of a vial and move it to a vacuum lock. A separate vacuum pump is provided to evacuate the vacuum lock after the sample is removed. Sample thieves are generally limited to the removal of vials from one shelf and may not reach to all areas of the shelf. Of course, lids on the trays prevent the use of a sample thief.

VI. FREEZE DRY EQUIPMENT

A freeze drying system for production of pharmaceutical dosage forms consists of a chamber containing shelves through which a heat transfer fluid can be circulated; a system for pumping, heating, and cooling the fluid; a vacuum pumping system; a condenser for trapping water vapor; and a refrigeration system for cooling the condenser. In recent years, a system for sterilization of the chamber/condenser has also become mandatory. In addition to these essential components, pharmaceutical freeze dryers may also incorporate systems for stoppering vials within the chamber, automatic clean-in-place (CIP) equipment, and, more recently, sophisticated mechanisms for automatic loading and unloading of vials. Computerized monitoring and control of freeze dryers has become widespread in the last 10 years. A modern pharmaceutical freeze dryer requires a large capital investment, with the cost of large production units approaching $1 million each. On the other hand, the value of a batch of product has increased drastically with the development of therapeutic proteins derived from recombinant DNA technology. The value of one freeze dryer load of a product such as tissue plasminogen activator or erythropoietin may well be more than the cost of the equipment itself; thus it is important to design freeze dryers with adequate redundancy in both equipment and control systems. Below is an overview of some of the important equipment used in freeze drying as well as some general design considerations.

A. Vacuum System

By far the most common type of vacuum pump in freeze drying is the rotary oil pump. The pump consists of a steel cylinder rotating eccentrically within a round casing. The gas being pumped is admitted into the casing via an inlet valve, compressed, and forced out a discharge valve. Oil serves both as a lubricant and as a sealant to prevent back diffusion of gas past the rotating cylinder.

There is generally a trade-off between pumping speed and attainable vacuum—the higher the attainable vacuum, the lower the pumping speed. For this reason, pumps with very high attainable vacuum, such as diffusion pumps, are backed by one or more "roughing" pumps that discharge directly to the atmosphere.

Rotary oil pumps are designed to discharge at atmospheric pressure and are able to achieve vacuum as low as about 1 μm Hg. Thus compression ratios are very high, on the order of 10^3 to 10^6. Because of the high compression ratios, condensation or dissolution of vapor in the oil can result when water vapor is present, forming an emulsion. This causes a sharp reduction in pumping speed and the lowest attainable vacuum. This is a particular concern in freeze drying, since water is the predominant vapor. Therefore, effective trapping of water vapor by the condenser is essential to proper operation of the vacuum system. Even so, some water vapor will bypass the condenser and enter the pump. The most practical method for handling this problem is the use of gas ballast. This method consists of admitting air into the pump chamber after the chamber has been shut off from the inlet side of the pump. The result is to decrease the compression ratio and prevent condensation of vapor. Also, using gas ballast, the pumping speed decreases and the lowest attainable pressure increases.

The exhaust from a rotary oil pump contains a fine mist of oil droplets. The use of gas ballast increases the rate of oil loss from the pump, so more frequent addition of oil is necessary. Regardless of whether gas ballast is used, a trap on the outlet of the pump to collect the oil mist is advisable. Many users leave the gas ballast control on during primary drying, then turn it off during secondary drying to reach the lowest possible pressure in the chamber.

Since the vacuum pump is critical to the integrity of the freeze drying operation, redundant equipment is important. Since the main vacuum pump is usually a rotary oil pump, an extra pump should be designed into the system as a "live" spare.

Roots-type pumps, or Roots blowers, are frequently used on vacuum systems for freeze drying and comprise two figure eight-shaped rotors that counter rotate without touching each other or the chamber walls. There are no inlet or discharge valves, and the rotors do not require any oil or other fluid for lubrication. The function of the Roots pump is to increase the speed of the pumping system by about a factor of 10, and to also increase the lowest attainable vacuum. They will not discharge directly to atmosphere, so they are always used in combination with, or backed by, another pump such as a rotary oil pump. Roots pumps are not turned on until a rough vacuum has been attained; they typically "windmill" until a pressure of about 25 mm Hg has been reached, then are turned on automatically.

A more recent development in vacuum technology is the "dry" pump which is used primarily in the semiconductor industry, where an ultraclean environment is critical. Dry pumps are similar to Roots pumps except that an interlocking, claw-shaped rotor is used to form a more positive seal.

Water ring pumps are often incorporated into modern freeze drying systems, although they are not used in the freeze dry process per se but rather are used for steam sterilization operations. Water ring pumps are the primary vacuum system for autoclaves and other "wet" applications. They consist of a rotor mounted in a circular casing, where the clearance between rotor and casing is larger at the top than at the bottom. The rotor blades are shrouded at the sides to form a series of chambers. At the point in a revolution where the rotor blades are nearly touching the housing, the chamber is filled with water. Because of centrifugal force and the eccentric mounting of the rotor, the water in the chamber recedes as the rotor advances through a revolution until, at the top of the cycle, the rotor chamber is nearly empty. As the water in the chamber recedes, the inlet stream is drawn through an inlet port in the stationary housing. As the rotor turns and water is forced back into the chamber, the compressed inlet stream is discharged through another port in the housing. The water used as the compressant also forms the seal between the rotor and the casing and is referred to as the seal water. Constant replacement or external recirculation of the seal water is necessary in order to prevent overheating.

The attainable vacuum of a water ring pump is determined by the vapor pressure of the seal water, which in turn is determined by the seal water temperature. At 25°C, the vapor pressure of water is 23.75 mm Hg. This is nearly two orders of magnitude larger than the pressure needed for freeze drying but is still greater than 29 inches of mercury vacuum. This is more than adequate for sterilization applications. In practice, a water ring pump will begin to cavitate before it reaches the pressure determined by the seal water temperature. The pumping speed and the attainable vacuum of a water ring pump can be enhanced by using an air ejector between the system being evacuated and the pump. The air ejector is a simple device with no moving parts, consisting primarily of a drive nozzle and a diffuser. Air at atmospheric pressure is drawn into the ejector and accelerated in the diffuser at ultrasonic speed. This acts as an aspirator, creating a suction that accelerates the gas being pumped. The pressure at the outlet of the diffuser is in the range of 50 to 80 mbar.

B. Refrigeration

Refrigeration is required both for cooling the shelves during freezing of product and for cooling the condenser during drying. The condenser is generally cooled by direct expansion of the refrigerant, usually a fluorohydro-carbon, in the condenser coils. The refrigerant evaporates in the condenser coils, withdrawing the latent heat of sublimation from the condenser. Vapor is drawn from the freeze drying condenser by a compressor and pumped to a condenser at a higher pressure. In the condenser, cooling water causes the compressed vapor to liquefy, and the condensed refrigerant is collected in a receiver. The liquid refrigerant is returned to the cooling coils via an expansion valve and the cycle is repeated.

The temperature of the cooling water required for condensation of the compressed vapor depends on the type of refrigerant used; care should be taken to assure that the available cooling water is compatible with the requirements of the refrigerant. Cooling of the heat transfer fluid to the shelves is accomplished by one or more heat exchangers in the circuit. Generally, refrigeration can be switched from the condenser to the heat transfer fluid during freezing of product, and back to the condenser during drying.

Redundant compressors are necessary for reliability of production freeze drying equipment. If the refrigeration load requires four compressors, for example, at least two additional units should be included as live backup in the event of compressor failure.

As the concern over the use of chlorofluorocarbons increases, alternative compounds will be introduced. This may necessitate changes in the type or capacity of compressors currently being used. When purchasing a new freeze dryer or upgrading an existing unit, this issue should be discussed with the manufacturer of the equipment.

C. Heat Transfer Fluid

The most common types of heat transfer fluid are silicone oil, trichloroethy-lene (TCE), and Lexol, an oil similar to kerosene. Silicone oil is by far the most common. Trichloroethylene has been phased out, for the most part, due to safety concerns.

D. Condenser Design

There are two basic types of condenser configuration, internal and external. For the internal design, condenser plates or coils are mounted either along the side walls of the chamber or in the bottom of the chamber. In the external arrangement, a separate condenser chamber, again containing either refrigerated plates or coils, is connected to the dryer chamber by means of a very short, large diameter pipe containing a valve to isolate the chamber from the condenser.

There are some advantages to an internal condenser design, including lower cost, less floor space required, and a less complicated system to sterilize. However, most production scale freeze dryers use an external condenser.

There are several reasons for this. First, placing the condenser between the product and the vacuum pump allows for more effective trapping of water vapor by the condenser and minimizes the quantity of water vapor that gets to the pump. For the same reason, this design helps to minimize the quantity of backstreaming hydrocarbons from the pump to the freeze dryer. Second, the external design allows for more uniform buildup of ice on the condenser and thus more efficient use of condenser surface area. Internally mounted condenser plates tend to collect ice only on the side of the plate toward the product. Third, use of an external condenser allows more than one lot of product to be freeze dried before the condenser is defrosted, provided that the condenser is adequately sized. Finally, an external condenser is necessary if certain in-process tests like the pressure rise test for residual moisture, discussed above, are to be used.

E. General Construction Considerations

Pharmaceutical freeze dryer chambers and condensers are usually constructed of type 304 or 316 stainless steel, and they should be pressure-rated vessels to accommodate steam sterilization. Internal surfaces should be mechanically polished (320 grit) for cleanability and passivated for improved corrosion resistance. All internal surfaces should be free draining to eliminate standing water after either cleaning or steam sterilization. Most freeze dryers have hydraulically movable shelves to insert lyostoppers into vials after drying is complete (internal stoppering). Several designs are available, including a single piston that enters the chamber from either above or below to push the shelves together. Shelves may also be drawn together by pulling shelf support rods out of the chamber from above. Regardless of the design used, it is important that no nonsterile element be allowed to enter the sterile chamber while product is present. All drains must incorporate a break in the drain line to prevent the contents of a drain from backing up into the chamber or condenser.

F. Sterilization of Freeze Dryers

The most common method of sterilization of freeze dryers is steam under a pressure of about 15 psi, which corresponds to a temperature of about 121°C. Some units are sterilized by ethylene oxide (EtO), but this agent has come under increased regulatory scrutiny, with respect to both residual ethylene oxide (or its byproducts) in the product and exposure of workers to ethylene oxide. Most companies are seeking to eliminate EtO in all pharmaceutical manufacturing operations. Some older freeze dryers are not pressure-rated vessels and will not withstand steam sterilization. These units are generally sanitized by a chemical sanitizing agent. The principal objection to the use of chemical sanitization is that many internal surfaces are not easily reached by manual application of a disinfectant solution. Also, the piping for introduction of air or nitrogen is not easily sanitized. FDA inspection guidelines concerning freeze dryers state the following: (1) Freeze dryers should be steam sterilized prior to every lot, including both the chamber and condenser. (2) Validation of freeze dryer sterilization should follow the same approach as validation of an autoclave. Two independent temperature recording systems should be used, one to monitor and control temperature and the other to monitor the cool point in the system. (3) Provisions should be made for sterilizing the lines used for the introduction of air, nitrogen, or other gas. (4) Provisions should be made for sterilization and integrity testing of vent filters. (5) Sterilization should include the shelf support rods.

Given the high temperatures of steam sterilization, equipment cool-down time has a large impact on equipment turnaround time. This can be minimized by the use of cooling jackets on the chamber and condenser. Water cooling of the freeze dryer door is particularly important, since the door is the slowest component to cool.

G. Vacuum Integrity Testing

The vacuum integrity of the freeze dryer chamber/condenser should be monitored routinely, since a leak of nonsterile air into the system will compromise asepsis. Monitoring is easily done by evacuating the system to a known pressure (for example, 100 μm), closing the valve between the vacuum pump and the freeze dryer, and measuring the increase in pressure for at least 15 min. Ideally, this should be done when the freeze dryer is first put into service to establish baseline data. An increased leakage rate can indicate the need to replace such components as door gaskets and seals. Leaks in the system are generally located by means of a helium leak detector.

VII. CASE STUDY: DEVELOPMENT OF A FREEZE DRIED PROTEIN FORMULATION

The theoretical aspects of lyophilization provide the basis for efficient and effective development of freeze dried products, including formulation development and identification of processing conditions that result in a product that is quickly and easily reconstituted, recovers full potency on reconstitution, and is stable during storage as a freeze dried solid. The following case study illustrates the sequence of activities in the development of a freeze dried product: (1) determination of the freezing characteristics of the formulation, (2) selection of conditions for primary and secondary drying, and (3) process scale-up.

A formulation of a therapeutic protein to be freeze dried contains 1.0 mg/mL of protein in 0.05 M phosphate buffer at pH 7.5. The formulation also contains 0.05% Tween 80 and 6% sucrose, both of which are stabilizers. Human serum albumin (HSA) at 1.0 mg/mL is also in the formulation to minimize loss of the protein due to surface adsorption.

The purpose of formulation characterization is to determine the maximum allowable product temperature during primary drying. For this formulation, analysis by DSC reveals a glass transition at −34°C. This indicates that sucrose is the predominant component in determining the physical characteristics of the formulation, since sucrose alone has a glass transition at this temperature. This means that product temperature must remain below about −34°C during primary drying in order to avoid product collapse.

When the maximum allowable product temperature is determined, the freezing temperature can be specified. Because of the low collapse temperature, freezing the product to −40°C or below is indicated. In order to provide an adequate safety margin to guard against potential loss of product, keeping the product temperature at least 3 to 4°C below the collapse temperature throughout the cycle is necessary.

Next, temperature and pressure conditions during primary drying must be established. While the above discussion of process monitoring has pointed out the limitations of product temperature measurement as a routine process monitoring technique, measurement of product temperature is essential for cycle development and scale-up in order to establish the relationship between shelf temperature, chamber pressure, and product temperature. The product temperature resulting from a given shelf temperature and chamber pressure depends on the relative rates of heat transfer from the shelf to the product and mass transfer of water vapor from the sublimation zone to the condenser. Relative rates of heat and mass transfer depend on the system geometry, including the depth of fill in each vial, the type of vial (tubing or molded; molded vials, because of the more concave bottom surface, have a higher interfacial, or contact, resistance to conductive heat transfer than tubing vials), whether metal trays are used, the type of material used for the trays, and the condition of the trays (warped or flat).

Estimates of this relationship can be obtained by monitoring the product temperature during lyophilization at a given shelf temperature and chamber pressure. The chamber pressure can be changed stepwise at constant shelf temperature, allowing time for equilibration between changes in set point and observing the resulting change in product temperature. A plot of product temperature as a function of shelf temperature at different chamber

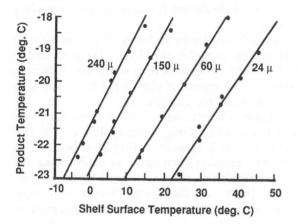

Figure 18 Product temperature vs. shelf temperature at various chamber pressures.

pressures is illustrated in Fig. 18. It should be remembered when doing this type of experiment that once the sublimation front passes the temperature measuring element, the accuracy of the product temperature data becomes questionable. From these data, product temperature isotherms can be constructed for any combination of shelf temperature and chamber pressure. As expected, the higher the chamber pressure, the lower the shelf surface temperature necessary to obtain the desired product temperature. For this example, there was a 1°C increase in product temperature during primary drying for every 4 to 5°C increase in shelf temperature at constant chamber pressure, and a 1°C increase in product temperature for every 0.17 log unit (base 10) of chamber pressure at constant shelf temperature.

In order to establish the end of primary drying, product temperature data can be used, where the end of primary drying is indicated by a sharp increase in product temperature. Other methods discussed above may also be suitable for determining the end of primary drying.

As discussed above, it is customary to increase the shelf temperature during secondary drying. The extent of secondary drying that is necessary depends on the nature of the active entity and on the formulation. A formulation such as the one in this example, with a relatively high sucrose content, would be expected to require considerable secondary drying time since the sucrose remains amorphous and has a high concentration of unfrozen water. The secondary drying temperature should be as high as possible without causing collapse during secondary drying. The effect of chamber pressure during secondary drying, if any, should be established during cycle development studies.

For protein formulations, the level of residual water after drying may be critical with respect to stability of the biological activity. The appropriate level must be established empirically using sequential stoppering, comparative pressure measurement, electronic hygrometer output, product temperature, or residual gas analysis to monitor the process and stop at several levels of residual water. An alternative approach is to dry the product to the lowest practical level of residual water, then subdivide the vials and reequilibrate the dried product at several different relative humidities to create samples with different residual water levels. Limited stability studies should then be carried out in order to determine whether residual moisture is a critical product attribute and, if so, what level of residual moisture provides an adequate shelf life for the product.

Historically, process scale-up has been based on trial and error, and to a large extent it still is, although progress is being made on modeling of the freeze drying process. However, until a predictive model is available, the data collected during the development of the lyophilization cycle can be very useful in predicting scale-up. Nonpredictivity of scale-up is accounted for largely by design and performance differences between small scale and large scale lyophilizers. This includes system geometry factors discussed above, system design features, such as internal vs. external condenser configuration, and system performance parameters such as time required to heat the shelves to a given temperature. Differences in materials of construction and surface finish may also account for small scale-up errors, largely because of the effect of materials and surface finish on thermal emissivity of the surface, which can change the relative contribution of heat transfer by thermal radiation. Monitoring of product temperature during scale-up is important in order to determine the reproducibility of process conditions established during laboratory scale cycles. Sampling of vials for residual moisture measurement should be extensive, and it should cover all areas of the freeze dryer in order to locate any "cold spots," which cause local high residual moisture levels after the bulk of the batch is adequately dry.

Frequently, cost or availability of the active component may prohibit use of actual product for process scale-up studies. If the active component has no measurable effect on the physical properties of the formulation during freezing and drying, the placebo (everything in the formulation minus the active component) may be suitable for process scale-up studies. In order to gather stability data from scale-up lots, it is common practice to include enough actual product in the batch along with placebo to provide the necessary stability samples.

VIII. SUMMARY

Freeze drying provides a valuable tool to the formulation scientist by permitting dehydration of heat-sensitive drugs and biologicals at low temperature. The final product is quickly and easily reconstituted, and the process is compatible with aseptic operations.

Freezing is a critical step, since the microstructure established by the freezing process usually represents the microstructure of the dried product. The product must be frozen to a low enough temperature to be completely solidified. If the solute crystallizes during freezing, this temperature is the eutectic temperature. If the solute remains substantially amorphous with freezing, the relevant temperature is the collapse temperature. Understanding the physical form of the solute—crystalline or amorphous—after freezing can be important from the standpoint of drying characteristics, appearance of the final product, and even product stability during storage. Supercooling is a significant factor in freezing of formulations intended for freeze drying—prior to both primary and secondary (eutectic) crystallization.

The driving force for freeze drying is the difference in vapor pressure of ice between the sublimation zone and the condenser. Because the vapor pressure of ice increases sharply with increased product temperature, it is important from the standpoint of process efficiency to maintain product temperature as high as possible during primary drying without damaging the product. The upper limit of product temperature during primary drying again depends on the physical form of the solute. Exceeding either the eutectic temperature (crystalline solute) or the collapse temperature (amorphous solute) results in loss of the desirable properties of a freeze dried product.

Freeze drying is a coupled heat and mass transfer process, where either heat transfer or mass transfer may be rate limiting with respect to the overall drying rate. Heat transfer is often the rate-limiting transfer operation because of the high heat of sublimation of ice and the inefficiency of heat transfer. Conduction is the primary mechanism of heat transfer, as opposed to convection or thermal radiation. The rate-limiting resistance to heat transfer is usually the interfacial, or contact, resistance caused by poor contact between materials—the heated shelf, metal trays, and the bottom surface of glass vials. Since the thermal conductivity of a gas is directly proportional to pressure in the free molecular flow regime, the chamber pressure during primary drying is an important determinant of the overall heat transfer rate. As a result, the drying rate for a heat transfer-limited process increases sharply with chamber pressure up to a pressure where free molecular flow conditions no longer apply.

The amount of water to be removed during secondary drying also depends on the physical form of the formulation. For materials that are crystalline after freezing, the only water vapor remaining after primary drying is the small amount adsorbed to the surface of the solid. For formulations that remain substantially amorphous, a relatively large amount of "unfrozen" water remains after sublimation of ice. Because of the high concentration of water to be removed during secondary drying of amorphous materials and the fact that mass transfer must take place largely by diffusion of water vapor within a glassy matrix, secondary drying can be the most time-consuming phase of freeze drying for amorphous systems. Because of the importance of temperature and pressure in defining the relative rates of heat and mass transfer in freeze drying, both variables are critical and should be monitored and controlled throughout the process. Either thermocouples or resistance temperature detectors (RTDs) may be used for accurate temperature measurement. The capacitance manometer is considered the instrument of choice for accurate pressure measurement in freeze drying.

The trend in parenteral manufacturing toward developing technology that removes operators from direct interaction with products suggests that the pharmaceutical scientist should be alert for opportunities to use methodology for monitoring the status of the product during freeze drying that does not involve placing probes directly in vials of product. Such methods include comparative pressure measurement, pressure rise measurement, use of an electronic hygrometer, and residual gas analysis. Modern pharmaceutical freeze dryers are well suited to GMP operations, including sanitary design concepts, cleanable surfaces, and sterilization capability. Critical system performance criteria include lowest attainable vacuum, ability to hold a vacuum, uniform shelf temperature distribution, redundancy of vacuum pumps and refrigeration compressors, and ability to sterilize the chamber, condenser, and piping used for introduction of air or inert gases.

REFERENCES

1. Castellan, G. W. (1971). *Physical Chemistry*, 2nd ed., Addison-Wesley, Reading, Mass., p. 333.
2. Campbell, A. N., and Smith, N. O. (1951). *The Phase Rule and Its Applications* 9th ed., Dover, New York, Chap. 17.
3. Pikal, M. J. and Shah, S. (1990). The collapse temperature in freeze drying: Dependence on measurement methodology and rate of water removal from the glass phase, *Int. J. Pharmaceutics*, *62*: 165.
4. MacKenzie, A. P. (1976). The physico-chemical basis of the freeze drying process, *Dev. Biol. Std.*, *36*: 51.
5. Franks, F. (1990). Freeze drying: From empiricism to predictability, *CryoLetters*, *11*: 93.
6. Gatlin, L. A., and DeLuca, P. P. (1980). A study of phase transitions in frozen antibiotic solutions by differential scanning calorimetry, *J. Parent. Drug Assoc.*, *34*: 398.
7. Pikal, M. J., Lukes, A. L., Lang, J. E., and Gaines, K. (1978). Quantitative crystallinity determinations for betalactam antibiotics by solution calorimetry: Correlations with stability, *J. Pharm. Sci.*, *67*: 767.
8. Koyama, Y., Kamat, M., De Angelis, R. J., Srinivasan, R., and DeLuca, P. P. (1988). Effect of solvent addition and thermal treatment on freeze drying of cefazolin sodium, *J. Parent. Sci. Tech.*, *42*: 47.

9. Nail, S. L., and Gatlin. L. A. (1993). Freeze drying: Principles and practice, *Pharmaceutical Dosage Forms*, vol. 2 (K. E. Avis, H. A. Lieberman, and L. Lachman, ed.) Marcel Dekker, New York, p. 163.

10. Gatlin, L. A. (1991). Kinetics of a phase transition in a frozen solution, *Develop. Biol. Standard.*, *74*: 93.

11. Nail, S. L., and Gatlin, L. A. (1985). Advances in control of production freeze dryers, *J. Parent. Sci. Tech.*, *39*: 16.

12. McCrone, W. C., and O'Bradovic, S. M. (1956). Microscope cold stage for controlled study over the range −100° to + 100°C, *Anal. Chem.*, *28*: 1038.

13. MacKenzie, A. P. (1964). Apparatus for microscopic observations during freeze drying, *Biodynamiea*, *9*: 213.

14. Freedman, M., Whittam, J. H., and Rosano, H. L. (1972). Temperature gradient microscope stage, *J. Food Sci.*, *37*: 492.

15. Flink, J. M., Gejl-Hansen, F., and Karel, M. (1973). Microscopic investigations of the freeze drying of volatile-containing model food solutions, *J. Food Sci.*, *38*: 1174.

16. Flink, J. M., and Gejl-Hansen, F. (1978). Two simple freeze drying microscope stages, *Rev. Sci. Instrum.*, *49*: 269.

17. Pikal, M. J., Shah, S., Senior, D., and Lang, J. E. (1983). Physical chemistry of freeze drying: Measurement of sublimation rates for frozen aqueous solutions by a microbalance technique, *J. Pharm. Sci.*, *72*: 635.

18. Kochs, M., Schwindke, P. and Koerber, C. (1989). A microscope stage for the dynamic observation of freezing and freeze drying in solutions and cell suspensions, *CryoLetters*, *10*: 401.

19. Dushman, S., and Lafferty, J. M. (1962). *Scientific Foundations of Vacuum Technique*, 2nd ed., John Wiley, New York, p. 14.

20. Nail, S. L. (1980). The effect of chamber pressure on heat transfer in the freeze drying of parenteral solutions, *J. Parent. Drug Assoc.*, *34*: 358.

21. Pikal, M. J. (1985). Use of laboratory data in freeze drying process design: Heat and mass transfer coefficients and computer simulation of freeze drying, *J. Parent. Sci. Tech.*, *39*: 115.

22. Pikal, M. J., Roy, M. L., and Shah, S. (1984). Heat and mass transfer in vial freeze drying of pharmaceuticals: Role of the vial, *J. Pharm. Sci.*, *73*: 1224.

23. Simatos, D. (1981). Transfer of heat and mass during freeze drying, Parenteral Drug Association Annual Meeting, November.

24. Quast, D. G., and Karel, M. (1968). Dry layer permeability and freeze drying rates in concentrated fluid systems, *J. Food Sci.*, *33*: 171.

25. Ho, N. F. H., and Roseman, T. J. (1979). Lyophilization of pharmaceutical injections I: Theoretical physical model, *J. Pharm. Sci.*, *68*: 1170.

26. Rey, L. (1964). Fundamental aspects of lyophilization, *Aspects Théoriques et Industriels de la Lyophilization* (L. Rey, ed.), Hermann Press, Paris, p. 23.

27. Sarvacos, G. D., and Stinchfield, R. M. (1967). Effect of temperature and pressure on the sorption of water vapor by freeze dried food materials, *J. Food Sci.*, *30*: 779.

28. Pikal, M. J., Shah, S., Ray M. L., and Putman, R. (1990). The secondary drying stage of freeze drying: Drying kinetics as a function of temperature and chamber pressure, *Int. J. Pharmaceutics*, *60*: 203.

29. Pristoupil, T. I., Kramlov, M., Fotova, H. and Ulrych. S. (1985). Haemoglobin lyophilized with sucrose: The effect of residual moisture on storage, *Haematologia, 18*: 45.
30. Hageman, M. J. (1988). The role of moisture in protein stability, *Drug Dev. Ind. Pharmaceutics, 14*: 2047.
31. Wang, J. (1988). Parenteral formulations of proteins and peptides: Stability and stabilizers, *J. Parent. Sci. Tech., 42* (Suppl. 25): 1.
32. Zografi, G., and Kontny, M. J. (1986). The interactions of water with cellulose and starch-derived pharmaceutical excipients, *Pharm. Res., 3*: 187.
33. Ahlneck, C., and Zografi, G. (1990). The molecular basis of moisture effects on the physical and chemical stability of drugs in the solid state, *Int. J. Pharmaceutics, 62*: 87.
34. Considine, D. M., ed. (1985). *Process Instrument and Controls Handbook*, 3rd ed., McGraw-Hill, New York, p. 247.
35. Armstrong, J. G. (1980). Use of the capacitance manometer gauge in vacuum freeze drying, *J. Parent. Drug Assoc., 34*: 473.
36. Pikal, M. J., and Nail, S. L. (1989). Freeze drying of pharmaceuticals: A short course for the Parenteral Drug Association, Parenteral Drug Association, Philadelphia, p. 2.
37. Nail, S. L., and Johnson, J. W. (1992). Methodology for in-process determination of residual moisture in freeze-dried products, *Dev. Biol. Std. 74*: 137.
38. Pikal, M. J., Roy, M. L., and Shah, S. (1984). Mass and heat transfer in vial freeze drying of pharmaceuticals: Role of the vial, *J. Pharm. Sci., 73*: 1224.
39. Roy, M. L., and Pikal, M. J. (1989). Process control in freeze drying: Determination of the end point of sublimation by an electronic moisture sensor, *J. Parent. Sci. Tech., 43*: 60.
40. Jennings, T. A. (1980). Residual gas analysis and vacuum freeze drying, *J. Parent. Sci. Tech., 34*: 62.
41. Leebron, K. S., and Jennings, T. A. (1982). Determination of the vacuum outgassing properties of elastomeric closures by mass spectrometry, *J. Parent. Sci. Tech., 36*: 100.

Index

Analytical considerations, 11–36
  accuracy of protein assays, 13–14, 30
  amino acid analysis, 14
  bacterial sterility assays, 30
  biochemical assays, 20–21
  biological activity of impurities, 29
  biological activity of proteins, 16–23
  biological assays, 12–13, 15–23, 32
  blank run for assay of in-process impurities, 31
  carbohydrate analysis, 28
  cell culture-based assays, 19–20
  contaminants, 24
  electrophoretic methods, 23, 26–27, 32
  electrospray HPLC, 28
  ELISA assay for host cell contaminants, 31, 33
  growth enhancement assays, 20
  growth proliferation assays, 23
  high performance capillary electrophoresis (HPCE), 27

high-pH anion exchange chromatography, 28
host cell protein assays, 31, 33
HPLC, 17, 23, 27–28, 33
immunoassays, 15, 31–32
impurities, 13, 24–32
  antibody derived, 30
  deamidation caused, 26–28
  DNA, 25, 31
  endotoxin, 25, 31
  glycosylation protein variants, 26
  host cell proteins, 31, 33
  introduced by chemical synthesis of peptides, 25
  Limulus Amoebocyte Lysate (LAL) assay for pyrogens, 31
  major, 25
  minor, 25
  proteolysis caused, 26
  pyrogens, 31
  rabbit assay for pyrogens, 31
  related to product, 25–29
  unrelated to product, 29–32

[Analytical considerations]
inhibition assays, 23
interfering substances, 14–16
isoelectric focusing, 26–27, 32
mapping of tryptic fragments, 28
mass spectrometry, 27–28, 33
mass spectrometry on line with
    HPLC, 28
potency, 12–13, 32
precision of protein assays, 13–14,
    30
pretreatment of samples, 15
product variants, 25
proteolysis in biological assays, 16
purity analysis, 21, 23–32
purity requirements, 23
receptor-binding assays, 17–19
scintillation proximity assays, 18
SDS-PAGE, 23, 26–27, 32
sensitivity of protein assays, 13, 15
size exclusion chromatography, 28
specificity of protein assays, 13,
    15, 30
TLC, 23
validation of analytical methods,
    13, 23, 30, 32
whole animal assays, 17
yield assay, 21

Bead mills, 46–52
design considerations, 48–52
    agitator, 48
    bead loading, 49–51
    bead size, 48–49
    cell concentration, 51
    chamber, 48
    comparison of different
        organisms, 49
    feed rate, 51–52
    speed of agitator, 48
    temperature, 52
process kinetics, 46–47
product denaturation, 52
residence time distribution, 47, 51

scale-up, 52
Biospecific affinity chromatography,
    259–316
activation and coupling methods,
    266–267
basic concept, 262–264
binding kinetics, 284
cost, 284, 288
cyanogen bromide activation,
    266–267
diffusion of protein to ligand, 284
dyes as ligands, 269
economics, 288
fluidized bed adsorption, 284, 289
future prospects, 289
glycoproteins, 262, 275–277
high-performance (HPAC),
    282–283, 289
hydrophobic interaction ligands,
    277–281
IMAC in the high-performance
    (HP) mode, 273, 283
immobilized metal ligands,
    259–262, 273, 283, 289
large-scale, 281–288
ligand:
    applications, 272
    commonly used, 269–272
    leaching, 267
    selection, 269
magnetic fields to stabilize
    fluidized bed adsorber, 284
magnetic polymers as ligand
    supports, 286
matrices, 269
monoclonal antibody ligands, 259,
    274
nonspecific protein binding, 268
peptide part of fusion protein
    purfied, 289
polyclonal antibody ligands,
    264–266, 274
processing modes, 266

[Biospecific affinity chromatography]
    protein matrix interactions,
        267–268
    receptor ligands, 260, 264, 266,
        275, 289
    scale-up, 285
    selectivity, 260
    spacer arm, 262, 266–268
    steps in general process, 262–264
    tails introduced by genetic engineering, 289
    types, 264–266
    of various proteins and enzymes,
        259–262, 269–277, 282,
        286–288

Cell breakage, 37–55
    chemical methods, 38
    comparison of different
        organisms, 39, 41, 44, 52
    dependence on physiological state
        of organism, 39
    enzymatic lysis, 38
    high-pressure homogenizer,
        38–46, 52–53
    high-speed agitator bead mill,
        38–39, 46–53
    of hybridomas, 37
    laboratory-scale, 38
    of mammalian cells, 37
    of microbial cells, 38
    product denaturation, 44, 52–53
    ultrasonication, 38–39
Chromatography, 209–316
    activation energies, 227
    adsorbent:
        compressibility and swelling,
            233–237, 240
        fouling, 228, 236
        lifetime, 236
        mechanical strength, 236
        particle size, 218, 227, 231,
            232–233

pore size, 232, 235
properties, 230–237
shape, 232–233
stability toward chemical and
    microbial attack, 235–236
type, 230, 236
adsorption isotherm, 227
adsorption process, 224–225
affinity, 211–212, 215
affinity elution, 213
air trap, 242
automation, 249–251
axial dispersion, 225–227
backmixing, 228
basic design equation, 218–219
binding kinetics, 225–227, 229
biospecific affinity, 259–316
breakthrough, 214, 225, 230–232
buffer pK, 228
capacity of adsorbent, 210–216,
    219–220, 223, 230–232, 235
chromatofocusing, 211, 215
clean-in-place procedure, 247
cleanrooms, 251
column:
    cycles per day, 220
    diameter, 237, 239
    geometry, 237–240
    height, 218, 222–223
    hygiene, 245–249
    material of construction,
        238–240
    prefilters, 240
    productivity per cycle, 219–220
comparison of elution and displacement chromatography,
    215
computer modeling, 225
conditioning of feed, 228
conductivity monitoring, 242
control of ionic strength and pH,
    228
convective flow through particle,
    229, 235

[Chromatography]
cost, 210–212, 214, 217, 228, 230, 236, 284, 288
Current Good Manufacturing Practices (CGMP) regulations, 251
dead volume, 229, 242
detectors, 241
displacement, 214–215, 281
displacer, 214
documentation, 249
dynamic capacity of adsorbent, 230, 232, 235
eddy diffusion, 228
effect of extreme purity requirements on, 217
effect of feed potency on number of columns required, 223
effect of flow velocity on column efficiency, 229
effect of process variables, 227–237
elution, 212–213, 216, 218, 223
elution volume, 221
FDA regulations, 248–249, 251
final design equation, 222
flowmeters, 243
flow velocity, 219–221, 228–229, 232
fluid film mass transfer resistance, 225–227, 229
formulation of the design problem, 218–224
fouling of adsorbent, 212
fractions collectors, 243
frontal, 214, 216, 218, 223
gel permeation, 149, 158, 210, 215, 218, 223–224, 228, 234, 237, 240, 260
gradient elution, 213, 221, 223
guard column, 228
haziness of feed, 228
height equivalent of a theoretical plate (HEPT), 229, 245

HPLC, 211–212, 215–217, 223, 227–228, 233, 260
hydrophobic, 210–211, 213, 215, 230, 277–281
improvement of resolution, 222
ion exchange, 149, 210, 215, 228, 230, 237, 260
isocratic elution, 213, 223
lab-scale, 215–217, 230–231, 238, 241–244, 249
ligand leaching, 212
liquid distributors, 237–238
liquid maldistribution, 229
long-term storage, 247–248
mass transfer limitations, 232
mathematical model of, 217–218, 224–227
mechanical design and operation, 229, 237–245
membrane, 229
modes of operation, 212–216
nature and composition of feed stream, 227
on-off, 213–214, 216, 218–227
optimization of individual steps, 237
packing the column, 244
Peclet number, 226
pH monitoring, 242
pilot plant scale, 238, 242–244, 249
piping, 242–243
pore diffusion, 225–227, 229, 232
preliminary lab-scale experimentation, 215–216
pressure drop, 228–229, 232–235, 237, 243
pressure gages, 243
pressure of operation, 238–239
production scale, 238, 241–245, 250–251
protein denaturation, 211
pulse input to column, 226
pumps for use with, 241

[Chromatography]
purity of product, 216
pyrogen removal, 210, 236, 245–247
rate controlling step determination, 224–227
ratio of adsorbent diameter to column diameter, 231
record keeping, 250
recovery of product, 230
regeneration volume, 221
salting-in, 149–150
sanitary design to 3A standards, 240, 247
sanitization, 236–237, 247–248
scale-up, 209, 211, 215–237, 251, 285
sizing of columns to production needs, 217–237
stability of protein, 230
stepwise elution, 213, 221
sterilization, 247–249
superficial velocity, 220, 228–229, 231
tanks for use with, 240
temperature, 229–230, 233, 237
thermodynamic capacity of adsorbent, 230
transfer units, 226–227
types of, 210–212, 215–216
undesired mixing, 229
usual rate determining step, 227
UV adsorption for protein detection, 241–242
validation, 249–251
valves, 242–243
vertex point or potency knee, 223
viscosity of feed, 228–229, 233
void volume, 235
water for injection (WFI), 247, 251
yield of product, 216, 230
Crossflow membrane filtration, 57–79

adsorption of proteins, 67
advantages compared to centrifugation, 71–72, 76
affinity membrane adsorption, 78–79
affinity membrane separation, 284–285
antifoaming agents, 67, 73
applications, 71–79
backflushing, 73–75
of bacteria, 72–73
of cell debris, 68, 75–76
cell separation and recycling, 71–75
cellulosic membranes, 59–60
cleaning of membranes, 67–68
concentration polarization, 62–67, 70, 73
coupled to fermentors, 73
of deformable and nondeformable cells, 65
effect of feed concentration, 70
effect of pH and ionic strength, 70
filtration modules and systems, 60–62
flat sheet membranes (thin channel), 60, 72, 75–76, 78–79
flow velocity, 67, 69–70
fouling of membranes, 62, 66–68, 70, 73
gel formation, 63, 65
hollow fiber membranes, 60, 75–77, 284–285, 289
hydraulic resistance of membrane, 64
of inclusion bodies, 57, 76–77
of mammalian cells, 71, 74–75
mass transfer coefficient, 63, 69
membrane structures and materials, 59–60
microfiltration membranes, 57–59, 62, 65, 67–76, 78, 284–285, 289

[Crossflow membrane filtration]
    operating conditions, 68–70
    osmotic pressure difference across
        membrane, 64–65
    performance characteristics, 62–70
    polymeric membranes, 59–60
    rejection coefficient, 62, 66
    reverse osmosis membranes,
        57–58
    rotary high shear filter, 61–62, 73,
        76
    spiral wound membranes, 60–61,
        72
    transient behavior, 65
    transmembrane pressure, 63–65,
        68
    tubular membranes, 60, 73
    ultrafiltration membranes, 57–59,
        62, 65, 67, 69–73, 76–78, 284
    vaccine production, 77
    of viruses, 57, 77–78
    wall shear rate, 61–62, 67–70, 73,
        76
    of yeasts and mycelia, 73–74

Denaturation of proteins, 44, 52,
        128, 130, 136–137, 147,
        152–154, 157, 173, 175, 211
Diafiltration, 158
Diameter of globular proteins,
        estimation, 235
Diffusion coefficient of a protein,
        prediction, 226–227

Electrodialysis, 149
Endotoxins, 25, 31, 245–246
Emulsions and microemulsions,
        105–108
    description, 105–106
    hollow fibers, 106–107
    liquid membrane systems,
        106–107
    scale-up, 106

FDA, 1, 4, 248–249, 251, 360
Freeze drying, 317–367
    advantages over products dried by
        alternative methods, 317
    air ejector with a water ring
        pump, 357–358
    amorphous phase, 328, 332, 339,
        343–345, 362, 364
    amorphous systems, 323–325, 331,
        365
    backstreaming of hydrocarbons,
        355, 359
    behavior of gases at low pressure,
        334–336
    bound water, 345
    bulk flow of water, 333, 341
    capacitance manometer for
        pressure measurement,
        351–353, 354, 365
    capital investment, 355, 359
    characteristics of dry products,
        317
    characterization of freezing
        behavior, 325–331
    clean-in-place (CIP) equipment,
        355
    collapse of product, 324, 332, 339,
        342–344, 361–362
    collapse temperature, 325, 333,
        364
    comparative pressure measure-
        ment for process monitoring,
        352–353, 365
    condenser design, 358–359
    conduction of heat, 336, 338–339,
        364
    contact between vials and shelf,
        336–338
    convection of heat, 336, 364
    cooling water use in refrigeration,
        358
    cost of, 319, 346
    critical process variables, 346

[Freeze drying]
crystalline material, 322–325, 343, 345, 364
crystallinity, 332
crystallization, 320, 322, 325, 326–328, 339, 343, 364
depth of dry cake, 341, 344
depth of fill in each vial, 361
differential scanning calorimetry (DSC), 326–328, 361
differential thermal analysis (DTA), 325–326
diffusion of water in secondary drying, 344
diffusive flow, 341, 342–343, 364
dominant heat transfer mechanism, 339
drains, 359
effect of chamber pressure on heat transfer in primary drying, 338–339
electronic hygrometer for process monitoring, 354, 365
endothermic transition, 325–328
equipment, 328, 355–360
error in pressure measurement, 350–351
error in temperature measurement, 347, 349
ethylene oxide sterilization, 359–360
eutectic, 322–324, 327, 364
eutectic melting, 327
eutectic point determination, 329
eutectic temperature, 323–324, 331, 333, 364
exothermic transition, 325–326, 328
FDA, 360
freezing of aqueous solutions, 321–325
freezing process, 320–332
gas ballast for rotary oil pumps, 356

general construction considerations, 359
glass transition, 327, 332
glass transition temperature, 323–325, 328, 331, 345, 361
good manufacturing practice (GMP) operations, 325
heat transfer, 346, 349, 361, 364
heat transfer fluid, 358
heat transfer-limited, 338
heat transfer in primary drying, 333–334, 336–339
instrument of choice for accurate pressure measurement, 365
irreversible thermal event, 326
Knudsen flow of gas, 342, 334–336
Knudsen number, 334–335, 341
latent heat of fusion, 322
leak rate of chamber, 354
leaks in system, 354, 360
limiting heat transfer resistance, 339
limiting mass transfer resistance, 340
manufacturing cost, 319
mass spectrometer for residual gas analysis, 354
mass transfer, 346, 349, 361
mass transfer-limited, 339, 343
mass transfer in primary drying, 333–334, 336, 339–342
mass transfer resistance, 340, 352
McLeod gauge for pressure measurement, 350
mean free path of a gas molecule, 334–335, 341
mechanical manometers for pressure measurement, 350–351
mercury manometer for pressure measurement, 350
microscopy, 325, 331–332
microstructure of product, 324, 364

[Freeze drying]
molecular conductance or
    permeability, 335, 338–339,
    341–342
molecular conductivity, 352
molecular diffusion of water, 333
molecular flow of gas, 334–336,
    338–339, 341–342, 364
most important objective of, 319
nucleation of ice, 321–322, 325,
    351
overall drying rate, 333
phase diagrams, 320, 323
Pirani gauge for pressure
    measurement, 350
pore diameters in the dry cake,
    341
pressure measurement, 349–351
pressure rise for process monitor-
    ing, 353–354, 365
pressure units commonly used,
    334
primary drying, 319, 332–344,
    351, 353, 361–362
process monitoring, 345, 351–355
process overview, 318–320
product temperature monitoring,
    361, 363
product temperature upper limit,
    364
protein formulation case study,
    360–363
radiation of heat, 336, 339, 364
rate of freezing, 342, 344, 352
rate-limiting mass transfer process
    for amorphous solid, 344
rate-limiting resistance to heat
    transfer, 364
redundant equipment, 356, 358,
    365
refrigeration, 358
relative resistances to mass
    transfer, 340
residual gas analysis for process

monitoring, 354, 363, 365
residual water, 344–345, 363
resistance vs. temperature curves,
    329–331
resistance temperature detectors
    (RTDs), 346–348, 351, 365
reversible thermal event, 326
sample thief for process monitor-
    ing, 355
sanitary design, 365
sanitization, 360
scale-up, 355, 361, 363
secondary drying, 319, 343–345,
    351, 361–362
sequential stoppering in process
    monitoring, 355
size of ice crystals, 342
soak times, 351
stability of product, 344–345
steam sterilization, 354, 359–360
sterility or sterilization, 352,
    354–355, 357, 359, 365
sublimation, 317, 319–320, 324,
    332–333, 336, 338–343, 347,
    355, 361–362, 364
supercooling, 320, 322, 325, 329,
    351–352, 364
temperature measurement,
    346–349
temperature of product vs. shelf
    temperature, 361–362
thermal analysis, 325–328, 332
thermal conductance, 338
thermal conductivity gauge for
    pressure measurement, 350,
    352–353
thermal treatments, 325, 342
thermistors, 346, 349
thermocouples, 346, 348–349, 351,
    365
thermoelectric or electrokinetic
    analysis, 328–332
thermograms of sodium chloride,
    mannitol, and cefazolin

[Freeze drying]
    sodium, 327–328
  transfer operations in primary
    drying, 333–334
  transition flow of a gas, 335, 341
  trap method for process
    monitoring, 354
  vacuum integrity testing, 360
  vacuum pumps, 356–358
  vacuum system, 356–358
  validation, 355, 360
  vapor flow in the dry cake, 341–
    342
  viscosity, 323–324, 328, 334, 344–
    345
  viscous flow of gas, 335–336, 341
  water adsorbed to surface of
    solute crystals, 343
  water of hydration, 343
  weight loss vs. time during
    primary drying, 337–338

Homogenizers, 40–46
  fluid interaction systems, 42–44
    comparison of different organ-
      isms, 44
    number of passes, 42, 45
    operating pressure, 42, 45
  product denaturation, 44
  scale-up, 44–46
    aerosol containment, 46
    cooling, 45–46
  valve-type, 40–41
    comparison of different organ-
      isms, 41
    number of passes, 40, 45
    operating pressure, 40, 45

Liquid-liquid extraction, 87–114
  centrifugal separators, 89
  columns, 89
  degradation of protein, 90
  differential extractors, 89

  emulsions and microemulsions,
    105–108
  of enzymes, 100–101, 107–108
  laboratory-scale tests, 89–90, 94,
    102, 108
  liquid membrane systems,
    106–107
  modeling and theory, 90–92, 100,
    107, 109
  optimum conditions, 108
  phase diagrams, 89
  reversed micelles, 107–109
  scale-up, 90, 99, 106–109
  supercritical fluid extraction, 88
  time of extraction, 90
  two-phase aqueous extraction, 87–
    105, 108–109

Organization and strategy, 1–9
  artificial intelligence in process
    synthesis, 6
  computer simulation of process, 6
  Current Good Manufacturing
    Practices (CGMP)
    regulations, 1, 4–5, 251
  economics of process, 1, 6
  equipment:
    explosion-proof specifications, 3
    laboratory, 2
    pilot plant, 2–3
  facilities, 2–3
  FDA, 1, 4
  importance of the biochemistry of
    the process, 7
  material balances in process
    development, 7
  practical considerations in
    development and scale-up,
    7–8
  proteolytic degradation of
    proteins, 7
  pumps, 3
  rules of thumb or heuristics for
    process synthesis, 6

[Organization and strategy]
sanitary design to 3A standards,
2–3
synthesis of process, 1, 6
teams for projects, 5
utilities, 3

Precipitation, 115–208
acoustic conditioning, 178–179
affinity, 162, 266, 283
aging of precipitate, 166–167,
169–170, 176–179, 182
by ammonium sulfate, 149–150,
158, 172–173
amorphous, 168
by anionic precipitants, 159–162
batch stirred tank reactor
(BSTR), 171–172, 174, 176,
179
by a bifunctional ligand molecule,
162
by carboxymethyl cellulose, 161
by cationic polyelectrolytes, 158
by cationic precipitants, 157–158
chemical nature of precipitant,
171–172
Cohn equation for salting-out,
141, 143, 171
Cohn process, 138, 154, 157, 172,
174, 177
continuous stirred tank reactor
(CSTR), 171–172, 179
continuous tubular reactor
(CTR), 171–173, 177, 179
denaturation of proteins, 152–154,
157, 173, 175
density of precipitate particle,
165–167, 169–170, 172, 174,
179
by detergents, 158
dialysis for desalting, 149
dialysis as method of reagent
addition, 174

effect of interfacial tension of the
solid phase, 165
euglobulins, 149, 154
excluded volume effect, 150–151
fluid shear, 168–169, 171–173,
175, 177, 179
general principles of precipitate
formation, 163–169
by group specific dyes, 162
growth, 163–165, 167–168, 170,
173, 176–179, 182
by heparin, 161
Hofmeister or lyotropic series for
effectiveness of salts in,
143–145, 280–281
hollow fibers, 174
from homogeneous solution, 166
hydrogen bonds in, 152
ionic strength in, 151, 153, 155,
158, 161
isoelectric, 155–156, 171, 173, 175
at isoelectric pH, 154–155
isoelectric point in, 156, 158,
161–162
large-scale, 175
by lectins, 162
by linear polyphosphates, 160
major problem, 165
by metal ions and complex
coordination compounds,
156–157
by metaphosphates, 160
methods, 148–162
by miscible organic solvents,
153–155
mixing, 169–171, 173, 175–177
mode of processing, 171–172
by natural anionic polymers, 160–
161
by nonionic polymers, 150–153
novel system designs, 179–183
nucleation, 163, 165–168, 177
objectives, 164–165
by organic bases, 157–158

[Precipitation]
orthokinetic aggregation, 164, 168, 169
orthokinetic growth, 177–178
particle formation, 163
particle size, 168–169
particle size distribution, 169–170, 173
by perchloric acid, 160
perkinetic aggregation, 164, 168–169
perkinetic growth, 177
physical state of the precipitant, 171, 173
pilot scale, 182
by polyacrylic acids, 161, 173
by polyethylene glycol (PEG), 150–153, 171, 173
by polysaccharide polysulfuric acids, 161
by polystyrene sulfonates, 161
primary perturbation affects the solute, 155–163
primary perturbation affects the solvent, 148–155
principles for obtaining good precipitates, 167
protein concentration, 171, 175
rate of addition of precipitant, 166–167, 169, 171, 173–175, 177, 179
reactor design, 171
reagent addition, 170–175
reagent concentration, 171, 175
ripening of precipitate, 166–167, 169
by Rivanol, 157–158, 177
salting-in effect, 154
salting-out, 136, 140–146, 149–150, 155, 171, 173
selectivity, 151, 153, 157–158, 174–175
by short chain fatty acids, 159
size of particles, 178–179

by small anions, 159–160
solid vs. liquid reagent, 173
of soluble affinity complex, 155
stability of proteins in, 152–153
staged addition of reagent, 174
strength of aggregates, 169, 172
by sulfated amylopectin, 162
by sulfosalicylic acid, 160
supersaturation, 163–168, 181–182
supersolubility limit, 163
by synthetic anionic polyelectrolytes, 161–162
by tannic acids, 160–161
temperature in, 151, 153–154, 158, 161
by trichloracetic acid, 159
unit operations, 170–183
zone, 150
Pyrogens, 31, 210, 236, 245–247, 251

Reversed micelles, 107–108, 286
affinity purification, 286
description, 107
enzyme purification, 107–108
microporous membrane system, 107
modeling, 107
scale-up, 107

Sanitary design, 2–3, 240, 247, 365
Solubility of proteins, 115–148
aggregation of apolar moieties in water, 125
amino acid composition, sequence, and protein conformation, 130–132
anions in medium, 134
basis for difference in solubility of charged and polar molecules, 117
Born equation, 117
Brownian bombardment, 116
cavity model, 125–126, 141

[Solubility of proteins]
chaotropic ions, 144, 146
charge transfer interactions, 121
Cohn equation for salting-out, 141, 143, 171
conjugation and binding, 132
Debye-Huckel theory of strong electrolyte solutions, 138–139
Debye induction interactions, 119, 127, 147
Debye polarization interactions, 120
denaturation of proteins, 128, 130, 136–137, 147
denatured globular proteins, 130
derived interactions, 121–125
dielectric constant of solvent, 135–138
dipole-dipole interactions, 120–123
distribution of apolar, polar, and charged moieties between surface and interior, 128
effects of solvents on dielectric constant, 136
electrodynamic dispersion interactions, 117, 119–121
electrodynamic polarization interactions, 117, 119
electrostatic interaction parameters other than charge, 135
electrostatic interactions, 117–118, 126–127
euglobulins, 138
excluded or effective volume of protein solute, 129–130
excluded volume of the solute, 126
folding of polypeptide chain, 128
forces of intermolecular interaction, 116–121
general principles, 115–127

halophobic effect in salting-out, 142
Helmholtz free energy for interactions, 117, 119
Hofmeister or lyotropic series for effectiveness of salts in precipitation, 143–145, 280–281
hydration, 123, 131
hydration layers, 118, 124, 131, 146
hydrogen bond, 122–123, 128, 131, 147
hydrogen bonding and the structure of water, 123
hydrophilic solvation, 118
hydrophobic bond, 125
hydrophobic effect, 124–126
hydrophobic hydration, 124
hydrophobic interaction, 122, 124–125, 147
hydrophobic structuration effect, 125
ionic strength, 132, 134, 138–143, 147
isoelectric point, 133, 134, 137, 148–149
Keesom orientation interactions, 117, 120, 127, 147
Kirkwood theory for salting-in effects, 139
kosmotropic ions, 144
Leonard-Jones potential, 121
Lewis acid-base interactions, 121–123, 127
London dispersion interaction, 119–121, 126–127, 147
membrane proteins, 131
miscible organic solvents, 137
molecular size and shape of the protein, 129–130
noncovalent interactions, 116, 126, 147

[Solubility of proteins]
  overview of globular protein
      structure, 127–129
  parameters of, 129–148
  pH of minimum solubility, 133
  protein charge, 132–135
  repulsive interactions, 121, 126
  salting-in, 134, 137–138, 140–142,
      144
  salting-out, 136, 140–146
  Setschenow equation for salting-
      out, 141
  solvation interactions, 122–124
  solvophobic interactions, 125, 128
  specific ion effects, 140, 143–147
  stability of proteins, 128, 144–146
  structure-breaking ions, 147
  structure-making ions, 146
  structure of water, 145
  surface tension of salts, 142
  surface thermodynamics theory,
      126–127
  temperature, 136–137, 147–148
  theory of protein solubility and
      salting-out, 141–142
  van der Waals interactions, 120,
      127–128, 132, 135, 137
Strategy (*see* Organization and
      strategy)

Two-phase aqueous extraction,
      90–105
  affinity partitioning, 102–103, 105,
      266, 283
  of broken yeast cells (clarified),
      92–99
  Bronsted equation to describe
      partitioning, 91
  centrifugal separator, 101
  centrifuge manufacturers, 103
  charged polymers, 102
  countercurrent centrifugal
      chromatography, 99
  coupled to adsorption, 100, 103

  dextran concentration effect, 95
  dextran substitute, 103
  effect of order of addition of
      polymers, 95
  of enzymes, 100–101
  equipment, 101–102
  goals of early process research, 91
  hollow fibers, 99
  integrated with fermentation, 104
  laboratory scale tests, 94, 102
  larger scale systems, 103–104, 109
  modeling, 100
  molecular weight dependence, 91
  monitoring of parameters, 104
  phase diagrams, 100
  pH effects, 102
  polyethylene glycol (PEG):
      with bound hydrophobic groups,
          102
      concentration effect, 96
      -dextran systems, 89, 93–97
      reducing molecular weight of,
          99
      removal, 97, 104
      -salt systems, 89, 97–103
  problem areas, 104
  product stability, 94
  protein partition coefficients from
      a thermodynamic model, 100
  reactive extraction systems, 103,
      105
  recovery or yield, 93
  scale-up, 99
  solvent reuse, 104
  surfactants, 96, 99, 103
  temperature effects, 91, 102
  theory, 90–92
  time for phase separation, 101
  toroidal coil planet centrifuge, 99
  Triton X-100 effect, 96, 99
  vaccine purification, 92–100, 104

T - #0031 - 111024 - C0 - 229/152/23 - PB - 9780367402259 - Gloss Lamination